1995

W9-ACE-868

Ever since Plato, human reproduction has been a subject for philosophical speculation. The present time is no exception. Quite the contrary: the present technological revolution within the field of human reproduction has provoked among philosophers reflection and ongoing controversies.

In his pioneering book, Kurt Bayertz provides a comprehensive analysis of the philosophical deep structure behind the ongoing controversies. He strikingly relocates some of the central ethical issues concerned with human reproduction and its technological control. The central aim of the book, however, is not to solve the many ethical problems within the field, but to understand the nature of these problems. Such an understanding remains impossible until we realise that technology does not reduce to external power. Control over human reproduction is perhaps the most impressive example of technology as a part of ourselves. We have to face the conclusion that, by changing technology, we change ourselves.

GenEthics

KURT BAYERTZ

GenEthics

Technological Intervention in Human Reproduction as a Philosophical Problem

Translated into English by
Sarah L. Kirkby

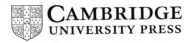

CAMBRIDGE
UNIVERSITY PRESS

Published by the Press Syndicate of the University of Cambridge
The Pitt Building, Trumpington Street, Cambridge CB2 1RP
40 West 20th Street, New York, NY 10011-4211, USA
10 Stamford Road, Oakleigh, Melbourne 3166, Australia

Originally published in German as *GenEthik* by Rowohlt Taschenbuch Verlag GmbH,
Hamburg, 1987, and © Rowohlt Taschenbuch Verlag GmbH.

First published in English by Cambridge University Press 1994 as *GenEthics*

Printed in Great Britain at the University Press, Cambridge

A catalogue record for this book is available from the British Library

Library of Congress cataloguing in publication data

Bayertz, Kurt.
[GenEthik. English]
GenEthics: technological intervention in human reproduction as a
philosophical problem / Kurt Bayertz; translated into English by
Sarah L. Kirkby.
p. cm.
"Originally published in German as GenEthik by Rowohlt Taschenbuch
Verlag, Hamburg, 1987"–T.p. verso.
Includes bibliographical references and index.
ISBN 0 521 41693 0
1. Human reproductive technology–Moral and ethical aspects.
2. Genetic engineering–Moral and ethical aspects. I. Title.
RG133.5.B3913 1994
176–dc20   94–15919   CIP

ISBN 0 521 41693 0 hardback

TAG

Dedicated to my daughter, Charlotte

Contents

Foreword

GenEthics springs from the recognition that our technology has turned upon ourselves and made us and our biological future a moral problem. The Roman Catholic Church has been right about contraception. Artificial interventions into reproduction are unnatural in changing our relationship to our own biology and our customary understandings of sexuality. Artificial contraception has shaped the character of contemporary society in which women can be sexually active and engaged in the workplace. Simple ways of controlling our reproductive biology have had vast impacts on the experience of what it is to be human. They have given issue to divisive moral controversies. However transforming these changes have been, knowledge about human genetics and the development of the technology to change both genes and their expression will even more dramatically alter our self-understanding and our selves. The central question is now not simply how to reproduce or what values should direct reproduction. It is rather how we should evolve, how we should make our own evolutionary choices.

We will be able to change our heredity with ease. Third-party assisted production, such as artificial insemination by donor, has been followed by high-technology artificial reproduction, genetic counselling, prenatal diagnosis, and now the prospect of technologically driven autoevolution. Eugenics and proposals for the improvement of human heredity have until recently presupposed selective breeding augmented at times by genetic selection through abortion. We stand on the brink of unprecedented knowledge about our own genetic inheritance and a rapidly increasing capacity to engineer ourselves technologically. The various technologies, current and envisaged, have spawned many and often impassioned moral and public policy debates about somatic and germline genetic engineering. This book gathers these various debates together under the rubric of GenEthics to identify a cluster of moral controversies and reflections that will become ever more central to our culture. Ideas, tools and moral controversies are tied together; technology shapes moral debates. As we increase the scope of our technological power over ourselves, it will become ever more necessary to be clear about how we should use it. This volume explores not just the issues, but the presuppositions and pre-decisions that underlie secular moral, in particular philosophical, debates on GenEthics. In so doing, it names an already substantive area of moral concern.

For many readers, this volume will more than justify itself through its map of the arguments, questions and conflicts that are part of assessing the morality that should guide our genetic technologies. This volume offers a fine-grained exploration of the philosophical issues that frame the debates on the control and fashioning of our genetics. It combines reflective breadth and depth with a perspective that has been well informed by discussions not just in North America, but in Europe and across the globe. However, the volume's special strength is its recognition of (1) the centrality of GenEthics for our future self-understanding and yet (2) the impossibility of GenEthics pulling a guiding normative moral vision as a philosophical rabbit out of the hat of reflection. As Kurt Bayertz shows, just as we can do more with our heredity, we have less certainty regarding the guidance that philosophy can provide.

Our choices must be made in the absence of a secular ethic that can deliver concrete instruction. Philosophical approaches can disclose maps of arguments and different weightings that can be given to various considerations. In our post-Christian, post-communist world, one encounters the stark truth: secular morality provides analyses, but not concrete moral direction. As we move from breeding to engineering, abandon guidance from revelation, and turn to holiness found in a secular reverence for nature, we find that GenEthics not only systematises, explains, and justifies existing moral norms that might guide technological interventions into human reproduction, but calls these into question. Even if much of conventional morality is not seen to be in jeopardy, the unconventional character of our new technological opportunities leaves uncertainty where moral instruction is passionately sought.

For those who are believers such as I, this book will underscore the immense cultural gap between the secular morality of GenEthics, which will develop in the face of the new genetic technologies, and the traditional understandings of the Judeo–Christian heritage. The book provides not just a philosophical map, but a guide to a cultural challenge that will not have a unique resolution. For any reader, this book is an indispensable introduction to GenEthics as an area of pressing moral dialogue, an unavoidable domain of philosophical and cultural inquiry. The volume, however, is more. It recognises that we must take possession of a morality for our self-fashioning. Yet, responsibility requires asking questions about goals for ourselves that neither nature nor subjectivity can provide. The scientific challenges involved in understanding our GenEthics give rise to moral challenges regarding how to use our new knowledge properly. As we look to a future of self-transformation, Bayertz discloses the cardinal difficulty: content for moral guidance cannot be found in reason alone.

H. Tristram Engelhardt Jr

Preface to the English edition

I was very tempted to use the English edition of this book as an opportunity to rewrite some of it. Since the German edition appeared in 1987, some of my views have changed. And yet, although I now see many things more clearly and could probably formulate them more poignantly, the central message of this book does not seem to be in need of correction. Most of all, I believe that the main intention behind this book is still relevant today. I did not set out to find a practicable 'solution' for each of the problems raised by modern gene and reproduction technology, but far more to *understand* philosophically the nature of these problems.

This understanding includes the insight that the progress of technology is more than just a growth in knowledge and in the viable options available to us. Gene and reproduction technology is one of the most impressive examples of the way in which technology is part of ourselves. By changing it, we change ourselves. The crucial changes throughout human history are always those which involve the human being itself. This insight shatters the illusion that there could be simple 'solutions' to such problems. The concept of solution, such as we are familiar with from the field of mathematics, presupposes precise criteria. In this case, however, there are not any. Criteria are proposed by human beings, and alter with them. Instead of finding solutions, we can only *deal with* the technological options available to us – and this means ourselves – more or less adequately, more or less humanely.

I would like to conclude by expressing my heartfelt thanks to everybody who helped to make this English edition possible. A special mention goes to Mikulas Teich, who gave me the original idea, and to Sarah Kirkby, who was faced with the difficult task of finding solutions to the problems raised by the translation.

Münster, Summer 1993   *Kurt Bayertz*

1

At the start of a technological revolution

*The ancient mode of procreation
Is quite absurd, we now declare*
Johann Wolfgang von Goethe

July 25th, 1978, the day on which $5\frac{3}{4}$ lb Louise Brown was born in an English hospital, marked the opening up of a whole new continent of possible human actions. Louise Brown was the first 'test-tube baby' in human history: the result of a technique which is known as *in vitro fertilisation* because fertilisation takes place outside the mother's body in a small, flat, glass dish. There can be no doubt that this birth signified a medical breakthrough, not limited merely to its *technological* success. Its symbolic dimension alone – a process which was previously restricted to the darkest regions of the human body has been exposed to the laboratory lights and subjected to technological control – is good reason for *in vitro* fertilisation to assume a position well beyond the criteria by which technological innovations are usually measured. At the same time, it marks the start of a development which sees technology gradually gaining access to the entire process of human reproduction. It is no coincidence that in recent years, and in connection with *in vitro* fertilisation, there has been talk of a *technological revolution* within the field of human reproduction.

Biological breakthroughs

This technological revolution should be viewed against a background shared by all the modern biological sciences, namely a stormy developmental phase. In the last fifty years, theoretical knowledge about human reproduction has bounded ahead at the same rate as the interventions made possible within practical medicine. Investigation of the hormones regulating the female cycle, of physiological mechanisms of fertilisation, and of the complex processes involved within embryogenesis has rendered these processes not only easier to comprehend, but also easier to control. Only part of this progress has been made within the bounds of pure medical research; other parts stem from transferred knowledge and skills from other disciplines within the biological sciences. Much of what we summarise today as 'human reproduction technology', for example, originated in connection with animal production: techniques such as artificial insemination or embryo transfer were tested on animals and then developed for the breeding of high quality cows and sheep.

This is especially the case regarding our understanding of the molecular mechanisms involved in human genetics, and the technological possibilities this understanding has led to. In 1953, Francis Crick and James Watson unravelled the molecular structure of DNA and shed light on one of Nature's innermost 'secrets'. 'The phoenix-like rise of molecular biology' (Mayr 1982, p. 574) had begun, which was later to unearth a plethora of fundamental discoveries about the structures of life's processes. For example, in 1961 – less than a decade after the worldwide enlightenment regarding the structure of DNA – the genetic code was cracked. In connection with this development, the character of biological research has undergone a fundamental alteration; in its formation of methods and theories, it has changed to become much closer to the 'hard' sciences. In the last few decades, the dynamics of theory development have acquired a new dimension; it seems safe to suppose that we are in the middle of a phase of deep structural alterations, taking place within the entire scientific system, at the end of which biology will assume a position of equal importance, as far as technological significance and the type of research are concerned, as that held by physics, considered to be the leading science since the 17th century.

This refers not only to the expectation that one of the sciences of complexity – biology – will prove to be paradigmatically more fruitful in the future than physics, traditionally more reductionistically orientated, but also to the close connection in modern biology between theory and practice. Firstly, molecular biology, and especially molecular genetics, may be distinguished from traditional biology due to a quantitative and qualitative expansion in its use of the experimental method as an intra-scientific field of practice. Of course, traditional biology has always carried out experiments and processed the results theoretically, too; and yet the collection, classification and formation of concepts and models were always the most prominent methods of obtaining theoretical knowledge. Today this relationship has turned around; theoretical progress is directly dependent upon the technology available.

> At this point more is being learned about molecular evolution by the application of new techniques than by the development of new concepts.
> (Mayr 1982, p. 576)

In addition, these technologies are not only there in order to allow the scientist access to vital microscopic processes, not available to the 'unequipped' eye; the application of these technologies to the object in question often implies constructive access to that object. In 1961, H. Mattaei and M. Nirenberg successfully deciphered the first codon of the genetic code by *synthesising* an artificial molecule of ribonucleic acid. They created the molecule, consisting only of the base thymine, and proved that each tri-combination of this base produced the code for phenylalanine. The crux of this procedure with regard to the philosophy of science is that the traditional relationship between understanding and construction has been inverted: nature is understood via its scientific *construction*. This brings molecular biology into line with a development in chemistry which started to become noticeable in the 19th century: a transition from analytical to synthetical science.

The consequences of this development are not limited to the epistemological structure of the research process. They cast just as much doubt upon the traditional differentiation between *science*, which discovers the world, and *technology*, which changes it, as

upon the differentiation between pure research and applied science. It has become impossible to separate biological research from
biological technology: the acceptance of research in this field
necessarily implies acceptance of is potential application. The connection between pure research, applied science, technological
development and industrial exploitation has never been as close,
nor the transition between these as rapid, as is the case within the
field of molecular biology. Constituting 'synthetic biology' implies
a change not only in the significance of intra-scientific practice for
the acquisition of knowledge, but also in the structure of the former's relationship to external practice. Whilst none of the scientific revolutions in the past – Copernicus, Galileo, Darwin or
Einstein spring to mind – bore a direct influence on technological
practice, the theoretical breakthroughs in biology within the last
four decades have coincided with a biotechnological revolution.
Many theoretical discoveries have proved to be directly relevant to
practice, and have rendered living material accessible to an extent
previously unthinkable. The fact that we are presently experiencing the historical ascent of a new branch of industry, whose products are created not by physical, mechanical machines, but by
genetically manipulated microorganisms, is the direct result of the
theoretical progress being made in the field of molecular genetics.
The dimensions – in the main as yet prospective – of this new
technology are apparent if we compare it to nuclear physics. One
of the pioneers – and subsequent critics – of gene technology,
Robert Sinsheimer, used this line of argumentation during a hear-
ing of the American Senate public health committee (quoted from
Kieffer 1979, pp. 106–7):

SENATOR KENNEDY: Do you agree that in terms of magnitude
this is of as great significance as the splitting
of the atom?

SINSHEIMER: What this technology does is to make available to us the complete gene pool of evolution. We can take the genes of one organism
and recombine them with those of others in
any manner we wish. To my mind this is an
accomplishment as significant as the splitting
of the atom.

SENATOR SCHWEIKER: Are you saying that all that has gone before,

we now have the power to change in some
way – the evolutionary process?
SINSHEIMER: Yes.

Self-knowledge and self-control

Since Darwin, we have been aware that human beings are part of
the evolutionary process, a process which, with the help of modern
biology, human beings have been learning to alter, step by step.
All the theoretical knowledge which we obtain about the mechanisms of evolution and inheritance, and all the possible ways of
controlling these mechanisms which we develop are, if not always
directly, also applicable to ourselves. The progress made within
the biological sciences over the past few decades has thus explo-
sively increased our theoretical understanding and possible technological options not only with regard to *external* organic nature,
but also with regard to our *own nature*. The basic laws behind the
coding and transferral of genetic information are the same for all
organisms. Research into bacterial genetics therefore provides
additional information about the human genetic process; and since
within modern science the discovery of nature and control over
nature are inseparable, the ability to control bacterial genetics
opens up possibilities for controlling the human genetic process.
This does not mean, of course, that the genetic constitution of
human beings can be manipulated in the same way as that of *E.
coli* bacteria; it would also be missing the point to reduce the connection between research into, and control over Nature on the one
hand, and that of our own nature on the other, to the spectacular
successes of gene technology. Important is the close relationship
between (a) theoretical progress within various fields of the biological sciences, (b) connected biotechnological breakthroughs and
(c) the resulting possible applications to the human race, in turn
leading to a fundamental change in the medical field.

The human race is thus affected by the revolution within the
modern biological sciences not only as a result of its acquired ability to control Nature, and of the consequences of this for industry,
but also as a result of its acquired ability to 'control itself'.

According to the euphoric visions of some observers, we are currently on the threshold of a 'biotic age', in which human beings
will gradually succeed in exercising total control over their own
natural constitution.

> In this new biotic age our human fortunes are far more influenced by
> those we might call 'intranauts' than by the astronauts. These explor-
> ers of the inner spaces of man are the biochemists, immunologists,
> embryologists, placentologists, teratologists, geneticists, fetologists,
> and so on. They are much more important in our lives and we are
> affected far more by their discoveries than by what mere moon walk-
> ers and rock collectors do for us. Yet even the intranauts' labels and
> language are unfamiliar, while the astronauts' lingo is on the front
> pages. The public has been catching up only very slowly with the
> meaning of organ transplants, antibiotics, mechanical organ valves and
> pumps, artificial tissues, myoelectric prostheses (artificial limbs),
> machine supports such as kidney dialysis, respirators, and pacemakers,
> chemotherapy, transistorized electronic monitors, and cryonics.
>   (Fletcher 1974, pp. 9–10)

There really does not seem to be even the tiniest corner of our
'inner space' left as yet unexplored by 'intranauts', and as yet not
under the – slightest – technological control. The human reproduction process is no exception; theoretical explanations and technological interventions are penetrating this as much as all other
physiological processes. Perinatal medicine investigates its end,
gynaecology, reproduction physiology and reproduction medicine
its beginning, and embryology its middle.

Artificial procreation

It makes sense to speak of a technological revolution of the human
reproduction process if (a) the quantitative increase in our practical options is emphasised, leading to (b) access to at least several
processes previously beyond the realms of our influence, and if (c)
attention is drawn to the fact that we are presently at the start of a
development which has not yet reached its climax. Categories such
as 'revolution' should not, however, obscure the fact that not even
revolutions bring about things *ab ovo*: they are processes with a

history, the roots of which are often entangled in a long line of tradition. What is new about the present development is not that it enables human nature to be accessed and human reproduction to be manipulated – this has been the case for thousands of years; what is new is far more that, through scientific and technological innovation, these options which are thousands of years old are raised to a totally different niveau. This is especially the case for contraceptive interventions, which represent the type of manipulation most commonly practised to date. Most important here is the Pill, but also the sheath, the intra-uterine pessary, the coil and sterilisation. A central characteristic of the present revolution is apparent here already: the more or less explosive expansion in technological options.

Besides this quantitative expansion there are also numerous noteworthy qualitative breakthroughs which have led to new practical options. This is especially the case where interventions are not contraceptive, but 'proceptive'. Of course, even here the efforts are all but new, as we are aware from the fertility rituals practised by early primitive peoples, later the appropriate prayers and offerings within Christian tradition, the family remedies passed down from mother to daughter, not to mention the recipes favoured by herb ladies, midwives, etc. Not even the search for substitute solutions, known today as 'surrogate motherhood' is new: in the First Book of Moses several cases of this kind are mentioned (Genesis 30: 1–6; 16: 1–4). Other techniques aimed at the therapy or compensation of fertility problems, foremost artificial insemination, were not developed until well into the modern age: the first successful homologous insemination took place in 1799, the first heterologous insemination in 1884 (Jüdes 1983, p. 18). Nevertheless, this technique was not able to gain acceptance straight away; not until the past few decades has it been able to achieve the status of a therapy recognised and accepted by the medical profession as well as the public, now applied to *c.* 7000 to 15 000 couples worldwide every year.

In vitro fertilisation is the most spectacular achievement within this field, and without doubt the one with the most consequences. Various myths exist which tell of the transfer of embryos from one woman to another (Diedrich & Krebs 1983, pp. 25–6), yet prior to the 19th century no practical attempts in this direction were made.

In 1978, the gynaecologist Steptoe and the physiologist Edwards finally carried out the first successful extracorporeal fertilisation. Whilst artificial insemination serves to compensate certain cases of male infertility, *in vitro* fertilisation can be applied in cases of female infertility stemming from faulty or blocked Fallopian tubes. About 15 per cent of all couples are sterile; in about one half of these cases it is the female partner who is infertile, of which about one half again are due to a Fallopian tube defect. Thus *in vitro* fertilisation is a possible option for about one quarter of all sterile couples, that is for about 3–4 per cent of all couples. Its significance is therefore, on the one hand, due to the high number of potentially interested subjects: in Western Germany alone the figure is around 100 000 couples. On the other hand, it permits laboratories access to the embryo in its earliest phases of development, thus fulfilling the conditions for its direct manipulation. This renders it the focal point for a whole series of further techniques, such as the cryo-conservation of embryos, or the transferral of fertilised egg cells to other women (surrogate mothers). In this manner, all possible combinations of genetic parents, surrogate mother and social parents (guardians) are thinkable, including the possibility of rearing a child with five 'parents'.

In addition to the techniques already being practised today, there are those which for now may only be regarded as projects. These include *cloning*, a form of asexual reproduction, common in lower forms of life such as bacteria or plants, where reproduction takes place via dividing or budding. In higher forms of life, which usually reproduce sexually, cloning can be introduced by transplanting the nucleus of a body cell into a denucleated egg cell, in order to gain a complete organism. This organism is then genetically identical with the donor of the body cell. A clone therefore has only one 'parent', and what makes this technique so fascinating is the possibility of creating 'identical twins' of different ages, or of copying particular genotypes. This procedure was initially carried out in frogs and has already been applied to lower mammals (mice). The cloning of human beings is presently still confronted with difficulties; yet it should be assumed that, even with human subjects, there will be a successful breakthrough in the future.

Another technique which never fails to occupy numerous

authors is *ectogenesis*: breeding human embryos in artificial surroundings from start to finish. In the mid-term this technique is hardly likely to be realised, and many embryologists consider ectogenesis to be a fundamentally unrealistic concept. On the other hand, control over embryogenesis is being driven forward from both ends all the time: extracorporeal fertilisation of egg cells and cultivation of the resulting embryos, at least during their earliest stages, has already been successful in connection with *in vitro* fertilisation; at the same time, advances in perinatal medicine are forever decreasing the minimum age at which an embryo has reasonable chances of surviving. It would thus be wrong to consider ectogenesis solely within the realms of science fiction.

Genetic prognostics

Although there has always been a strong desire to discover the characteristics of future children before their birth, there was no way of doing so until very recently. In the past few decades, the situation has undergone drastic changes: due to sophisticated discoveries within the field of human genetics and a manifold of technological aids, modern medicine now has access to a wide spectrum of methods for predicting certain, especially clinical characteristics of future children. Of course, these various forms of genetic prognostics are not themselves *interventions* in human reproduction, but in many cases they are a prerequisite for such interventions; in this sense they are an integral part of technological control over human reproduction. The advantage of this kind of prognostics is its ability to provide information either about *future* diseases or about disease *dispositions*, thus enabling prospective action. The number of diseases which can be determined using the various methods available is forever increasing; *c.* 150 congenital metabolic diseases can be diagnosed with the help of amniocentesis alone. The same techniques allow some non-clinical characteristics (e.g. sex) to be determined, and a deepening of our knowledge within the field of human genetics will no doubt lead to the prenatal recognition of countless additional, genetically (co-)determined characteristics and dispositions.

1. *Genetic counselling* is usually sought by couples who, due to a family predisposition, are worried that their children could be born with a disease, and who would like information about the possible risks before embarking on a pregnancy. Central to such counselling is the taking down of a family history: a family tree including all immediate relatives and their diseases, miscarriages, stillbirths, etc. This family tree enables conclusions to be drawn about possible increased risks for potential children of the couple in question.

2. *Prenatal diagnostics* enable diseases to be determined in an already existing foetus. The methods applied most often are ultrasonic examination and amniocentesis, especially recommended for mothers over the age of 35, whose children suffer an increased risk of Down's syndrome. A further method, which is not yet used everywhere, is trophoblast centesis, which can be carried out much earlier on than amniocentesis: if a grave disease is diagnosed, an abortion may be carried out in the 10th week – instead of (at the earliest) in the 18th.

3. *Genetic tests* enable genetic peculiarities to be determined in adults. A difference must be made here between medically motivated examinations, aimed at the diagnosis of genetic diseases, and tests for non-medical purposes; the latter might be for paternity suits, for example, or in order to determine genetic dispositions relevant to particular environmental burdens which the subject is exposed to at work.

4. *Genetic screening* is a possible way of gaining records about complete sections of the population, within the framework of a preventive public health policy. In the 1970s, obligatory screening programmes for certain diseases were introduced in several States of the U.S.A. At the present time in Germany, only newborn children are routinely screened, and only for five congenital diseases.

Quality control

Technological intervention in reproduction is not limited to the prevention or creation of offspring, but may be extended to include the manipualtion of congenital characteristics. This means

measures aimed either at preventing particular, undesirable characteristics ('negative eugenics') or at creating or increasing particular, desirable characteristics ('positive eugenics'). We have already
seen that measures of this kind have a long tradition, and that they
were practised at early stages of civilisation. We now have access
to *selective abortion*: whenever grave foetal damage is prenatally
diagnosed, the pregnancy may be terminated; even countries with
restrictive legislation in this matter (including Germany) permit
abortion when such 'eugenic indications' are present. Considering
the stormy development of the modern biological sciences and
biotechnology, some authors harbour the expectation that, in the
near future, a much larger number of practical options will be
available, enabling a precise influencing of our descendants. Joseph
Fletcher has introduced the term 'quality control' with a mind to
all these options. Considerable hopes are being set on the possibility of reproducing 'qualitatively' exceptional genotypes through
cloning: would it not be an enrichment for humanity if great
artists such as Mozart or Picasso, or important scientists such as
Darwin or Einstein could be reproduced again and again? Or
entertainers such as Bobby Charlton or Marilyn Monroe? Even
the more futuristic possibilities offered by *gene manipulation* are
called upon to improve the quality of future generations, whether
through ambitious plans for an increase in intellectual, artistic and
moral abilities, whether through an elimination of congenital diseases and defects. Emerging is the prospect of an evolution consciously controlled by human beings, in which the biological fate
of our species is forcibly removed from the blind chance of mutation and selection, and placed in the hands of deliberate guidance.

  Whilst the reality of many of these ideas does not extend beyond
the realms of science fiction, the 1990s have seen the ascent of
somatic gene therapy to a medically viable option. In contrast to
genetic engineering, which deals with the genetic constitution of an
entire organism, gene therapy aims at replacing a defect or missing
gene within the cells of a particular organ, in order to enable the
latter to function normally; intervention does not extend to the
germ line, but is limited to one organ in one individual. Gene therapy of this kind has opened up possibilities for the treatment of a
strictly defined group of genetic (and other) diseases. This branch
of technology may be considered as a continuation of traditional

medicine: its goal is not an improvement of the human race, but
the therapy of its disease. Whilst gene therapy may be considered
separately from the projects involving control over human evolution with a mind to changing the species, it nevertheless forms a
half-way mark in the long-term development of possible ways of
controlling the quality of our descendants.

Moral problems

The technological revolutionisation of human reproduction, of
which we are at the start, has today already led to a massive
increase in our practical options. It is obvious that these possibilities are just as ambivalent as other scientific and technological
innovations to date. As a matter of fact, opportunities and risks
seem to be closer to each other here than anywhere else: on the
one hand, the prospect of medical aid for infertility and congenital
disease, on the other the nightmare of tailor-made, test-tube people like those we all know from Aldous Huxley's much quoted
book, *Brave New World*. Since the birth of Louise Brown in 1978,
there has been much intensive debate in the specialist biomedical
world, and in public, about the *moral* problems raised by reproduction technology. In this debate, fascination surrounding the
possibilities offered by science and technology is confronted by
great uneasiness concerning the technological revolution of human
reproduction and possible abuse of this technology. Countless
manuscripts have been written, congresses held and committees
formed, all intent, with varying perspectives, on finding a solution
to these moral problems; they are all an indication of the great
need for a reliable, normative orientation in the field of gene and
reproduction technology. The institutionalisation of *GenEthics*, as
applied moral philosophy and a new sub-discipline of biomedical
ethics, is called for, picking up on the theoretical problems surrounding this branch of technology and, most importantly, formulating the norms and principles according to which responsible
interaction with the new practical options may be measured.

Within the debates dealing with GenEthics, two fundamental
positions may be distinguished. The advocates of these two

positions base their views on diametrically opposed assumptions, their considerations – if not always, then often – coming to diverging conclusions. The first position assumes a very positive attitude to the new technologies; it especially emphasises the increase in individual freedom of action, enabling many people to escape the constricting fate of unwanted childlessness and/or to protect their offspring from suffering due to congenital diseases. However, new options also imply new decisions; and this pressure to decide is often related to burdens, particularly when the matter to be decided upon is encumbered with established habits and traditional prejudices. Sexuality and reproduction are just such an area, and for this reason the new technologies bring with them great uneasiness.

> Major ethical isssues arise directly or indirectly from the new genetic knowledge and correlated technologies... The conscious guiding of human procreation from start to finish is becoming more and more dependent on the parent's desire to have normal children. But availability does not imply use. Some of the major obstacles to implementing reproductive improvements are psychological and ethical, based on traditions which are sometimes hard to break. The classical sanctity-of-life ethic, for instance, is still preferred by some over a quality-of-life one.
>
> (Kieffer 1979, p. 128)

The obvious central message of this passage is that gene and reproduction technology opens up new practical options, as well as creating new responsibility. Thus the new technologies arouse the need for an amendment of, and an extension to traditional morality, in the sense of 'ethics of genetic responsibility', teaching people early perception of possible risks and conscious interaction with new possibilities.

Whereas the GenEthics aspired to by the advocates of the first position will be rooted in a revision of traditional morality and its adaption to achievements within the field of reproduction technology, the advocates of the second position are striving towards the very opposite.

> The biological control of man, especially genetic control, raises ethical questions of a wholly new kind for which neither previous praxis nor previous thought has prepared us. Since no less than the very nature and image of man are at issue, prudence becomes itself our first ethical duty, and hypothetical reasoning our first responsibility.
>
> (Jonas 1974, p. 141)

There is agreement with the advocates of gene and reproduction technology that this new branch of technology gives rise to moral problems which present ethics is not capable of solving. Yet consensus regarding the necessity of modern GenEthics stops at the point where the content of this ethics is to be determined: it is no longer an adaption of morality to technology which is demanded, but a recollection of the fundamental values of our culture, and effective protection of the human beings within it from the erosion threatened by science and technology. In making human nature accessible to technology, the new ways of manipulating reproduction break through a moral sound barrier: in dealing with human beings

> the absolute comes to the fore and raises, beyond all calculations of benefit and harm, ultimate moral, existential, indeed metaphysical aspects.
>
> (Jonas 1985, p. 211)

Thus, according to the second point of view, a GenEthics worthy of this label cannot originate from an adaption of traditional morality to new technology, but must instead radically question the technology itself.

Aims of this book

The following considerations attempt to draw a balance between the two fundamental positions outlined above. They do not aim to discuss in detail possible solutions to individual problems. Questions such as:

- Is surrogate motherhood morally permissible or not? If so, under which circumstances?
- What should be done with the numerous embryos which are often the 'by-product' of *in vitro* fertilisation? May they be used for research purposes, for example, later to be discarded?
- Would the cloning of famous people be morally permissible, or would this contradict human dignity?

will be referred to and discussed on many occasions in the pages to follow, but they will not be clearly answered. Extensive literature attempting to provide answers of this kind already exists; most importantly, various bodies of people with extensive interdisciplinary specialist competence, commissioned by diverse governments, parliaments, medical and legal organisations, have dedicated their time to these individual problems, sometimes coming up with completed suggestions for precise regulation. There can be no doubt as to the importance and necessity of such suggestions; such a multitude of differing technologies can only be ruled via detailed norms. However, the fact that such regulations always contain a great many implicit pre-decisions and presuppositions should not be overlooked. It is precisely these pre-decisions and presuppositions which are the object of a *philosophical* debate on GenEthics, and precisely these pre-decisions and presuppositions are and remain controversial. This book therefore concentrates on ever controversial questions of principle, such as: are there any reasons to reject gene and reproduction technology *on principle*? And can *human nature* be the justification for such a rejection? Of course, philosophical questions of principle such as these can never be 'worked out' in the same sense as mathematical questions can, and yet it would be wrong to conclude that every attempt to approach the former rationally and analytically is totally useless. The following considerations take three main directions.

1. Individual technologies are not to be presented as much as their overall coherence is to be made apparent. As different from each other as they might be, they all focus on technological access to human nature, with respect to the same delicate, as well as strategic point: control over reproduction and, ultimately, the prospect of conscious control over human evolution. This is not at all new, as human beings have been influencing their evolution for thousands of years. The concept is nevertheless Utopian since in the foreseeable future – if ever – evolution will not be totally controlled by human beings. This is, however, not the end to, but merely the formulation of the philosophical dimension of the problem. Part I of this book demonstrates the profound historical dimension of the present phase of development, from both sides: it presents the temporary finishing point of a long tradition of technological intervention in human reproduction, as well as the prelude to future technologies which, at present, we can only

speculate about. Special attention will be drawn to the mutual connection between real, possible technologies and the technological concepts, projects and Utopias involved in each case.

2. One of the key concepts in the debate to date is that of human nature. This concept determines the unity of various gene and reproduction technologies, as well as their link to other biomedical technologies; it also forms the focal point for the convergence and divergence of all the various ethical lines of argumentation. The core of Part II is a critical summary of those GenEthical approaches which consider the concept of human nature to be not only an analytical category, but also a normative category, and which postulate a holiness, demanding respect, for human nature.

3. Since the attempt to deduce moral principles from human nature raises a whole series of meta-ethical problems, the question of the efficiency of the alternative conception of GenEthics, favouring human subjectivity as its key concept, arises. Part III examines the extent to which a moral evaluation of gene and reproduction technology based not on human nature, but on the concepts of 'autonomy' and 'self-determination', can hold water.

Part I
Towards autoevolution

2

Reproduction 'according to philosophical principles'

*Nicht nur fort sollst du
dich pflanzen, sondern hinauf!*[1]
Friedrich Nietzsche

With the recent developments in reproduction medicine and
GenEthics in mind, the impression may well arise that technology
is penetrating a field which, until now, was always beyond the
grasp of human manipulation. In their euphoria regarding the
prospect of complete control over human reproduction, the scientistic protagonists of this technology, as well as the critics, tend to
assume that technological intervention in human reproduction
represents a practical option which has only been opened up as a
result of most recent scientific and technological innovations. In
actual fact, human reproduction has never been a pure and
unscathed field. It has a basis in the history of medicine, in
Utopian dreams and human hopes.

Tradition and Utopia

Even with regard to terminology this is the case. If 'nature' is

[1] *Translator's note*: This is a German play on words, appealing to the human race to
reproduce not only quantitatively, but also qualitatively. 'Thou shalt not only have
offspring, but also enhance it!'

taken as being a process uninfluenced by human beings, then reproduction is no more part of this concept than any other human action. The reproductive process does, of course – like every other physiological process – have a natural aspect, which until very recently remained uninfluenceable; nevertheless, human beings have been intervening in the reproductive process since the earliest epochs of their history. This is true first of all with regard to the various social controls over reproduction, including all the customs, habits and institutions which regulate human reproductive behaviour: the ban on incest and exogamy, marriage barriers between different ethnic groups, social classes or, above all, between family members.

> It is extremely difficult to think of any social habit or act of legislation that has *no* genetic consequences. Penal, fiscal social, moral, medical, political or educational laws, schemes, treatments, habits or observances will all make *some* mark on our genetic structure.
>
> (Medawar 1961, p. 58)

Within Western culture, Christian morality has had the most trenchant consequences for sexual and reproductive behaviour; the same goes for a profound transformation of sexual drive with the progress of civilisation. This social and cultural regulation is all the more effective for its internalisation by individuals, leading them to view it not as the result of external pressures, but as 'natural' expressions of sexuality. As Elias (1981) states, the individual is conditioned by society to curb his/her sexual drive in public, even to avoid all mention of it, and this to such an extent that it becomes a habit, dominating even within the intimate and private spheres. This social behavioural code is in fact so overbearing that it becomes a part of the individual ego.

Non-intentional repercussions of control over Nature are a second mechanism affecting the human reproductive process. However far back we go in the early history and even the prehistory of *Homo sapiens*, we find a being which, more or less consciously, regulates its 'metabolic exchange' with the natural surroundings, and which uses various tools in an attempt to control this exchange. Technology is as old as the human race itself. The conscious and deliberate character of this technological control over Nature does not mean, of course, that its side-effects have

always been obvious, and that in good time, or that its repercussions for the human race have always been anticipated. Far-
reaching influences upon human reproduction have sometimes
been due to non-intentional repercussions from actions which
were 'actually' directed at Nature. The consequences for human
reproduction of the Neolithic revolution, for example, can hardly
be made clear enough: the development of an artificial environment through the erection of protective buildings and villages –
later towns – and the transformation of these residential areas and
their surroundings, in connection with the development of agricul-
ture and farming, led to fundamental changes in the process of
natural selection (Vogel & Motulsky 1986, p. 456). Quantitatively,
this development provided the first real chance for a population
expansion; qualitatively, the structure of the human gene pool
changed, with social and cultural factors gradually reforming the
conditions for natural selection.

Thirdly, as early as prehistoric times, the seemingly so intimate
processes involved in human reproduction became the object of
deliberate technological manipulation. In all the societies known to
man, human beings have always tried to control not only Nature,
but also their own, human nature. Shaman practices are evidence
of efforts to manipulate elementary, biological mechanisms within
the human constitution in accordance with human interests. Magic
rituals play an important rôle here as technological predecessors,
as well as 'genuine' mechanical and especially chemical manipulations, such as the introduction of drugs in order to bring about a
state of intoxication, or to relieve pain. Early interventions in
human reproduction are to be viewed within this context.
However primitive the means may have been: the *attempt* to exercise control over human reproduction is as old as the human race
itself. This is especially true of birth control (Himes 1970, p. 422).
Besides magical techniques, *coitus interruptus* has always been common practice; also important are the drawing out of lactation (thus
delaying the recommencement of oestrus subsequent to giving
birth) and exploitation of the infertile days within a woman's
cycle; just as significant again are abortion and infanticide (ibid.,
p. 55). Ethnology has made us aware of peoples where the women
give birth only between the approximate ages of 34 and 37, prior
to which all pregnancies – up to 16 – are aborted (Devereux 1976,

p. 9). We are also aware of the practice of killing newborn babies, not only common amongst primitive peoples, but also possessing a long tradition in Europe; in Ancient Greece and Rome it was a measure taken legally and as a matter of course (Feen 1983) and, despite the Christian ban on killing, it was common in most European countries until well into the second half of the 19th century (McKeown 1976, pp. 75–6, 106–7).

Interventions of this nature served not only to limit the number of offspring, but also to regulate the latter's *quality*. Infanticide was a very common European strategy in this respect. The best known example within European history is Ancient Sparta, where all the newborn babies whose health did not meet the norms of this militarised State were abandoned or killed (Feen 1983). Aristotle's comment in *Politics* that it should be *'law that no mutilated being is raised'* (Book VII) shows that infanticide for eugenic reasons was also common in Athens. In Ancient Rome, children born handicapped or diseased were thrown over the Trapejic cliffs (Cavalli-Sforza & Bodmer 1971, p. 754). Other cultures followed strategies of positive eugenics by allowing certain individuals with superior characteristics the privilege of having more children (Haldane 1967).

The present development within the field of gene and reproduction technology is therefore 'revolutionary' only with regard to its *means*. If we view it with the needs underlying it in mind, then a more appropriate term must be 'evolutionary', the consistent continuation of a long tradition of direct and indirect reproduction. As long as there have been human beings, and as far back as our information about them extends, they have always tried to prevent unwanted offspring or somehow to realise the desire, unfulfilled by Nature, to have children. Viewed this way, modern gene and reproduction technology thus appears revolutionary only because it promises the fulfilment of human desires and needs which have existed for thousands of years.

However, human beings do not simply have needs which they adhere to, or try to adhere to in practice; they also reflect upon these needs, and often endow them with an independent, spiritual existence in myths, ideas or theories. This sort of independence has also been bestowed upon the desire to determine autonomously one's number of offspring and the timing of their arrival, as well as their characteristics. Ever since human beings began to give theoretical structure to their needs and hopes, to heighten their daydreams to Utopias, they have attempted to disregard possible contemporary ways of influencing the reproductive process in favour of anticipatory models of complete control over reproduction. A future perfection of medicine is exceeded by a perfection of human nature. To be included are all the projects concerned not with individual healing, but with attempts to remove evils affecting the entire genus. They are: sex determination, artificial choice breeding, removal of the ageing process. This kind of *eugenic Utopia* is even used to herald social and political goals, such as the breeding of an élite ruling class or, conversely, of a race of industrious and humble servants, regardless of which individual goals have been aspired to using such Utopias: they have always been for the design of an 'ideal reproductive process', which should result in a race of perfect human beings, free from all imaginable afflictions and limitations.

Plato

One of the earliest known eugenic Utopias is to be found in Ancient Greece: in Plato's *Republic*. Founded on the conviction that the best Republic is the one in which the ruling positions are held by the best men, Plato gives voice in his major political work to detailed considerations concerning racial[2] selection of the class predestined to rule. The notion of deliberately breeding human beings has a spiritual tradition in the class morality of the Ancient Greek nobility, which rejected all marriages with members of other social ranks; above all, it is an extension of the cautionary poems about Theognis, who, according to tradition, was the first to declare racial selection, of the sort familiar to us from animal breeding, to be proof of the necessity of consciously maintaining purity within the human master race (cf. Jaeger 1973, pp. 840–1).

[2] The term 'race' as used here is not to be confused with the irrationalistic concept of race as began to emerge towards the end of the 19th century; it does not yet refer to a particular ethnic minority (Jaeger 1973, p. 845). For the present concept of race, cf. Vogel & Motulsky 1986, p. 534; Cavalli-Sforza & Bodmer 1971, pp. 698–700, 792–4; Dobzhansky 1962, pp. 251–80.

Plato's thoughts obviously found additional orientation in the eugenic strategy practised in Sparta, which had already been portrayed in an exemplary light by his uncle, Kritias. Although he assumes that, in general, the offspring of the élite ruling class will possess the same excellent characteristics as their parents, he is not keen to rely on the spontaneous effects of the hereditary mechanism. Firstly, a certain 'social mobility', i.e. the social degradation of incapable and unworthy members of the aristocracy on the one hand, and the admission into the ruling classes of particularly capable lower-class individuals on the other, is to guarantee that the élite always remains a combination of the best citizens at any one point in time. Secondly, Plato conceives of a system of Republican-controlled spouse selection, for the breeding of optimal offspring: in a well-ordered Republic, 'disorder and promiscuity' (Plato V, 458d) would be unhallowed and could not be suffered by the rulers. Referring to the practice of animal breeding, Plato demands that

> the best men must cohabit with the best women in as many cases as possible and the worst with the worst in the fewest, and that the offspring of the one must be reared and that of the other not, if the flock is to be as perfect as possible.
>
> (Plato V, 459d)

In order to realise this breeding concept, marriage as a social institution for the breeding and raising of offspring has to be abandoned; its place is to be taken by a temporary union of men and women for reproductive purposes. The individuals of each sex which come together in this manner are to do so seemingly as the result of drawing lots; in actual fact, the lots will be prepared by 'the rulers' in such a way that the best men come together with the best women, and the worst men with the worst women. This deception is a precautionary measure

> so that the inferior man at each conjugation may blame chance and not the rulers . . . And on the young men, surely, who excel in war and other pursuits we must bestow honours and prizes, and, in particular, the opportunity of more frequent intercourse with the women, which will at the same time be a plausible pretext for having them beget as many of the children as possible.
>
> (Plato V, 460a–b)

With their control over the quality of the Republic's offspring, the seniors also exercise control over its quantity, by adjusting the number of 'weddings' to meet demand. The final eugenic measure to be taken in Plato's concept is a critical examination by the seniors of all newborn babies:

> The offspring of the good, I suppose, they will take to the pen or crèche, to certain nurses who live apart in a quarter of the city, but the offspring of the inferior, and any of those of the other sort who are born defective, they will properly dispose of in secret, so that no one will know what has become of them.
>
> (Plato V, 460c)

As early as Plato's *Republic*, guidelines are visible which are to determine eugenic thinking right through to the present century. More than anything, this includes transferring the principle of selection, empirically investigated and tested within the framework of animal breeding, to human reproduction (Plato V, 459a). Selection is to be carried out by appropriate Republican bodies: the realisation of a eugenic strategy requires a 'strong Republic', in possession of enough power to be able to assert 'common', 'racial' or 'gene pool' interests over individual interests, usually of a contrary nature, regarding sexual autonomy. In contrast to the eugenics of the 19th and 20th centuries, Plato's only concern is reproduction of the élite; his breeding strategy is conceived only for this class of citizens, and not for the lower classes within the Platonic Republic.

Campanella

Two thousand years later, the Dominican monk, Tommaso Campanella, takes up some of Plato's eugenic ideas and develops them further in his *City of the Sun*, first published in 1602. He too assumes that reproduction may not be regarded as a private affair: there is no natural human right to a relationship with a partner, entered into according to individual tendencies, to an own home or own children. The premises for his considerations are much more that children are bred for the preservation of the species and not for individual pleasure, as St. Thomas also asserts. Therefore the breeding of children has reference to the commonwealth and not to individuals, except in as far as they are constituents of the commonwealth. And since individuals for the most part bring forth children wrongly, and educate them wrongly, they consider that they remove destruction from the state, and therefore, for this reason, with most sacred fear, they commit the education of the children, who as it were are the element of the republic, to the care of the magistrates; for the safety of the community is not that of a few. And thus they distribute male and female breeders of the best natures according to philosophical principles.

(Campanella 1885, pp. 235–6)

Again following the example of Ancient Sparta, exercises of a sporting nature are to be carried out in Campanella's *City of the Sun*, during which the male and female participants are naked; the 'most senior officials in matters of reproduction'[3] controlling the exercises thus have the opportunity to establish which individuals are capable of reproducing, and who is best suited to whom. On the one hand, tall and beautiful women will be joined with tall and competent men, on the other hand, fat women with thin men (and vice versa) in order to balance out these characteristics in the resulting offspring. Campanella does not believe the manipulated process of drawing lots favoured by Plato to be necessary in his Republic, since regular physical exercise will see to it that there are no ugly and misformed citizens. Behind this concept lies the conviction that a human being's 'natural characteristics' are fundamental to its social qualities, and that they can only be acquired genetically. He therefore emphasises

that a good disposition, the origin of all virtue, cannot be acquired through any kind of effort, and that the naturally bad human beings may act well, out of respect for God and the Law, but as soon as this respect vanishes they will destroy the Commonwealth, whether unobtrusively or publicly. This is the reason why matters of reproduction

---

[3] *Translator's note*: I have translated this and the remaining Campanella quotations myself. In his introduction to *Ideal Commonwealths* (1885), Henry Morley states that he has omitted from his translation a few passages which we can all well do without . . . Needless to say, it is precisely these censored passages which are of prime interest within the context of this book.

should be tended to above all else, and why it is natural characteristics which should be taken into account, and not deceiving dowries or aristocratic titles.

Campanella's Utopian breeding also contains elements which signify later developments. Efforts to regulate the business of breeding according to scientific principles are worthy of note:

> They sleep in two separate chambers until the appointed time of consummation. Then the supervisor gets up and opens both doors from the outside. The time is appointed by the astrologist and the doctor, who endeavour to choose the time when Venus and Mercury are in a favourable house east of the Sun, in conjunction with Jupiter, Saturn and Mars, or in no conjunction with them at all. The Sun and the Moon, which are often at odds with one another, are taken into particular consideration. The preferred star-sign is Virgo.

Whereas Plato stops at the transfer of experience gained from selection within animal breeding, Campanella goes a step further by wanting to subject human reproduction to the principles of the scientific theories contemporarily available – astrology and medicine – and thus to the control of the relevant experts.

Homunculi

The time which followed was not to see a break in the chain of Utopian breeding philosophies. Alongside the biologically orientated concepts, an additional line of speculations could be observed very early on, tending more towards the contemporary chemistry and physics; in different variations, usually taking up mythical and literary visions of living statues, golem, homunculi and androids, the notion of artificial human beings was propagated. In the 18th century, this notion was given a magnificent boost; in *d'Alembert's Dream*, Denis Diderot describes 'human polyps' which dissolve into an atomic state and then turn themselves back into complete organisms.

> Man splitting up into myriads of men the size of atoms which could be kept between sheets of paper like insect-eggs, which spin their own cocoons, stay for some time in the chrysalis stage, then cut through

their cocoons and emerge like butterflies, in fact a ready-made human
society, a whole province populated by the fragments of one individual, that's fascinating to think about . . . a warm room, lined with
little phials, each one bearing a label: warriors, magistrates, philosophers, poets – bottle for courtiers, bottle for prostitutes, bottle for
kings.

(pp. 172–3)

The notion of breeding human beings which is outlined here
remains episodic in *d'Alembert's Dream*, as it does in Diderot's
other works; and yet it signifies – twofold – future variations on
this notion, thus anticipating important tendencies which are not
to unfold in their entirety until later concepts. Firstly, it is no
coincidence that the notion of breeding appears in connection with
general philosophical discussion on the transformation of sensitive
matter to organismic systems and, in particular, on the problems
connected with reproduction; it is thus closely connected to the
attempt to explain theoretically the reproductive process, and may
be seen, to a certain extent, as a by-product of this attempt.
Secondly, the notion of breeding human beings has proved to be
extremely effective for certain social functions and activities; it is
evident – albeit in modern form – in numerous 19th and 20th century concepts.

In Part Two of *Faust*, Goethe takes up the alchemist concept of
the homunculus anew, ironically letting Faust's practical assistant,
Wagner, complete his creation in a bizarre laboratory – 'after the
manner of the Middle Ages; extensive, clumsy apparatus for fantastic purposes' (p. 211). As Mephistopheles enters, the following
dialogue unfolds (p. 212):

MEPHISTOPHELES (*in a still lower tone*):   What is it then?
WAGNER (*as above*):   A man's being created.
MEPHISTOPHELES: A man? And pray, what amorous pair
                                  Hath in your smoke-hole found a habitation?
WAGNER: Nay, God forbid! The ancient mode of procreation
                    Is quite absurd, we now declare.
                    The tender speck which was life the source
                    The joy that issued from that tender force
                    And took and gave, for self-manifestation,
                    First near then foreign stuff, just by appropriation,
                    Is now despoiled of all its dignity

> And, though the beast may still delight therein,
> Man is so gifted that in future he
> Must have some purer, nobler origin.

At about the same time – albeit without Goethe's irony – Mary Shelley takes up the same alchemist tradition, reminding us expressively of Paracelsus and Albertus Magnus, and reveals in her novel *Frankenstein or The Modern Prometheus*, which appeared in 1818, the drama of a researcher who succeeds in uncovering the 'arcanum of life'.

> Some miracle might have produced it, yet the stages of labour were distinct and probable. After days and nights of incredible labour and fatigue, I succeeded in discovering the cause of generation and life; nay, more, I became myself capable of bestowing animation upon lifeless matter.
>
> (p. 52)

And once again, this time with the intention to warn, the idea emerges of breeding a new, better human race:

> A new species would bless me as its creator and source; many happy and excellent natures would owe their being to me.
>
> (p. 54)

The end of the novel – biological engineer Frankenstein is unable to dispose of the bloodthirsty creature of his own making: he dies, whilst the monster is left, so we fear, to roam – bathes this Promethean hope in the wan light of failure.

Schopenhauer

Yet Mary Shelley's warning went unheeded. It is true that the idea of chemically creating human beings lost significance with the triumph of the positive sciences during the 19th century; but the notion of breeding human beings was just entering its heyday. Again it was the philosophers who, right at the beginning of that century, provided some of the key terms for the entire future discussion on breeding. Arthur Schopenhauer wrote

> that a real and thorough improvement of the human race might be attained not so much from without as from within, thus not so much

by instruction and culture as rather upon the path of generation. Plato had already something of the kind in his mind when in the fifth book of his Republic he set forth his wonderful plan for increasing and improving his class of warriors. If we could castrate all scoundrels, and shut up all stupid geese in monasteries, and give persons of noble character a whole harem, and provide men, and indeed complete men, for all maidens of mind and understanding, a generation would soon arise which would produce a better age than that of Pericles.

(Schopenhauer [1896] p. 331)

In his thoughts, Schopenhauer does not restrict himself to 'such Utopian plans', however; he prefers to discuss various practical applications of his theory that 'characteristics are inheritable'. Building on the theory that human beings inherit their intelligence from the mother – character, inclinations and heart from the father – one could consider, for example

whether, as regards results, it would not be more advantageous to give the public dowries which upon certain occasions have to be distrib- uted, not, as is now customary, to the girls who are supposed to be the most virtuous, but to those who have most understanding and are the cleverest; especially as it is very difficult to judge as to virtue, for, as it is said, only God sees the heart. The opportunities for displaying a noble character are rare, and a matter of chance; besides, many a plain girl has a powerful support to her virtue in her plainness; on the other hand, as regards understanding, those who themselves are gifted with it can judge with great certainty after some examination.

(ibid., p. 332)

The idea hinted at here of deliberately applying social and political means for the purpose of breeding intelligence anticipates many a eugenic notion to come.

Nietzsche: Great Politics

The rest of the 19th century saw an increasing interest in breeding notions, reaching a philosophical climax with Friedrich Nietzsche. One of the points introduced at this stage to the theories on breed- ing human beings is their connection to the problem of 'degenera- tion'. In his work *Der Fall Wagner* (The Wagner Case), which appeared in 1888, Nietzsche introduced this French term to the German-speaking world and employed it as a critical characterisation of Richard Wagner's conception of aesthetics. Yet here it is already clear that the literary, aesthetic meaning of this term forms merely a part of a far more general conception of decadence, for which Wagner can be viewed as a paradigmatical case:

> What is interesting about Wagner, if anything, is the logic with which a physiological disgrace conclusively and gradually develops as a practice and a procedure, as a renewal of principles, as a crisis of [good] taste.
>
> (*WAG*, p. 27)

Wagner's aesthetic decadence is, according to Nietzsche, not merely a sign of the cultural times, but expression of a 'physiological degenerescence' visible in many forms, including alcohol and anarchy, emancipation of women, music and acting, pessimism and tolerance. It is of fundamental importance that Nietzsche bases his assumptions on a primacy of physiological decay, and that he uses the terms 'décadence' and 'degenerescence' more or less synonymously. In the fragments written during the 1880s, degeneration appears time and again as a phenomenon comprising part of each epoch within human history (1887, p. 87): as the product of an excretory procedure accompanying every vital process, and thus as a 'necessary consequence of life' (ibid., p. 255). Nietzsche's theory of decadence and degeneration picks up on a mood of decline which was rife in the second half of the 19th century, and which was still on the increase at the *fin-de-siècle*, a mood which literary and cultural circles circumscribed using the term decadence, and which during that time became stylised as an attitude towards life. In the last third of the 19th century, flirting with decadence was a raging fashion all over Europe; so, too, the biologistic vocabulary employed to interpret this decadence by many, including Nietzsche.

Since the 1850s, psychiatrists such as Bénédict August Morel and Valentin Magnan had been delivering biological explanations for the 'degeneration' of individuals, families and entire peoples; and in his *Versuch über die Ungleichheit der Menschenrassen* (Essay on the Inequality of the Human Races), Arthur Comte de Gobineau had related the degenerative decline of the most advanced cultures and peoples to the mixing of blood from higher and lower races, a 'dilution' of the more valuable blood from culture-bearing races being the consequence. In contrast to these theories of decline, Nietzsche did not stop at diagnosis, preferring to take it as the basis for his deliberations regarding a *therapy* for degenerative tendencies. Whereas Gobineau declared degeneration to be an unavoidable fate, Nietzsche introduced a kind of activism, heralded in his treatment of Wagner: Wagner is a 'case' for Nietzsche, not so much because of his decadence, but because he has accepted his decadence instead of attempting to fight it (*WAG*, pp. 11–12). The notes stemming from the late 1880s include much more obvious comments regarding the necessity of actively fighting degeneration. These notes emphasise the biologistical character of the concept of degeneration, as well as Nietzsche's strategy of how to fight it. A fragment written in December 1887 and bearing the characteristic title *Große Politik* (Great Politics) includes the words:

> Great politics want to make physiology the mistress above all else. They want to create a power which is strong enough to *breed* humanity, complete and elevated, ruthless towards the deformed and parasitical in life – towards everything which spoils, poisons, slanders, destroys . . . and which perceives the destruction of life as the emergence of an elevated type of soul.
>
> (1887, p. 638)

Underlying these 'great politics' is the – seemingly contradictory – theory that degeneration is unavoidable. Nietzsche views the *décadents* in parallel – between the vital process of the individual and that of the species – as 'the *excrement* of society' (ibid., p. 503), believing the décadents to be just as necessary as the excrement. Consistently maintaining the analogy of the individual organism's metabolic process, he manages at the same time to provide a solution to this contradiction between the unavoidability of the excrement and the fight against it: degeneration is just as unavoidable as 'excretion', but it is also just as harmless, providing that its products are consistently discarded. Thus the problem is not so much degeneration *per se*, but the 'unnatural' protection of those affected by it:

> Décadence itself is not something *which has to be fought*: it is absolutely necessary and part of each epoch and each people. What we

do have to fight with all our strength is contagion to the healthy parts of the organism. And do we? We do the *opposite*.

(ibid., p. 427)

Following this concept, Nietzsche developed his programme for the breeding of human beings, aimed neither at ensuring the health and well-being of the entire human species, nor at raising its average *niveau*; for presuming degeneration to be an unavoidable excretory process, a strategy of this kind must be doomed to fail. In place of worries about the future of the species, characteristic of Schopenhauer's considerations, the breeding of excellent *individuals* now emerges. Nietzsche conceives of a dichotomic breeding concept, envisaging two radically different types of human being: a small class of select 'overmen'[4] opposes a de-individualised mass, whose only reason for existing is to serve the 'strong'. In the Autumn of 1887, in a long fragment entitled *Die Starken der Zukunft* (The Strong of the Future) he calls for 'rift, distance, ranking', in order to protect the future 'master race' from contamination through the weak, as well as to guarantee it the total freedom to unfold:

> a race with its *own vital sphere*, with an excess of power for beauty, courage, culture, manner, to the most spiritual; a *positive* race which can allow itself every luxury.
>
> (1885, pp. 425–6)

Nietzsche: Breeding Strategy

It is not possible here to provide an interpretation of the 'overman' concept, controversial within secondary literature to the present day (Benz 1961; Kaufmann 1974). Fundamentally important is the close connection between this concept and that of breeding. Nietzsche emphasises time and again that the chance to create consciously and deliberately what nature has produced only occasionally and coincidentally has now arrived, as well as the necessity of doing so, and that this – the idea of breeding – is central to

---

[4] Regarding this translation of the German term *Übermensch*, cf. Kaufmann 1974.

his philosophy. He does not stop at a general discussion of 'breeding', instead clearly formulating the principle which should underlie it: an artificial increase in selection. In addition, he develops
numerous practical suggestions for a breeding strategy of this
kind. Of course, it would be naïve to expect a detailed and systematically worked out programme from a philosopher as aphoristic as
Nietzsche; yet even if a philosophical idea was of primary importance to him, and not the construction of a socially and technically
worked out catalogue of measurements, pieces and elements of
such a catalogue are nevertheless to be found within his works and
can be smoothly incorporated into the eugenics programmes of
later years. These elements may be summarised as three major
groups.

1. First of all, fragments come to our attention which at least
suggest a direct killing of the diseased and the degenerated, for
example when Nietzsche calls for 'the pathetic, misshaped,
deformed *to die out*' (1880, p. 250). It remains open whether a
mere generative extinction or a direct killing is the intention here;
and yet some passages definitely point to the latter possibility,
especially the fierce polemic against the Biblical ban on killing,
repeated in various notes more than once, sometimes directly cited
(1887, pp. 594, 599–600, 611–12). Similarly, in *The Gay Science* –
albeit carefully formulated as a question – Nietzsche proposes
infanticide to deal with diseased children.

2. This kind of deliberation is, however, more infrequent than
those aimed at a *generative* destruction of the 'dregs of humanity',
in other words, at preventing a further transfer of genetic defects
from one generation to the next. The idea with which Nietzsche
was to prove himself as a pioneer in eugenics, a field which was
not to be established in Germany until the turn of the century,
involves excluding from reproduction the diseased, the 'degenerated, the 'weak' and the 'disadvantaged'.

> In all cases where it would be a crime to have a child, for the chroni-
> cally ill and the third-degree neurasthenics, and yet where vetoing the
> sexual drive would constitute little more than a pious wish (this drive
> has a repulsive irritability in the disadvantaged), we have to call for
> *reproduction to be hindered*. There are few demands known to society
> which are as urgent and as fundamental. Contempt or social infamy
> will not be a sufficient means of deterring such a despicable weakness

of character. It will be necessary to punish this kind of crime with the highest of penalties, maybe even with the loss of 'freedom', with enclosure, regardless of status, rank or culture . . . A syphilis sufferer who begets a child is the cause of a whole chain of unsuccessful lives; he creates an objection to life; he is a pessimist *in the act*: he actually causes the value of life to be reduced indefinitely.

(1887, pp. 401–2)

Castration (p. 599), called for alongside detention and financial penalty, is to be seen within this context; so too the 'ennoblement' of prostitution (p. 402) as an outlet for those banned from reproducing. As early as 1880, obviously believing it unrealistic to limit the sexual activity of (and especially of) the ill, Nietzsche had called for sexuality and reproduction to be separated, later to become a key point within eugenics programmes:

It is necessary to *separate* the aphrodisiac stimulus from the consequences of satisfying it for the reproduction of the race . . .

(1880, p. 207)

3. A further complex of measurements concerns the institution of marriage. Since the randomness of betrothal renders 'all progress made by individuals' pointless (1880, p. 103), Nietzsche calls for a functionalisation of marriage, for generative purposes. He is convinced that the nobility has 'kept so well' due to its not entering into marriage for reasons of *amour passion* or *amour physique* (ibid., p. 120). Taking this as an example, all marriages in the future should be entered into 'for the purpose of higher development':

We should not render satisfaction of the [sexual] desire a practice inducing the race to suffer, in other words, one in which selection no longer takes place, instead each pairing up with the next and producing children. The *extinction* of many types of human being is just as *desirable* as any reproduction . . . In addition: marriage should only be (1) for the purpose of higher development, (2) in order to produce fruit from this kind of humanity. – For all others, concubinage should suffice, combined with the prevention of conception. – We have to put an end to this dull thoughtlessness. These geese should not be allowed to marry! There should be *far fewer* marriages! Take a walk through the cities and ask yourselves whether this people should be allowed to reproduce! They should all go visit their whores!

(ibid., p 189)

In a fragment bearing the title *Zur Zukunft der Ehe* (On the Future
of Marriage) and written eight years later, Nietzsche again suggests institutionalising marriage for generative purposes. New criteria are brought into play which are especially conspicuous in
their concreteness:

> – a *tax increase* at times of inheritance, etc., also an increase in mili-
> tary service for bachelors, starting at a particular age and increasing
> with time (within the community);
> – *advantages* of all sorts for fathers producing a wealth of sons:
> possibly a majority of votes;
> – a *medical certificate* preceding each marriage and signed by the
> committees within a community: in which both the engaged couple
> and the doctors have to answer a number of defined questions ('family
> history');
> – as an antidote to *prostitution* (or as its ennoblement): marriages
> with expiry dates, legalised (for years, months, for days), with a guar-
> antee for the children;
> – responsibility for and advocation of each marriage by a particular
> number of confidentials within a community: as a community affair.
>
> (1887, p. 495)

Even though evidence suggests that the idea of breeding human
beings has been a topic and a problem for philosophers and the
Arts ever since Ancient times, Nietzsche nevertheless assumes a
special position within this tradition in that he marks the crossover
from philosophy to science. On the one hand, his philosophy relies
on the theory of evolution: not only because his emphasis on
'becoming' adopts basic evolutionary theory or because he made
this one of the central points of his philosophy (Kaufmann 1974).
Far more important in the context here is that Nietzsche does not
base his concept of breeding human beings on the experiences
gained from animal and plant breeding, but on a theoretical principle: on the Darwinian principle of artificial selection. This is not
altered by the fact that wherever he explicitly mentions Darwin
and his theories, he usually does so dismissingly and despisingly.
Nietzsche may certainly be considered a pioneer in the field of
eugenics, anticipating the genetic programmes to come more than
a decade and a half in advance, often with astonishing accuracy.
On the other hand – and this is part of the reason for his discrepancy regarding eugenics – Nietzsche's philosophising is not really

aimed at *scientification* of the idea of breeding human beings. However important the adoption of various elements from contemporary biological theories may have been for his philosophy, a claim to having a scientific nature, as pointedly staked by the eugenicists, would have contradicted not only his style of thinking, but also his key intention: a 're-evaluation of values', as he was aiming at, could only, as far as he was concerned, remain a purely philosophical project.

3

The evolution of eugenics

Racial breeding as politics
is the kidnappers' love of children
Gottfried Benn[1]

The 19th century took up the idea of breeding human beings,
which had been around for two thousand years, and steered it in a
radically new direction: in the second half of the century, a new

---

[1] This excellent formulation (Benn 1968b, pp. 858–9) should not lead one to assume
that the famous poet was a fundamental opponent of 'racial breeding'. Before
Fascist *reality* changed everybody's views on breeding, Benn's were as follows: 'The
fact that this purfication of the people has to come about – not only in order to
shape up the race, but also for socio-economic reasons – becomes obvious when one
hears that the average number of children in Germany, low enough as it is, is only
achieved through the feeble-minded, who exceed the average by as much as 64%,
and that their offspring, which is usually also feeble-minded, costs the State enormous sums of money: whereas a normal child costs the State 120 Marks p.a., a feeble-minded schoolchild costs 250 Marks and an imbecilic, institutionalised child 900
Marks... The criteria according to which German eugenicists – very representative
of the new German *Weltanschauung* – want to breed the German type provide a significant orientation. I would like to emphasise that the following comments do not
stem from Parliamentary reports, nor from political essays, but from scientific publications. These publications state that a public department of genetic health is to be
established with branches all over the country, classing and registering the entire
population according to a kind of points system, whereby the total number of points
for each individual is to be calculated not only from his/her personal constitution,
but also from an exact investigation of his/her ancestors. This points sytem would
then be taken as the basis for marriages. Marriages would be carried out or prevented, approved of or particularly sanctioned by the State. It seems that some marriages, particularly desirable to the State for being in a position to preserve and continue the population's most precious genetic matter, is to be encouraged by subsidy'
(Benn 1986a, pp. 797–9).

scientific discipline bearing the name *eugenics* emerged, claiming to investigate systematically the possibilities of rational control over human reproduction, thus guiding procreation away from Utopian projects. There is no direct historical or theoretical continuity between this movement and the older conceptions of Plato or Campanella. The eugenicists have often referred to Ancient Sparta and its exemplary nature, and have on occasion extolled Plato as a predecessor of their convictions; sometimes there is also agreement about the content of policies and objectives. Yet there is a difference between the fundamental problem, that is the theoretical foundation underlying the discipline of eugenics, and the ancient Utopian notions of breeding already mentioned; more than anything, with the foundation of societies and magazines, with its far-reaching efforts to popularise and politically to realise its ideals, eugenics extends beyond the limits of (more or less) fantastic plans and programmes, to become a scientific, social and political *movement*.

Degeneration

It seems appropriate for this 'realistic' turnaround in the notion of breeding that eugenics based itself on a problem which was – so its advocates believed – empirically evident, as well as crucial for the entire future fate of humanity: the problem of degeneration. Contrary to common prejudice, belief in progress, which was chided as naïve during the 19th century, certainly did not escape from a consciousness of decline, until then staged as a decadent desire for decay, but frequently as a naked fear of visions of an apocalyptical future as well. The prophecy of a 'physical degeneration' threatening civilised humanity played a key rôle in the apocalyptic visions of the *fin-de-siècle*, as already shown in the discussion of Nietzsche. The historical background of this fear of degeneration was industrialisation, fulfilled under Capitalist conditions, and with trenchant social consequences. The accumulation of ever increasing masses of human beings in the towns, the renowned living conditions in those towns, the poverty and the inhuman working conditions of the industrial proletariat all had grave consequences for the health of large sections of the population: death rates in infants and children within the towns were alarmingly high; the physical constitution of those who had had to survive a twelve to fourteen-hour working day since the age of children, with insufficient nutrition, usually catastrophic hygiene and in cramped living conditions, was often pitiful. During the second half of the century, impressed by the progress of evolutionary and genetic theory, with a professionally limited perspective – many of the eugenicists were doctors – and under the spell of political and social prejudices, the historical and social causes of this development were pushed into the background; degeneration appeared as a purely biological process.

This biologistical interpretation was confirmed theoretically by Darwin's theory of evolution, at that time gaining all the dimensions of an intellectual and ideological fashion. The phenomenon of degeneration could be deduced from this theory, for if (1) it is correct that natural selection is the driving force behind evolutionary progress; if (2) it is true that this natural selective mechanism does not have the same effect within human society as it does within Nature, that a large number of human actions are directed at slackening or even abolishing natural selection; then we may conclude (3) that humanity in a state of civilisation cannot progress, but can only degenerate. It is not possible here to investigate in detail the tacit and, biologically speaking, partly untenable premises for this deduction. The fact that Darwin himself, who was otherwise very reticent regarding the application of his theory to human history, had just as little doubt in this respect as most of his contemporaries is more than significant evidence of the degree to which it was unquestioningly accepted. In his book *The Descent of Man and Selection in Relation to Sex*, which first appeared in 1871, he writes:

> With savages, the weak in body or mind are soon eliminated; and those that survive commonly exhibit a vigorous state of health. We civilized men, on the other hand, do our utmost to check the process of elimination; we build asylums for the imbecile, the maimed, and the sick; we institute poor-laws; and our medical men exert their utmost skill to save the life of every one to the last moment. There is reason to believe that vaccination has preserved thousands, who from a weak constitution would formerly have succumbed to small-pox.

Thus the weak members of civilized societies propagate their kind. No one who has attended to the breeding of domestic animals will doubt that this must be highly injurious to the race of man. It is surprising how soon a want of care, or care wrongly directed, leads to the degeneration of a domestic race; but excepting in the case of man himself, hardly any one is so ignorant as to allow the worst animals to breed.

(Darwin 1974, pp. 130–1)

Darwin was not the first person to make a connection between the problem of degeneration and the principle of natural selection; moreover, he was not to be the last. We can understand the conclusiveness which the tracing of degeneration back to the principle of selection was to acquire if we consider that the problem of decline, physically, spiritually and morally, of civilised humanity had been an established part of the European history of ideas at least since Rousseau's *A Discourse on Inequality*, and had become very obvious around the middle of the century in connection with the problems of industrialisation and urbanisation mentioned above. For the first time ever, Darwin's theory made it possible to provide a scientific explanation for a phenomenon which had been diagnosed many a time, but which had never been understood theoretically. In natural selection – or, more precisely: its exclusion from civilised societies – the causal mechanism responsible for degeneration seemed to have been found at last.

Artificial selection

Darwin's theory is also fundamental to eugenics in another respect. Revealing the causal mechanism of degeneration can be regarded as one of the central achievements of the 19th century, not only for theoretical reasons, but also for practical ones. A theory of the type common to the modern sciences does not only permit explanation of phenomena; at the same time, it provides the intellectual prerequisites for their technological control. Whereas Darwin – together with theoreticists such as Ernst Haeckel or Herbert Spencer – was content to stop at the regrettable conclusion that 'degenerative' tendencies are one of the consequences of reduced selective pressure upon the civilised human being, younger generation evolutionists now emerged with the idea of putting the selection theory to practical use, in order to halt the degenerative process, and maybe even turn it around. As early as the 1860s, Darwin's nephew, Francis Galton, had published his thoughts on how the quality of the human race could be improved; in the years to follow, he systematically expanded upon these considerations, pushing measures for increasing intellectual quality into the foreground; it was also Galton who introduced the term 'eugenics' – derived from the Greek 'eugen'es' = 'of noble origin'. In the 1890s, following on from Galton, the scientific movement which developed under this name also found protagonists in Germany, with the work of Alfred Ploetz and Wilhelm Schallmayer (cf. Weingart, Kroll & Bayertz 1988). Darwin's theory revolutionised not only biology, but also the social sciences; as the most significant 'theoretical reformation' of the 19th century, it opened up a field of practical options which until then had been barred:

> The mission of the 20th Century seems to be to deduce the practical use of the theory of descendence and apply it to life in practice.
>
> (Schallmayer 1903, p. X)

The central idea of the eugenic strategy is based on an attempt to break through the causal mechanism of degeneration, outlined in the deduction above: if modern civilisation strips natural selection of its powers, and if this causally leads to degeneration, then natural selection must be replaced by consciously controlled *artificial selection*. In the first chapter of his *Origin of Species*, Darwin describes and explains the procedure of artificial selection as it has been practised in plant and animal breeding for thousands of years. In practice, from a given population (e.g. a flock of sheep) those individuals are selected which come closest to the breeding aim in question (e.g. lots of wool), and only these individuals are allowed to reproduce; if this selection is repeated over generations, it leads to a gradual increase in the desired characteristic. This procedure is the rôle model for the eugenic concept of procreation. Further degeneration of the human species is to be prevented by, on the one hand, excluding genetically 'inferior' individuals from reproduction, thus preventing them from passing on their defects to the next generation and, on the other hand, by giving individuals with desirable characteristics the opportunity to have as many off-spring as possible.

It is not necessary to examine eugenic policies in detail here; apart from a great many Utopian projects, the considerations of the eugenicists concentrate on two criteria complexes: firstly, control over marriage, whether by voluntary marriage guidance, or by making it law for couples wishing to marry to have to exchange health certificates in which suitability for marriage and reproduction (to be medically ascertained beforehand) are confirmed according to eugenic criteria; secondly, the sterilisation of criminals, of the mentally ill, the blind, deaf and dumb, and all other 'inferior' individuals. Besides these disqualifying criteria, there exists a catalogue of social and political privileges, intended to encourage the healthy and 'able' to reproduce actively: e.g. tax benefits for families with many children, and an improvement in the salaries of high-ranking civil servants, officers and teachers, in order to proliferate their especially valuable generative disposition.

Eugenic strategies have never enjoyed consistent and complete realisation. Insofar as individual parts have been put into practice, they have – significantly – not been the social and political, but the authoritative segments of eugenic policy: as early as 1907, laws to enforce sterilisation were introduced within the U.S. State of Indiana; several other U.S. States followed, as well as various European countries, including Denmark and Sweden. On 14 July 1933, a 'law to prevent genetically diseased offspring' was passed in Germany, following which a complete system of State sanctions was built up, for the purpose of 'keeping the race pure' (cf. Weingart *et al.* 1988), and smoothly paving the way to subsequent extermination machinery in the concentration camps.

Rationalisation

The brutal consequences of eugenic philosophy under Fascist rule, its – partial – link, formed long before, with irrational racial ideology and Utopian ideas of procreation should not conceal the fact, however, that eugenics was an emerging movement borne from the spirit of science, and with a bold claim to being scientific.

The historical 'success' of eugenics really would have been impossible without its scientific foundations. More or less realistic notions of breeding human beings have existed, as we have seen, at least since Plato's time, without any one of them extending beyond the status of a theoretical project. None of them did much more than to extrapolate to human beings the knowledge gained from plant and animal breeding; it was Darwin who first managed to gain a theoretical understanding of this practice, and it was his theory which made a scientification of the notion of breeding possible. Progress was theoretical as well as 'ideological': if eugenics had any hope at all – however small – of being realised, then more than anything because of its support from the *scientific authority* of Darwin's theory and the scientistic *Zeitgeist* of the 19th and 20th centuries.

In more than one respect, eugenics has proved to be a specific manifestation of that 'occidental rationalism' which, according to Max Weber, rules all of Western European history. First of all, eugenics, together with its theoretical foundations, the theory of evolution and inheritance, may be regarded as a perfect example of science's tendency to 'destroy the mystique' within our world. The occidental nature of rationality

> is essentially characterised through the *calculability* of technically crucial factors: of the basis for accurate calculation. Yet this really means: through the uniqueness of Western science, especially the mathematically and experimentally accurate, rationally founded natural sciences.
>
> (Weber 1947, p. 10)

One of the things which the theory of evolution has rendered calculable and 'lacking in mystique' is sexuality. Science had previously had little to say about it, describing it in its many forms but never attempting even the slightest explanation of it:

> Here was a fact for which, as Buffon put it, 'there was no other solution than the fact itself'. It was not until the theory of evolution that sexuality acquired a scientific status. It then became possible to discuss sexuality not only in terms of its origins, but in terms of its function.
>
> (Jacob 1983, p. 17)

This process can be interpreted as 'rationalisation' inasmuch as scientific discourse has conquered a new, previously impenetrable field and acquired additional parts of reality. It is not by chance that the emergence of eugenics at the end of the 19th century coincided with a strong scientific interest in 'sexual matters': the writings of Galton, Ploetz and Schallmayer are contemporary with those of Richard von Krafft-Ebing, August Forel and Sigmund Freud.

The rationalisation process is not limited, however, to an understanding of the world, theoretically or scientifically; far more, it includes the 'human ability and disposition towards certain kinds of practical and rational *lifestyles*' (Weber 1947, p. 12). In this sense, eugenics may be interpreted as a movement towards rationalising human sexual and reproductive behaviour. Numerous statements from eugenicists certify that this interpretation is fully in line with key eugenic notions. The actual state of randomness and individual arbitrariness – 'Krethi and Plethi get married for the hell of it' (Ploetz 1895, p. 149) – are desperately in requirement of fundamental change; procreation may not be left to chance, but must be controlled according to principles 'which science has drawn up for time and other conditions' (ibid., p. 144). At any one time, the scientific and technological state of the art exerts continually increasing normative pressure upon mankind; in the same way as in other areas of life, human reproduction is no longer to be left to the natural course of events and routine, traditional behaviour, but is to be planned and controlled in accordance with the scientific and technological options available.

Revising morality

This claim to rationalisation evidently opposes governing moral norms. One of the key elements within Western morality is the equality of all human beings, a principle which can be traced back to the Christian conviction of having been created in God's image. The principle of equality does not maintain that all human beings are factually equal, but that they are morally equal in the sense of being entitled to equal rights: it postulates equal treatment. Eugenics questions just this. For the eugenicists, biological inequality in human beings amounts to human inequi*valence*. By being able to transfer his defect to community, people or race via reproduction, the carrier of a genetic disease or other genetic defect renders himself 'inferior'. Like the Social Darwinists before them, who had rejected the principle of equality favoured by Western ethics because of its contradiction of the biological facts, the eugenicists also view this principle as an obstacle to be removed in the fight against degeneration. In this respect, human beings appear as mere members of the genus, to which they, as carriers of good or bad biological characteristics, are indebted, but without rights.

Eugenic policy and existing morality are thus insurmountably contradictory. Firstly, the problem which eugenics claims to solve has itself been created by this very morality. In the programmatic title of his most major work, Alfred Ploetz confronts 'protection of the weak' with 'the fitness of our race'. Running through his entire line of argumentation is the notion that the triumph of 'the idea of humanitarian equality' (Ploetz 1895, p. 194), as created by Christian religion and adopted by both modern democracy and socialism, has to be made (at least partly) responsible for the degeneration of humanity. Ploetz is by no means alone in this opinion:

> One characteristic of Christianity is its promotion of the interests of the *weak* and *unfortunate*: this is not at all helpful to the social organism or the interests of our race . . . Judging without prejudice and independently of any particular tendency... it is hardly possible to overlook the fact that *Christian views, insofar as they are effective at all, do not tend to improve the selection process, neither consciously nor unconsciously, but rather – unconsciously, of course – the reverse.*
> (Schallmayer 1903, p. 227)

Secondly, Christian morality is an obstruction to the central eugenic goal: excluding the genetically 'inferior' from the reproductive process. From a eugenic perspective, the notions of individual self-determination and natural human rights, including the right to have children, represent probably the most decisive obstacle to a 'rationalisation' of human reproduction for the purpose of advanced generative development.

The eugenicists are forever demanding 'a partial change in current moral views' (Schallmayer 1903, p. X), aimed at overcoming

Christian and individualistic morality in favour of 'developmental ethics'. Nietzsche is cited as a pioneer of such ethics, his main objection to Christian morality also concentrating on its principle of equality for all human beings and its welfare for the diseased and weak.

> If we view all individuals as equal, we cast doubt upon the entire genus, favouring a practice which can only end in its ruin: Christianity is the opposite principle to *selection*. If the deformed and the diseased 'Christian' is to be as worthy as the healthy 'Heathen', or even worthier, according to Pascal's judgment of disease and health, then the natural course of development is crossed, and *unnature* made Law.
>
> (Nietzsche 1887, p. 470)

In their criticism of Western morality, the eugenicists are able to refer to Nietzsche,[2] whose bitter campaign against Christian religion and humanistic morality coincided with the goals of the eugenicists in two major points: in its demand that human inequality and, especially, human inequivalence be recognised, and in its demand that all special welfare for the 'weak' be renounced, replacing it with strict selection.

Selection according to 'stud farm' principles

There are also contemporaries who see eugenics, with its call for a comprehensive rationalisation of sexual activity, with its notions – part socially and technologically rational, part Utopian and irrational – of a breeding State (Weingart 1984), and with its opposition to Western Christian morality, as an outrage or as a political and moral challenge. Although it must be taken seriously, biological

---

[2] Schallmayer, for example: '*Yet in theory, there can be no denying that the theory of descendence leads to the postulate for ethics to be improved in the sense of a developmental ethics.* This was also recognised and voiced hundreds of times by *Nietzsche* in his philosophical, poetic manner . . .'. Following several citations from *Also sprach Zarathustra*, Schallmayer hints at probably the greatest difference between the eugenics programme and Nietzsche's breeding concept: 'But his hyperaristocratic sense leads him to underestimate social capabilities. He focusses far more upon individual improvement than upon that of society' (Schallmayer 1903, p. 243).

and ethical criticism of eugenic theories and policies has been astonishingly weak. In 1918, the German zoologist Oscar Hertwig published a work entitled *Zur Abwehr des ethischen, des sozialen, des politischen Darwinismus* (A Rejection of Ethical, Social and Political Darwinism), in which he scathingly attacked contemporary eugenics, especially emphasising the consequences which would ensue should these policies ever be realised.

> It has to be clear from the very beginning that a breeding State cannot be established successfully without passing compulsory laws, and without outrageous interventions in one of the first and strongest natural rights of every individual, the preservation of its species, and the right to self-determination practised within it . . . Just as the institutions of the Church accompany its members through life, a Christening symbolically accepting them into the Christian community, Confirmation sending them into their working lives, marriage entered into as a holy sacrament and, ultimately, the comfort offered to them and their relatives in times of approaching death and at funerals, in a breeding State – according to the Utopias of some Social Darwinists – a committee would receive the newborn babies and subject them to a medical examination in order to determine whether they should be fit to be brought up, or whether, because of a weak constitution or, far more likely, because of being genetically unsuitable for the breeding of a noble race, a useless burden on the State, it would be better to weed them out immediately, with a dose of morphium or a similarly mild alternative method. A board of educational governors would then monitor the young people's physical and mental development, and would test the reproductive worth of each individual. The highest and ultimately decisive Government body would then use this most valuable preliminary work to select candidates for marriage according to the principles of a stud farm, with every instance of reproduction marking a gradual improvement to the human race.
>
> (Hertwig 1921, pp. 89–91)

Whilst Hertwig's far-sighted criticism was to have no influence on eugenic developments in Germany, unable to prevent rapid descension to a system of State controls, the same development took a very different direction in the Anglo-Saxon countries. As early as the 1920s, a group of theoreticists came together which, on the one hand, firmly believed in Darwin's theory and the eugenic notion regarding the necessity – not to mention feasibility

– of rationally controlling human reproduction yet, on the other hand, distanced itself from the 'classic' eugenics prevalent in England and the U.S.A. at that time. In a short, Utopian work entitled *Daedalus*, J. B. S. Haldane makes no attempt to conceal his mockery:

> The eugenic official, a compound, it would appear, of the policeman, the priest and the procurer, is to hale us off at suitable intervals to the local temple of Venus Genetrix with a partner chosen, one gathers, by something of the nature of a glorified medical board. To this prophecy I should reply that it proceeds from a type of mind as lacking in originality as in knowledge of human nature. Marriage 'by numbers', so to speak, was a comparatively novel idea when proposed by Plato 2,300 years ago, but it has already actually been practised in various places, notably among the subjects of the Jesuits in Paraguay.
>
> (1924, pp. 40–1)

More so than the German eugenicists, Haldane and his colleagues were aware that eugenic policies could have a chance of succeeding only if they were capable of strongly motivating the majority of the population to participate voluntarily; they spent no time on the establishment of an authoritarian breeding State in the manner often conceived by German eugenicists. Influential was not only the background of a liberal and individualist Anglo-Saxon culture, but especially the political orientation of this group, the members of which were mainly Socialists, with an open ear for Marxism. In 1936, in his book *Out of the Night*, the American radiogeneticist Herman J. Muller, one of the leading brains behind 'left-wing' eugenics, published a comprehensive vision of the biological future ahead of the human race, as well as a new eugenic strategy which he was continually to modify and develop throughout the subsequent three decades. First of all, Muller firmly distances himself from the eugenic concepts prevalent before then, and especially from their often reactionary political background, as expressed in the Social Darwinist supposition that the members of the upper classes and particular races are *eo ipso* genetically 'superior' to the average members of other classes and races (1936, pp. 149–50). Indisputably with humanist intentions, and without losing sight of the deterring example of eugenic politics within Fascist Germany (ibid., p. 11), he rejects all forms of State control and bases his suggestions on the principle of strict voluntarism towards all eugenic criteria (pp. 146–7). In addition, his eugenic strategy differs from the more technocratic concepts, such as those proposed by Schallmayer, mainly due to the fact that it declares a profound social, political and economic revolution of society to be a key requisite for its own success: without alterations, in the sense of a stronger cooperative structuring of society, any eugenic strategy is doomed to fail under the given Capitalist circumstances. This is expression of the Socialist conviction held by Muller at this time – as by many of his contemporary British eugenicists. A key element within a social reform of this kind has to be a change in the position of women: through general distribution of contraceptives, through alleviation of labour pains, through an unburdening of women from sole responsibility for the raising and bringing up of children and through overall improvement in their social status. This could pave the way to the prerequisites for deciding reproductive matters in accordance with the aspects of love and common sense, and in the interests of future generations on the one hand, and the partners involved on the other (ibid., p. 134).

Mutation

Yet why eugenics in the first place? The main reason for Muller's adherence to the necessity of scientific control over human reproduction is a premise shared by the rest of the eugenics community: the conviction that the human race is degenerating. It is no mere postulation that the mechanism of natural selection undergoes severe limitations and alterations under civilised circumstances, and the question of which alterations will result in the long term for the human biological constitution is a scientific and, of course, political problem which has to be taken seriously. On the other hand, Muller does not simply adopt the concept of degeneration from traditional eugenics, preferring to reformulate the problem on the basis of the latest achievements within the field of genetics.

Following the rediscovery of Mendel's rules, the field of genetics entered a stormy period, on a theoretical level (emergence of the theory of chromosomes and mutation, as well as population genetics) and on a methodical level (in particular, *Drosophila* research), during which genetics ventured further and further into the micro-regions of the hereditary mechanism. This was not irrelevant for the science underpinning eugenics, not least because Muller's decisive step lay in the shifting of the degeneration problem to a molecular level. Whereas eugenics had formerly related its diagnosis of degeneration to more often than not imprecisely definable, physical, phenotypic characteristics, Muller refers to the molecular hereditary mechanism itself, emphasising the importance of the problem of mutation for his concept of degeneration. Based on the assumption that the number of new mutations within the two gametes from which a human individual originates ranges from 1:2 to 1:10 (i.e. one mutation to 2–10 gametes), he comes to the conclusion that every human individual carries several heterozygotic genes which, if they were homozygotic, would be lethal. Since, on the one hand, natural selection is at least partly excluded from modern societies and the harmful genes are not eliminated but steadily reproduced and since, on the other hand, additional new mutations repeatedly occur, the amount of harmful genes is forever increasing. Muller feared that the continual growth of this genetic burden had to reach a critical limit at some stage, beyond which the entire human genetic system would collapse, taking humanity down with it.[3]

The problem of degeneration becomes even more of a threat if we consider that, up until now, we have reviewed only spontaneous mutations. In highly developed industrial countries, the genetic burden is increased, however, by a second group of – exogenously induced – mutations. As early as 1927, Muller pioneered experiments in which the mutagenic influence of ultraviolet rays on *Drosophila* was demonstrated for the first time. Generally speaking, the result of these experiments, for which Muller received the Nobel prize in 1946, was proof that the rate of mutation may be drastically increased by exogenous influences. These environmental influences include the various energy rays (radioactivity, gamma and X-rays), as well as chemical substances

---

[3] Although the theory of a growing 'genetic burden' cannot conclusively be rejected, modern human geneticists no longer assume that genetic defects will rapidly increase in number, leading to a collapse of the entire human genetic system (cf. Dobzhansky 1962; Vogel & Motulsky 1986).

used in the industrial production process or found in waste products. The inhabitants of industrial countries are exposed to the effects of chemicals and radiation to a much greater extent than ever before in history, causing Muller and other biologists to express their fears very early on that the rate of mutation in these countries could increase dramatically as a result of increasing mutagenic factors.

Even if this process did not lead to a total collapse of the genetic system, the consequences would be threatening. The increasing genetic burden is leading to irreversible genetic damage in a growing number of individuals and to an increase in the defects affecting any one individual. They include not only grave, but also minor defects, not potentially fatal but cumulatively able to lead to serious limitations in quality of life. Prior to a final extinction of the human race, there would be a long period of decline to be reckoned with, during which the human race would exist mainly of diseased and crippled people, dependent for their lives upon a steadily expanding system of medical care and compensation. B. Glass describes the consequences of this process very clearly:

> . . . by surrounding ourselves with an ever more artificial environment, we unwittingly modify the rigor of natural selection in many ways. The price we must pay, in the end, for the mercies of medical care and surgical aid is a dysgenic [detrimental from a genetic viewpoint] increase in the frequencies of certain detrimental genes, the effects of which we have learned to ameliorate . . . No one, I think, would have it otherwise. Yet to contemplate the man of tomorrow who must begin his day by adjusting his spectacles and his hearing aid, inserting his false teeth, taking an allergy injection in one arm and an insulin injection in the other, and topping off his preparations for life by taking a tranquilizing pill, is none too pleasant. To say the least, medical science steadily increases the load it must carry.
>
> (quoted from Etzioni 1973, pp. 81–2)

Germinal choice

As is always the case when apocalyptical visions of the future are put into words, Muller's 'biological fire-and-brimstone prophecy' (Dobzhansky 1962, p. 295) is not an end in its own right, but is the starting point for a strategy intended to interrupt and, if possible, even revert a fateful development. Behind Muller's strategy is a critical analysis of traditional eugenic policies. On top of his political and ethical scepticism, he strongly criticises the scientific criteria of these policies. Carrying on from Haldane's research, Muller begins by demonstrating the hopelessness of one of the central points of traditional eugenics: the elimination of certain characteristics by sterilising their carriers. If we assume, as in Muller's mock calculation, that in the U.S.A. there are 300 000 feeble-minded people whose illness may be traced back to a recessive gene, then sterilisation would have to be carried out through eight generations in order to reduce the number of those affected by half; it would take another twelve generations (i.e. twenty in all – 600 years) to reduce the number to 75 000; further reduction would require even longer (1936, p. 97). This slight and, with time, ever slighter success is due to the fact that the genes responsible for feeble-mindedness are to be found not only in the 300 000 feeble-minded people, but also in about ten million apparently normal individuals; these 'carriers' have inherited the gene from only one parent, inheriting the normal, dominant gene from the other one. Totally healthy themselves, they can unknowingly pass on the gene in question to their children; not until two carriers come together will the children – although both parents are healthy – be born feeble-minded. Thus, according to Muller, as long as there is no control over the reproductive behaviour of all the carriers, most of the defect genes will be passed on to the next generation; even after a thousand years there would still be more than four million heterozygotic carriers and approximately 35 000 acute sufferers of the disease. Therefore, any eugenic strategy which does not include these heterozygotic carriers will remain largely unsuccessful.

> But if we could detect all the 'carriers', it is not unlikely that we should find the majority of seemingly 'normal' persons to be 'carriers' of some gross defect or other, or of several at once. It would then be obviously impracticable to advise that all 'carriers' refrain from reproduction . . .
>
> (ibid., p. 100)

For this reason, Muller's own eugenic strategy dissociates itself from sterilisation and essentially advocates the introduction of technological means not considered by 'classical' eugenics and which even Muller could only hope to see realised in the future. Such means include the transplantation of ripe or fertilised egg cells from one woman to another, the development of egg cells without fertilisation and the manipulation of embryos, in particular artificial insemination in connection with the selection of desired genetic material (ibid., pp. 135–6). In his later writing, Muller concentrated more and more on this technology. In his contribution to the Ciba Foundation symposium in 1962, which subsequently gained embarrassing publicity, he again emphasised the necessity of preventing defect genes from being passed on from one generation to another, thus limiting their ability to spread.

> It is probable that some 20 per cent, if not more, of a human population has received a genetic impairment that arose by mutation in the immediately preceding generation, in addition to the far larger number of impairments inherited from earlier generations. If this is true, then, to avoid genetic deterioration, about 20 per cent of the population who are more heavily laden with genetic defects than the average must in each generation fail to live until maturity or, if they do live, must fail to reproduce. Otherwise, the load of genetic defects carried by that population would inevitably rise.
>
> (Muller 1967, p. 252)

By strictly rejecting State control for political and ethical reasons, at the same time believing a call for voluntary abstinence from reproduction to be unrealistic – formation of large families from a small proportion of the population, whilst the rest, the far greater proportion, remains childless would, in his opinion, be generally considered unfair, and would have no chance within a democratic society – Muller develops a way out of this dilemma, based not on the idea of preventing the creation of offspring, but on that of preventing the transferral of defect genes. In concrete terms: a couple with the desire to have children, where a genetic incompatibility between the partners is suspected or where the man possesses a genetic defect would – following 'classical' eugenic notions – have to sacrifice this desire. Yet Muller sees no necessity for this; the sacrifice can be avoided with the help of artificial insemination. This technology allows the woman in question to be fertilised with the sperm of a healthy man, (hopefully) leading to the birth of a healthy baby. According to Muller, this process of 'eutelegenesis' or *germinal choice* 'turns out on closer inspection to be the most practical, effective, and satisfying means of genetic therapy' (ibid., p. 258); for it does not take away a person's right to form a family and have children. Of course, the resulting children are not always genetically one's own. In the cases where it is necessary to prevent dysgenetic characteristics being transferred to the next generations, biological parenthood (at least for the male partner) is to be replaced by social parenthood.

Technological dynamics

There are two points in Muller's strategy worth noting. Firstly, it begins to close the large gap between the postulates of a rationalisation of reproductive behaviour and reigning social values. Muller spends no time on a 're-evaluation of values' along the lines of Darwinist development ethics. He does call for a renunciation of traditional attitudes regarding procreation and parenthood, as well as 'a new code of ethics governing in a more intelligent fashion our reproductive behaviour' (1936, p. 145; cf. also 1967, p. 254); yet this is not aimed at a total revision of Western Christian morality, but – far more – a sort of compromise between traditional ethics and the (supposed) demands of science. In particular, it rejects inconsiderate subordination of individual interests below those of the species, expressed not least in the demand for voluntarism regarding all eugenic measures.

Secondly, however, this is obviously not only expression of a humanist standpoint, but also the result of new technological options. It is the artificial fertilisation technology which provides a way out of the dilemma between necessary exclusion from reproduction and the legitimate desire to have children. Not only this, but an appropriate distribution of artifical (heterologous) insemination requires that suitable sperm be universally available. In *Out of the Night*, Muller still had to describe the extracorporeal cultivation of male germ cells as a vision for the future; in his later works he was able to refer to the technology of deep-freezing sperm, which had made the establishment of sperm banks possible and with them the 'material' for artificial insemination available at all times. Yet these were technological achievements which were not available for previous eugenic concepts. The significance of such technologies for Muller's concept of eugenics gained at the same rate at which he turned away from his former Socialist convictions. Whereas at first he wanted to solve the social problems which unavoidably arose with aspired rationalisation of reproductive behaviour through a profound social revolution, he now had to look for more pragmatic ways of solving them: technological solutions. Rationalisation of reproductive behaviour is thus transferred to a *technologisation*. The more than two thousand year-old notion of breeding human beings takes a turn which is to define its continued fate to the present day: by replacing the extrapolation of pre-scientific experiences with a systematic and direct investigation of the reproductive process, this notion loses its Utopian character and becomes a scientific problem and then a technological project. As an applied science, eugenics aims at the technologically do-able. As from the second half of the 19th century, the 'logic' behind breeding programmes began to follow more and more closely the state of the art of the biological sciences and the practical options of biotechnology.

Once in the slipstream of this dynamic process, the breeding programmes become dependent upon a characteristic dialectic. On the one hand, the ever increasing range of options opens up numerous possible ways, through the introduction of new technologies, of circumventing manifest conflicts between technical 'requirements' and socially anchored values, or at least of moderating them. With his 'germinal choice' policy, Muller solves the conflict between the socially accepted right to have a family (with children) and the necessity of a generative elimination of the carriers of damaging mutations. This is a characteristic case of 'technological fix': the attempt to solve a moral, social or political problem not with moral, social or political means, but with technology. This 'technological fix' strategy is to the present day a fundamental feature of not only the developments within the field of eugenics, but also characteristic of human genetics and gene and reproduction technology in general (cf. Weingart *et al.* 1988). On the other hand, scientific and technological dynamics lead to a constant temptation to invert the relationship between normative values and technological options: the development of eugenic policies does not follow a gradual change in the values underlying them or the goals aimed at within them, but the ever accelerating rhythm of scientific and technological innovation. The achievements of the biological sciences and biotechnology no longer serve as means of realising given eugenic policies, but begin themselves to dictate content and structure.

4

Reconstructing humanity

The human species is in desperate need
of genetic improvement . . .
Julian Huxley

Modern science has left us in no doubt that human beings are
natural beings. Since at least Darwin's time, we have known that
the biological species *Homo sapiens* has developed from the animal
kingdom, via a long line of transformations. Darwin's contemporaries compared this discovery with the Copernican revolution:
in the same way that three hundred years earlier heliocentric
astronomy destroyed prejudices about the position of the Earth
within the universe, the theory of descent destroyed illusions
about the position of mankind within organic Nature. Ernst
Haeckel, with the pathos prevalent in the 19th century, viewed
Darwin not as someone who had put forward just another scientific theory, but as the person with an answer to the 'question of
all questions':

> The immense value of the Theory of Descent in regard to the
> Biological consists, as I have already remarked, in its explaining to us
> the origin of organic forms in a mechanical way, and pointing out
> their active causes. But however highly and justly this service of the
> Theory of Descent may be valued, yet it is almost eclipsed by the
> immense importance which a single necessary inference from it claims
> for itself alone. This necessary and unavoidable inference is the theory
> of the *animal descent of the human race.*
>   The determination of the position of man in nature, and of his rela-
> tions to the totality of things and this question of all questions for

mankind, as Huxley justly calls it – is finally solved by the knowledge
that man is descended from animals.

(Haeckel 1892, p. 6)

Naturalising humanity

Although this was only a scientific reformulation of the old philosophical insight that mankind is a part of Nature, thus also subor-
dinate to its laws, science's naturalisation of humanity in the 19th
century met with harsh opposition. Yet this was not to prevent
biological research during the hundred years subsequent to
Darwin's work from unearthing a cornucopia of views which sup-
ported his theory of anthropogenesis. Molecular geneticists were
able to prove large similarities between the human genome and
that of the primates, thus additionally demonstrating the relationship between humans and animals at the microscopic level of our
genotype's chemical structure.

> This becomes evident if we compare human macromolecules with
> those of a chimpanzee. The very slight differences in the structural
> genes of these two species cannot explain the significant anatomical
> differences between them. On average, a human chain of protein is
> more than 99% identical to the appropriate counterpart from a chim-
> panzee. Differences within the DNS sequence can usually be attrib-
> uted to redundancy within the genetic code or variations within DNS
> sections which have not been transcribed. In roughly fifty structural
> genes the middle genetic distance between the human being and the
> chimpanzee is very short; it is shorter than the middle distance
> between related, anatomically very similar species, and much shorter
> than the distance between any two species of the same class of species.
> Allan Wilson has shown that the organisational differences between
> the human being and the ape are sometimes attributable to mere
> changes in their regulatory genes.
>
> (Jacob 1983, pp. 61–2)

The scientific evidence of such findings is sufficiently over-
whelming to disavow any contradiction of the basic propositions
underlying the evolutionary theory of anthropogenesis. The
human race – excluding the exceptions – actually does seem in the

20th century to have got used to the fact that, in the light of new discoveries, traditional convictions may prove outdated and in need of revision. Modern societies orientate their view of the world according to science and not according to tradition; and since science is a dynamic enterprise, designed to criticise the old and make progress towards the new, there is no such thing within these societies as a right to intact prejudices and illusions. This is not only true of the view of the world in general; even our view of ourselves today as members of the human race cannot be, and is no longer to remain, immune to the results of empirical research. Thus naturalisation of humanity via the modern sciences has, by and large, imposed itself on even everyday consciousness. If, up until now, gene and reproduction technology has been accused of destroying the 'mystery' of reproduction by Kass (1972, pp. 21, 53), then this accusation is hardly more than the expression of individual uneasiness. In a world characterised by science, the term 'secret' does not signify a *noli me tangere*, but, far more, is a plea for further research.

> The human being is only 'mysterious' when we attribute it with having a personal creator; in this case, the numerous biological and psychological contradictions within human nature imply mysterious and incomprehensible motives on the part of this 'author'. If, however, we admit that we have emerged over millions of years as a result of the trials and activities of evolution, then the 'mysterious' is simply reduced to a catalogue of solutions which were able to be realised in the given evolutionary historical circumstances. We can then start deliberating the manner in which the processes involved in self-organisation could be altered in order that everything causing suffering to our genus may be eliminated.
>
> (Lem 1976, p. 641)

Indignation regarding the supposed disparagement of mankind first of all overlooks the fact that Darwin's theory in no way completely eliminates the special position of the human race: by declaring it to be the highest product of evolution, setting it at the top of its tree, it underlines the human race's extraordinary position within Nature. The supposed disparagement of humanity through the 'ape theory' is even more obviously the product of a rash and short-sighted interpretation of Darwin's findings if an attempt is made to formulate the historical significance of the theory of evolution in terms of its very own categories: as a product of evolution, mankind is aware of the evolutionary laws of which it is a result. It is possible to take this thought further, to the rhetorically impressive statement:

> We are privileged to be living at a crucial moment in the cosmic story, the moment when the vast evolutionary process, in the small person of enquiring man, is becoming conscious of itself.
>
> (Huxley 1967a, p. 1)

The reflexive structure of this idea is not limited to the theoretical fact of self-recognition of evolution within Darwin's theory. It also gives rise to a practical dimension. One characteristic of the modern sciences is that they open up the possibility of direct intervention in their subject matter. In contrast to philosophy of nature, for example, natural science is closely connected with technology; natural science is theory and practice in one. Even if it cannot always be factually realised – in astrophysics, for example – it is still true in principle that a scientifically understood process or event is also technologically controllable. This is also true of the theory of evolution. By applying it technologically and making it a means of controlling Nature, mankind gains the ability to intervene directly and consciously in the evolutionary process.

The breeding model

The *pointe* of this idea becomes clear if we consider that mankind is part of the evolution which recognises itself in mankind – and his theories – eventually beginning consciously to 'make' it. This is actually the central idea of eugenics.

> By proving that a gradual development has taken place from the lowest forms of life as far as the human race, the theory of descendence teaches that an improvement in the innate capabilities of human beings is also possible. And by tracing the conditions necessarily behind this development it also shows the way to a generative improvement in the human race, not only in the past, but also for the future . . . This is precisely what has caused so much interest in the theory of evolution since *Darwin*. Just as causal understanding, which the theory of

descendence owes to *Darwin*, and the rich assortment of facts with which he furnished his theory have since then drastically increased their persuasiveness, the theory of descendence sustains our interests most because the principles behind these teachings, which *Darwin* created by linking the theory of descendence with the idea of selection, are not only relevant to the past, but also to the present and the future. In other words, they permit conclusions regarding the future effectiveness of the conditions necessary in order for organisms to develop.

(Schallmayer 1903, pp. 94–5)

This passage lends clear expression to the two main eugenic ideas: (1) the idea of putting Darwin's theory to practical use, thus making it possible for mankind to control evolution, in particular his own evolution. After thousands of years of being a mere object of the evolutionary process, mankind has now acquired the theoretical knowledge and technological skills necessary to become the subject, planning and steering its continued course. (2) This planning and steering is to serve a 'generative perfection' of mankind. Previous evolution of the genus *Homo* has certainly led, via numerous crises and catastrophes, to advanced development; yet future progress of this genus can be accelerated and steered in the desired direction if mankind chooses to see to it.

Following the central position assumed by the concept of selection in Darwin's theory, improvement in the biological constitution of the human race is conceived as a selection carried out by the human race itself. The animal breeding model, referred to as early as Plato's *Republic*, retains its exemplary status for the idea of improvement, despite numerous alterations, right up to Muller and Huxley: only the best examples from each generation are to be allowed to reproduce. The eugenicists have mostly retained the goal of improving humanity even when viewing prevention of further degeneration as the most pressing goal. In the early 1960s, Julian Huxley declared:

The obverse of man's actual and potential further defectiveness is the vast extent of his possible future improvement. To effect this, he must first of all check the processes making for genetic deterioration. This means reducing man-made radiation to a minimum, discouraging genetically defective or inferior types from breeding, reducing human over-multiplication in general and the high differential fertility of various regions, nations and classes in particular. Then he can pro-

ceed to the much more important task of positive improvement. In
the not too distant future the fuller realization of possibilities will
inevitably come to provide the main motive for man's overall efforts;
and a Science of Evolutionary Possibilities, which today is merely
adumbrated, will provide a firm basis for these efforts. Eugenics can
make an important contribution to man's further evolution . . .

                                                              (1964, p. 252)

Thus negative eugenics is viewed merely as a first step on the
way to a much more ambitious and demanding goal, and in *Out of
the Night* Muller was already adamant that it is not enough to be
satisfied with preventing damaging characteristics: the prolifera-
tion of good ones must be aspired to. The prospects of such a
development are limitless. If it is possible within one or two
decades to attain in laboratory animals what evolution may have
needed ten millenia to attain, why should human evolution not be
party to such accelerated progress? And as Nietzsche's Zarathustra
calls out to the people:

> You have made your way from worms to human beings, and much of
> you is still worm. Once you were apes, and even now the human
> being is more of an ape than any ape is.
>   Even the wisest of you is only a conflict and a cross between plant
> and ghost. But do I tell you to become plants or ghosts?
>   Behold, I will teach you the overman!
>
>   (*ASZ*, p. 14)

Muller explains: led by science and technology, evolution will
extend beyond humanity in its present state to the same extent
that humanity extended beyond the amoeba. We may not yet
know in detail how this will be possible, but

> in time to come, the best thought of the race will necessarily be
> focused on the problems of evolution – not of the evolution gone by,
> but of the evolution still to come – and on the working out of genetic
> methods, eugenic ideals, yes, on the invention of new characteristics,
> organs, and biological systems that will work out to further the inter-
> ests, the happiness, the glory of the god-like beings whose meagre
> foreshadowings we present ailing creatures are.
>
>   (Muller 1936, p. 156)

Neither did Muller fail to demand in his later writing that germinal choice should not be restricted to preventing major genetic

defects, but that it should extend beyond preventing the bad to include increasing the good:

> It is but a short step in motivation from the couple who wish to turn their genetic defect to their credit by having, instead, an especially promising child, to the couple who, even though they are by no means subnormal, are idealistic enough to *prefer* to give their child as favourable a genetic prospect as can be obtained for it.
>
> (Muller 1967, p. 259)

But it is obvious that germinal choice can only be the first basic step. Even if we proceed from negative eugenics to positive eugenics, in other words, even if particular desirable characteristics are deliberately encouraged, reproduced and strengthened: accelerating evolution 'beyond humanity', as heralded by Muller in *Out of the Night*, is not possible along these lines. Despite far-reaching goals, and disregarding their remaining criticism of traditional eugenics, Muller, Huxley and others remain trapped in a central point of eugenic ideology: orientation of eugenic policies towards the practice of breeding. The common denominator in all the eugenic concepts so far discussed, from Plato to Muller, is indeed the transferral to human populations of the principle of artificial selection, first purely empirically transferred from animal and plant breeding, later confirmed by Darwin's theory. Via selective reproduction, the bearers of desirable characteristics are to have as many offspring as possible, the bearers of undesirable characteristics as few as possible.

The molecular option

As early as 1895, Alfred Ploetz introduced a completely different technological model into the eugenics discussion. Like most of his eugenicist colleagues, Ploetz was aware of the severe conflict between his policies and traditional Western Christian morality; although he did not hesitate to take the side of the – supposedly irrefutable – generative interests of the species, he perceived a ranking of the individual below these interests as a serious problem. In the last few pages of his book, he expresses hope that one day this conflict may be solved by shifting the focus of eugenic measures from the individuals alive at any one time to members of the future generations which are to be improved. The advantage of this kind of shift would be that even extremely 'inferior' individuals need not necessarily be excluded from the reproduction process: transferral of parents' defects could be prevented by appropriate manipulation of the offspring's genetic constitution. In the future, eugenics should thus be aimed at 'gradually learning to control the laws of variation until human need and misery all but disappear' (Ploetz p. 239). In the last decade of the 19th century, when variance was merely a known fact, and its mechanism was still totally unclear, not to mention that nobody had even the slightest idea how to exercise control over this mechanism with technological means, this was a shrewd speculation. Today the situation is very different indeed.

Following the progress made within the field of genetics since the turn of the century, in particular following the 1950s' enlightenment of the molecular structure of DNA and the breaking of the genetic code in the 1960s, we are familiar with the principles underlying the biochemical mechanism behind both the transferral of genetic information and the emergence of genetic variation. On top of this, following the discovery of the effects of restriction enzymes we are now in a position to dissect DNA molecules from any organism and put them back together in new combinations, or to combine viral, bacterial, plant, animal or human DNA sequences in any way we like. Since the beginning of the 1970s, a completely new scientific research procedure has been developed, practised in numerous laboratories throughout the world: *gene manipulation*. This process is by no means limited to research purposes; it forms the technical basis for a new branch of industrial biotechnology which is rapidly gaining in size and importance. 'Tailor-made' bacteria are already being employed in various areas of industrial production today, especially in the making of drugs; work is being carried out on genetically manipulated plants, some with exotic characteristics, and on the reconstruction of animals. Why should this technology not be applicable to and applied to human beings? Suddenly Ploetz's vision seems to be realisable: if we are capable of cutting out one particular section of the genome of a bacterium and putting back another, if in this way we can make a bacterium produce human insulin or remove certain types of waste – why should the same methods not place us in a position to remove a particular, defect gene from the genome of a human being and/or introduce another, useful gene?

One of the first protagonists of a branch of eugenics based on molecular biological achievements was the geneticist and Nobel prize winner, Joshua Lederberg. His eugenic strategy, presented at the Ciba Symposium in 1962, contains two fundamental characteristics of the new type of biological research and theory formation. Whereas the classical biological sciences always deal with entire organisms or their macroscopic parts, molecular biology goes far beyond the realm of visible wholes and ventures forward on a microscopic level. It sees the human being not as an organism which has achieved its present state via variation, selection and adaption to a particular environment, but – as Lederberg (1967a, pp. 263–4) put it, in a definition which has since gained dubious fame – as a sequence of various atoms with a definite length:

> We can now define man. Genotypically at least, he is six feet of a particular molecular sequence of carbon, hydrogen, oxygen, nitrogen and phosphorous atoms – the length of DNA tightly coiled in the nucleus of his provenient egg and in the nucleus of every adult cell, 5 thousand million paired nucleotide units long.

Such a definition lends a whole new meaning to 'improving' humanity. It is no longer a case of controlling the general 'external' framework of the evolutionary process of an organism, but one of deliberately modifying the 'interior' mechanisms which form such organisms. According to Lederberg, progress in molecular biology has given rise to an entirely new situation by opening up the possibility of direct intervention in the molecular mechanism of human genetics. At the moment this technology might well still be 'terribly clumsy'; yet if one considers the extraordinary rate at which scientific knowledge grows, one could presume that this will change within a short space of time.

> Surely within a few generations we can expect to learn tricks of immeasurable advantage. Why bother now with somatic selection, so slow in its impact? Investing a fraction of the effort, we should soon learn how to manipulate chromosome ploidy, homozygosis, gametic selection, full diagnosis of heterozygotes, to accomplish in one or two

generations of eugenic practice what would now take ten or one hundred . . . As further extensions of experimental cytology, we might
anticipate the *in vitro* culture of germ cells and such manipulations as
the interchange of chromosomes and segments. The ultimate application of molecular biology would be the direct control of nucleotide
sequences in human chromosomes, coupled with recognition, selection, and integration of the desired genes, of which the existing population furnishes a considerable variety.

(ibid., p. 265)

A molecular biologically orientated eugenic strategy thus
assumes less of a biological and much more of a chemical nature; it
is no longer based on the transferral to mankind of procedures
from animal and plant breeding, but on the direct manipulation of
the chemical structure of the human genotype. Its 'synthetic'
nature is therefore to be emphasised as its second characteristic.
Following the transition from analytical to synthetic biology, outlined in Chapter 1, this kind of strategy is no longer aimed at controlling the evolutionary process, but at a particular type of chemical construction.

Cloning

However unconcerned Lederberg's optimism may have been in
1962, a little while later he becomes sceptical regarding the possibilities of direct gene manipulation, and ironically comments on
the expectation of being able to achieve the desired improvement
of mankind on this basis, with the statement:

> We have merely to specify the optimum sequence of some 5 billion
> nucleotides – the DNA information of the fertilized egg – and we can
> define the ideal man.

(Lederberg 1970, p. 49)

In addition, the desired results could in some cases be attained
using simpler procedures, in particular transplantation.
Nevertheless, these technical difficulties are for Lederberg no reason to throw in the eugenic sponge. He has a new technique
handy which could help the biological progress of humanity to be

brought about much more simply than via the difficult process of – termed by Lederberg, in analogy to alchemy, 'algeny' – gene manipulation. In the 1960s, the British cell biologist J. B. Gurdon had used frogs to demonstrate the possibility of asexual reproduction in higher forms of life. Gurdon made frogspawn, in which the nuclei had been destroyed by radiation and replaced by body cell nuclei, grow normally; the tadpoles which emerged from this spawn were 'clones', that is genetically identical copies of the creatures from which the body cell nuclei were taken. Eugenicists such as Haldane, and Muller (1936, pp. 136–7), had speculated about the possibility of asexual reproduction long before these experiments took place. Lederberg is able, however, to take cloning as a technological fact to support his arguments, superior to 'algeny' just from the fact that the period of time between its development and practical use is much shorter than with other biotechnologies.

More than anything, it is one argument on which Lederberg bases his suggestion for the application of cloning to humanity. Since cloning presupposes one genotype, which is then multiplied, this procedure provides an opportunity to circumvent the incalculability of sexual reproduction. Cloning does not combine two previously existing genotypes to produce a new one, but produces an individual which is genetically identical with the original organism.

> If a superior individual – and presumably, then, genotype – is identified, why not copy it directly, rather than suffer all the risks, including those of sex determination, involved in the disruptions of recombination. The same solace is accorded the carrier of genetic disease: why not be sure of an exact copy of yourself, another healthy carrier, rather than risk an overtly diseased offspring; at worst, copy your spouse and allow some degree of biological parenthood.
>
> (Lederberg 1966, p. 9)

In this manner, any uncertainty as to how the new organism will fare in its environment, as is the case after every sexual reproduction, is avoided:

> The most immediate implication of cloning is the production of genetically homogenous groups of individuals, and particularly of propagating a genotype already tested in one generation for further trial in a second.
>
> (1970, p. 50)

Lederberg sees asexual reproduction technology as having an important status, yet for him it is closely connected with a cornucopia of further procedures and techniques (including hormone therapies, immunisation, transplantation), which only together make up his concept of *orthobiosis*, the 'correction or perfection of life and of man' (ibid., p. 29). This concept is characterised more than anything by the transition from indirect to direct intervention. Traditional eugenic strategy *à la* Muller or Huxley is indirect in two ways: it wants to improve the fate of future human beings by improving the gene pool of the coming generation; and it wants to improve the gene pool of the coming generation by controlling the reproductive behaviour of the present generation. Lederberg's suggestions, on the other hand, refer directly to the individuals whose fate is to be improved – whether by replacing their defective organs with new ones with the help of transplantation, whether by stimulating their brain growth via optimal nourishment, hormones, etc., or whether by – en route to cloning – equipping them with the best genomes available.

Autoevolution

This constructivist way of thinking has been adopted just as consistently and impressively by Stanislaw Lem. In his *Summa technologiae* he designed a model of technological development, the efficiency of which is to be proven by its projective possibilities. Lem does not spend long on the beginnings of technology and the state of the art today, preferring to dedicate his main interest to the future dynamics of technological development, which will enable the transition from control over single natural processes to control over greater and more complex areas of Nature. If this process is extended far enough into the future, a 'pantocreatic' stage is reached, in which new worlds, superior to our own in every respect, are created. Such technical worlds would still be created 'naturally', inasmuch as they are constructed from the natural materials available at the time; yet in their ultimate form they would be totally independent of Nature. However fantastic the vision of such a 'cosmogonic art of engineering' may already appear, technological evolution, as conceived by Lem, by no means ends here. The further the construction of artificial worlds proceeds, the more the human race seems to be a foreign body within them:

> The human being is left as the last relic, the last 'authentic work of Nature' within the world which it has created. There is a limit as to how long such a situation can last. The invasion of the human body by man-made technology is inevitable.
>
> (1976, p. 501)

Pantocreation is followed by a phase of direct and systematic self-alteration of mankind, which Lem terms *autoevolution*, a process which includes various, but not strictly separate stages. The first stage, to date the only one to be practised, is the medical stage; it starts out from the human organism and is restricted to preserving the latter via prophylaxis or, in the case of illness, taking curative measures to restore it. The basic dogma of this stage is the inviolability of the evolving human organism. Lem, however, considers a restriction to mere maintenance and repair tasks such as this as short-sighted and ultimately untenable. The defects inherent within the human organism, on the one hand, and the steadily increasing burdens and demands due to progressing civilisation, on the other, render exceeding beyond the scope of medicine unavoidable in the long term. At the second stage – which could be termed the eugenic stage – mere repairing is replaced by controlling, aimed at removing the evolutionary gradients of Nature step by step and substituting them with human goals. The strategic creation of increasingly perfect types of human being begins.

> Succinctly, this would be the plan to create over hundreds, maybe even thousands of years 'the next *homo sapiens* model', not all in one go, but through slow and gradual changes, reducing the differences between the generations.
>
> (ibid., p. 503)

Such alterations of the human organism may be aimed at reducing susceptibility to diseases or immunisation against growing environmental burdens; it is also possible to perceive an increase in efficiency of individual organs, particularly the brain of course, and lastly the formation of totally new organs and senses as yet possessed by no human being.

For all its boldness, this eugenic stage nevertheless includes certain limitations. It is based on a 'naturalistic' and 'somatogenic' trend which sooner or later, according to Lem, will be replaced by a 'bionic and physico-technological strategy'. Following on from the medical 'prosthetics' of our day, and consistently continuing with them, individual organs and parts of the body would gradually be replaced by more efficient prosthetic devices until, at the end of the day, a combination of organic material and physical apparatus is the result (1980, p. 230). A 'denaturalisation' or 'dehomogenisation' of the human organism such as this opens up a whole new world of possibilities. Employing materials with little or no wear and tear, such as stainless steel and certain plastics, would remove the site of action for numerous diseases and geriatric complaints, thus achieving a huge step forward towards one of the main aims of all the future visions of mankind: a drastic extension in life expectancy, maybe even immortality. Even a breakthrough in new dimensions of human intellectual capability is conceivable, via direct coupling of the brain with highly efficient computers. By storing human memory on computer, for example, significant cerebral capacity could be set free for productive, inventive purposes. Indeed, an extension in life expectancy would only make sense following the prerequisite that the memory function be transferred to external computers, since the memory capacity of the human brain is not sufficiently large to retain all the information acquired over thousands of years. Once the scope of the evolved organism has been exceeded, the third, constructivistic stage of autoevolution begins, which approaches the problem in a far more radical manner, discarding not only the given structure of the human organism, but also the stepwise developmental pattern of the evolutionary process.

> The constructivist solution which Nature has chosen to give to the problem of 'what should the reasonable being look like?' may just as plausibly be found inadequate as a solution which could be arrived at by adopting its autoevolutive means. Instead of improving or 'patching' the current model with regard to this parameter or that, new values for it may be established at will. Instead of a relatively modest biological lifespan, near immortality may be called for. Instead of strengthening Nature's construction within the limits which her chosen materials permit, the greatest level of withstanding which current technology is capable of providing may be called for. In short, instead

of a reconstruction, the present solution may be given up totally and a completely new one projected.

(Lem 1976, p. 503)

Such a completely new constructional solution could start with the choice of another aggregate state. Under the circumstances with which it was presented, evolution could create life only on the basis of watery solutions, giving rise to the question of whether, in addition to these colloid variations, crystalline or gaseous variations on life could not also be created. Even if we are still a long way from the realisation of such projects, Lem does not consider them impossible. Nature has created only those equilibria whose final state may be achieved via gradual development and in accordance with the general thermodynamic probabilities of the phenomena. Contrary to all the headwords concerning 'the rebellion of living matter against the second principle of thermodynamics', such step-wise processes of self-organisation are on no account unthinkable.

In general terms, large, material systems are always striving for states of greater entropy, but they come across so many other states along the way, not to mention the many different paths they take, and ultimately within a time-span which is so long, measured over many billions of years, that 'along the way' – and not at all 'at odds' with the second principle of thermodynamics – it may come to not one, and not ten, but to countless types of self-organising evolution. There thus exists a huge, as yet empty (we are not familiar with its elements) class of homoeostatic systems, which may *possibly* be constructed from a solid, a liquid or a gaseous material. This class of systems gives rise to a subclass, namely the set of all those homoeostases which can exist solely due to the effects of Nature, without external interference from a personal constructor. The obvious conclusion to be drawn from this is that the human race is in a position to excel over Nature: Nature is only capable of constructing some of the possible homoeostases, whereas we, having acquired the knowledge necessary to do so, can build all of them.

(ibid., pp. 532–3)

From breeding to engineering

Thus, from Plato to the present day, the breeding idea has been continually developing. However much individual breeding goals may have altered, the main aim has remained the same: control over the reproductive process, directed on the one hand at human self-determination regarding timing of birth and number of children, on the other hand at positively influencing their characteristics. Here it should not be forgotten that the formulation 'human self-determination' has more than one meaning: it may refer to the desires and needs of individuals, to the interests of the State or the – supposed – well-being of the people and the 'race'. Eugenic notions never develop in a vacuum and are thus never value-free; they adhere to particular socially anchored values and politically orientated goals. In addition, they follow a scientific and technological logic which begins with the transfer to human reproduction of experiences made in animal breeding. When, in the 19th century, Darwin's theory of evolution scientificated the empirical concept of selection, the Utopian philosophical breeding ideas were also transformed into scientific and rational strategies for controlling reproduction. The decisive gain through this scientification is not a growth in the objectivity and security of these strategies, but the possibility of reclaiming the authority of the natural sciences.

This drags eugenics into the slipstream of a new kind of dynamics. As a *science* it is subject to the rapid change of concepts and models; and as an *applied* science, dependent upon the availability of technological means, it becomes dependent upon the current state of technology. At least since the beginning of this century, the evolution of eugenics has been more prone to follow the rapid alterations in scientific theories and technical processes than changes in basic values and desired goals. This technological determination is particularly noticeable in the spectacular projects of Lederberg or Lem. These projects are no less Utopian than Plato's or Campanella's, yet they are differently so. Here the technological means have largely been freed from the context of political and social reform, of primary importance in previous Utopian notions. Technology no longer appears as the means of realising given needs, but in itself makes options available which prejudice the structure of action.

Whatever chances the autoevolutionary project may have, it is demonstrative of the fundamental change of biology from an analytical to a synthetic science. The object, the methods and the subject of eugenics have undergone a fundamental change: (a) its basis is no longer an image of the human being as a macroscopic organism, but as a biochemical machine constructed from molecular structures, the 'parameters' of which may be modified more or less as desired through skilled intervention; (b) technological methods are no longer orientated towards the practice of animal and plant breeding, but to the model of synthetic chemistry; (c) the altered concept of technology relates to a different image of the engineer: paradigmatical is no longer the breeder who increases the available characteristics of an organism, but the chemical engineer who takes various materials and synthesises a new material with desired characteristics. Evolution is replaced by construction.

5

The great uneasiness

*Not even the thought of exchanging genetic matter between human beings
and animals
– nothing less than the formation of human/animal hybrids –
is enough to put some people off, a thought which brings to mind
terms as old and forgotten as 'heinous' and 'iniquitous'*
Hans Jonas

Hardly anybody who chooses not simply to dismiss the notion of 'improving the human race', but to take it and reflect upon it, will be able to do so without sensing a certain uneasiness. There are few technological concepts imaginable which are more disturbing than that of a 'dehomogenised' human being: made up, on the one hand, from the biological organs which have stood up to the engineer's critical scrutiny and, on the other, Teflon coated joints, hard plastic bones and steel teeth, all of course connected to a powerful computer partly replacing, partly enhancing the human being's cerebral functions. Horror fiction also makes its profits from the repulsion and outrage aroused by such thoughts. One may recall how Mary Shelley describes the reaction of the biological engineer, Victor Frankenstein, when the creature he has created awakes and unexpectedly stands before him:

> I started from my sleep with horror; a cold dew covered my forehead, my teeth chattered, and every limb became convulsed: when, by the dim and yellow light of the moon, as it forced its way through the window shutters, I beheld the wretch – the miserable monster whom I had created . . . Oh! no mortal could support the horror of that countenance. A mummy again endued with animation could not be so hideous as

that wretch. I had gazed on him while unfinished; he was ugly then; but when those muscles and joints were rendered capable of motion, it became a thing such as even Dante could not have conceived.

(Shelley 1969, p. 58)

It is difficult to imagine a more vivid description of the emotional repugnance sensed towards artificial human beings. Even those reacting less dramatically than Victor Frankenstein are hardly likely to feel at home with the idea of breeding and 'reconstructing' human beings. The imagination of biologists and genetic engineers actually goes as far as Frankenstein's, seriously considering the creation of human/animal hybrids through an exchange of human and animal matter – a thought which brings to mind, and probably not just to Hans Jonas', terms as old and forgotten as 'heinous' or 'iniquitous'.

Futile reassurance

Joshua Lederberg's clones and Stanislaw Lem's dehomogenised human beings are, of course, just as much works of science fiction as Victor Frankenstein's outrage is a horror story. Another look at the current possibilities within the field of reproduction technology, outlined in Chapter 1, does show an explosive increase in our practical options, it is true; yet it would be exaggerating beyond all proportion to talk of a 'technological revolution' within human reproduction if this were to suggest merely the slightest possibility of realising the Utopian eugenic notions of the past. Let us look first at the notions of breeding. Some of the prognoses made by Muller in *Out of the Night* more than fifty years ago, for example, have since been fulfilled and, assuming that the speed with which biology and medicine are developing does not suddenly decrease, some of the other prognoses will become reality within the foreseeable future. And yet this increase in our options has not led to changes, prophesied and desired by Muller

in our methods and customs concerned with the production of children – changes permitting a much greater degree of control over our choice of these children.

(1936, p. 137)

There are sperm banks in the U.S.A. which enable ambitious mothers to bear children from Nobel prize winners and top sportsmen, and thus make their contribution to a 'genetic improvement' of the coming generation. We have even, more recently, become aware of national, Government programmes for the promotion of quantity and quality within a population, e.g. in Singapore. Yet in each case these are 'fringe' ideas and projects, which will never be far-reachingly effective. Paradoxically, we seem to have distanced ourselves from a social realisation of such programmes to the same extent with which we have grown nearer to their technological realisation. Interest in eugenics has never been as low during this century as it is today. The same is true for the idea of 'reconstructing human beings', dismissed as unrealistic as early as Muller. He was convinced that reconstruction could not be achieved without resorting to breeding methods, believing a technological, somatic improvement over centuries or even millenia to be impossible – and 'uneconomical'.

> It seems to me that for a long time yet to come (in terms of the temporal scale of human history thus far), man at his present best is unlikely to be excelled, according to any of man's own accepted value systems, by pure artefacts. And although artificial aids should become even better developed, and integrated as harmoniously as possible with the human organism, it is more economical in the end to have developmental and physiological improvements of the organism placed on a genetic basis, where practicable, than to have to institute them in every generation anew by elaborate treatments of the soma.
>
> (Muller 1967, p. 255)

These considerations do not, of course, include molecular genetic manipulation of the human genome, as made possible by genetic engineering technology; recombining human DNA and/or splicing foreign or artificial genes into the human genome would not be affected by Muller's objections, since reconstruction in this manner would be on a genetic basis – just as he called for. Yet this project is forever being deemed unrealistic by specialists, amongst them Jacques Monod:

> Modern molecular genetics offers us no means whatsoever for acting upon the ancestral heritage so as to improve it with new features – to create a genetic 'superman'; on the contrary, it reveals the vanity of

any such hope: the genome's microscopic proportions today and probably forever rule out manipulation of this sort.

(1972, p. 153)

Even a scientistic optimist like Joshua Lederberg had only a brief
flirtation with the idea of molecularly reorganising human beings,
before rejecting it as technologically impossible. Recent genetic
developments seem to confirm the renunciation rather than deny
it; the human genome is proving to be a lot more complex than
some Utopians wanted to believe. Molecular biological improvement of human beings remains a notion which seems, with the
advance of genetics, to be becoming further from, rather than
closer to, the status of a concrete project.

> Compared with our present-day knowledge of the molecular biology
> of higher organisms, and our ignorance of the genetics of much of the
> normal morphological variation in humans, these proposals are some-
> what analogous to the idea that a boy who has just been given his first
> electronic set for Christmas could successfully improve the latest IBM
> computer.
>
> (Vogel & Motulsky 1986, p. 636)

Thus all the notions of improving and/or reconstructing human
beings appear to be, at best, naïve fantasy and, at worst, irresponsible speculation, far removed from reality.

And yet realisations such as these are hardly capable of reassur-
ing us. It is certainly correct that eugenic concepts are not boom-
ing at present; but is it not possible that this disinterest could turn
around if the social and political climate should change? And is
this thought not all the more threatening when we consider that
the technological means needed to carry out eugenic strategies on
a grand scale will then be available as never before? With the present state of science and technology, it is hard to imagine molecular genetically reconstructed or 'denaturalised' human beings. Yet
the assurance that such projects cannot be realised with our present knowledge offers no guarantee for the future. On the contrary: the boy whose interest in electronics was aroused by the
Christmas present might soon become a student of informatics
and then a computer scientist, employed by IBM and before long
actually improving existing computers and designing their next
generation. The same could go for the field of gene and reproduc-

tion medicine; it is characteristic of the present situation that the scientific and technological breakthroughs within the last few decades have created the basis for making concrete technological projects out of Utopian ideas, thus paving the way to their future realisation. However long it may take: nobody today can discount the possibility of fundamental 'improvements' to the human race some day becoming technologically viable. In addition, at least a few of the trenchant measures could also become viable in the foreseeable future; this may be true of cloning human beings, and of creating human/animal hybrids.

Current problems

It would be a complete misinterpretation of the uneasiness mentioned above to attribute it solely to the idea of a total rationalisation of reproduction, of cloning human beings and human/animal hybrids, or even of the future vision of a reconstructed human race. Fear of an unstoppable trend in this direction is always involved, yet the uneasiness is aimed at options already available today. We already have access to a spectrum of technological options far exceeding the traditional methods of controlling human reproduction. A great deal of progress has been made in the last few decades, especially in the areas of artificial creation of human life and genetic prognostics, of which the 'test tube baby' is the highlight *to date*. From the very beginning, this development has inspired uneasiness and rejection. The hefty debates about artificial insemination during the first two decades subsequent to the Second World War have today largely been forgotten; as early as 1949, Pope Pius XII rejected the entire principle of artificial fertilisation. He believed that, whilst it would be wrong to discount new methods in advance just because they are new, artificial fertilisation merited not only extreme caution but total rejection. He referred to *in vitro* fertilisation, which at that time was still being discussed as a mere possibility, in similar terms, condemning this practice as immoral and totally inadmissible (cf. Gründel 1983, pp. 255–6). It is not only the Catholic Church which fundamentally condemns this kind of technological intervention in human reproduction, however; uneasiness regarding such intervention may have religious motives, but not necessarily so. The debates can also be totally profane, as shown by biologist Leon Kass's verdict on *in vitro* fertilisation:

> There are more and less human ways of bringing a child into the world. I am arguing that the laboratory production of human beings is no longer *human* procreation.
>
> (1972, p. 54)

Subject for debate here is neither a monster patched together from human and other genes, nor the future possibility of dehomogenised human beings; both artificial insemination and *in vitro* fertilisation are concerned with the creation of normal human beings – albeit along a different path, made possible by technological intervention. In other words, not only the futurist product of intervention provokes rejection and uneasiness, but just the intervention itself, the technological procedure.

We do not need shrewd visions of the future in order to perceive the technological revolution of our reproduction process as disturbing. Options already available today, such as one woman taking over a pregnancy for another, or the cryo-conservation of sperm, embryos and egg cells, break with matters which have been taken for granted for thousands of years. Already a problem *per se*, these technologies appear to be even more disturbing when applied in bizarre manners. (1) *Birth planning*: a young woman has some of her egg cells artificially fertilised (whether homologously or heterogously) and the resulting embryos deep-frozen. If later on she wishes to have a child, she can have the embryos defrosted and implanted, thus avoiding the increased risk in older mothers of bearing a handicapped child. (2) *Child with five 'parents'*: an egg cell is taken from woman A and fertilised extracorporeally with sperm from man B; the resulting embryo is then transferred to the uterus of woman C and the child eventually born is adopted by couple D and E. Neither of these cases has been documented; they are conceivable, but hypothetical. Yet independently of whether they are realistic beyond their technological viability, we are moved by the mere thought of such possibilities: not only do they contradict what we are used to viewing as 'normal', but they also appear to introduce an element of arbitrariness and randomness into an area least suited to one. All of a sudden, they render intransparent and confusing what used to be clear and simple, thus making room for complications where there had been none. It is obvious that such practical options might well become a source of complicated problems, unprecedented and thus as yet unanswered. One only has to open a newspaper or switch on the television to be confronted with these problems and the public debates on them. True, the natural course of reproduction occasionally gives rise to problems, too (we only have to think of the the old legal principle *pater sempus incertus*, or of adoption cases), and yet these are not nearly as confusing as uncertainties surfacing with the new technologies. Let us take a look at a few examples.

1. Fertilisation *post mortem*: in 1984, after months of legal debate, 23-year-old French widow, Corinne Paraplaix, is granted Court permission to be artificially fertilised with sperm from her husband, who has been dead for many months. Her husband suffered from cancer of the testes and had deposited sperm in a sperm bank prior to an operation. After his death, the sperm bank refused to surrender the sperm.

2. Prenatal orphans: during the same year, Victoria State Government decrees in Australia that two deep-frozen embryos, whose parents have died in a plane crash, be defrosted and implanted in sterile women. An ethics committee had previously deemed that the embryos be defrosted and allowed to die.

3. Who 'owns' the child?: in the U.S. State of Michigan, Judy Stiver is paid $10 000 to be artificially fertilised with Alexander Malahoff's sperm, and bears the child as its surrogate mother; following the birth, the child proves to be severely handicapped. Malahoff refuses to take the child and demands a paternity test; it turns out that he is not the father. Both parties sue. Several years later, a surrogate mother refuses to hand over the child to the people who 'ordered' it, who have also paid $10 000 for the artificial fertilisation and for the pregnancy to be taken over; a Court in New Jersey orders the surrogate mother to hand over the child. Other, similar cases are known to exist.

4. Prenatal sexism: it comes to light that prenatal diagnostic methods are being employed in India and Korea to recognise and then abort female foetuses. Pending the development at Keio

University in Tokyo of a procedure to differentiate between sperm with an X- or with a Y-chromosome, various institutions begin offering *in vitro* fertilisation with sex determination.

Some of the problems suggested here can be solved relatively easily: sperm and embryo banks can demand instructions from their clients concerning what to do with the deposited 'matter' in case of death, in order to avoid uncertainty and possible legal squabbles, as in cases (1) and (2). According to German law, situation (3) does not pose any problem: the woman giving birth is in every case the mother; contracts entered into beforehand are categorised 'immoral' and thus legally irrecoverable. With regard to case (4), it is possible to envisage a civil law ruling which prevents prenatal sex determination and/or the passing on of this information to the parents. Yet this would neither solve the root of the problem, nor dispel the uneasiness felt around the world. For even if the obviously 'bizarre', or even immoral, usages of these technologies were legally banned and the unclear cases sorted out, the question would still remain: do these usages not throw significant light on the technologies themselves, and are the unclear cases not merely extreme cases of problems which, in a weaker strain, also arise in the middle of the spectrum?

Explanation

On the other hand, does not every technological innovation give rise to problems? Wherever one cares to look, progress in science and technology questions well-loved ways of viewing matters and threatens well-respected ways of carrying them out. Are the problems mentioned proof of anything more than that we have not yet learned to cope with the new potential? It seems reasonable to interpret the uneasiness surrounding reproduction technology as emotional expression of a religious or profane conservatism which, criticising as much vehemently as unsuccessfully, has accompanied modern age scientific and technological development since it began. Wherever and whenever established institutions and traditional views have been questioned as a result of scientific progress and technological innovation, profound uneasiness has surfaced, sometimes hefty protest, and it is difficult to say whether this is more rooted in a clinging to the old and familiar or in a mistrust of the new and unfamiliar. Religious opposition to Copernicus, Galileo and Darwin springs to mind, as well as opposition to the railways, immunisation or anaesthesia. Would it not be surprising if reproduction technology were any different? Bearing in mind the long historical tradition of such uneasiness, as well as its opposition to practically every step in the march of progress, the theoretical problem it raises seems to lie mainly in discovering its psychological and sociological roots. The uneasiness needs to be *explained*, empirically and scientifically. First attempts at such an explanation have already been made.

One such attempt has been an interpretation based on Mary Douglas's anthropological theory of the meaning of classification systems of the repugnance felt over the production of interspecific hybrids (Glover 1984, pp. 38–40). According to this theory, every culture has its own system of categories, which it uses to classify the world. Phenomena which do not fit into this system of categories, which exceed or blur its boundaries, are often viewed as problematic, offensive or 'dirty'. Thus shoes are by no means dirty *per se*, although they appear so when placed on the dining-room table; neither is food dirty *per se*, although it appears so when found lying around in the bedroom or spilt on our clothes. To summarise: we view everything as 'dirty' which lies perpendicular to the boundaries and lines drawn through the ruling classification pattern. With this theory in mind, uneasiness regarding interspecific hybrids seems plausible:

> For the divisions between the species are the lines of *our* system of classifying animals, and disturbance at the thought of blurring them may be playing a part in our hostile response. And the division between our own species and others is even more important to our system of thought.
>
> (ibid., p. 40)

This approach could also explain the emotional reactions which the new technologies provoke towards confused family relationships: we feel strangely moved when we hear that the mother of a child is also its grandmother or sister. This would be the case if a remarried, older woman desired a child with her second husband,

and her adult daughter from the first marriage bore as surrogate mother a child from the stepfather.

However, there are objections to explaining the uneasiness in this manner. Why do we react with such a profound uneasiness to the idea of human/animal hybrids, whilst mules do not irritate us, although they are also interspecific hybrids? In the same way, new, genetically created hybrids – such as a cross between a tomato and a potato – seem to be more curiosities than anything else. All of these cases deal with phenomena which, according to our common classification system, are not 'allowed' to exist. If we react more strongly in one case than in another, then this is because in one case we ourselves are involved; in the other, 'only' other species. It is plausible that we react more strongly when personally involved, yet this is not explained by the approach outlined above. Confused family relationships are, in addition, possible through adoption. Nobody feels uneasy about a child being adopted by an aunt or uncle following the death of its parents, even though, here too, the aunt would at the same time become the mother and the uncle the father. Yet, independently of the possibilities and limits of this particular explanatory approach, we should be asking whether this kind of psychological or sociological explanation does not rule out from the start an important dimension of the problem which this uneasiness raises.

The considerations which follow are based on the theory that the feeling of uneasiness may and should actually be endowed with a *moral meaning*, for which the exposure of its psychological or sociological causes does not compensate. From a moral philosophical point of view, it cannot be sufficient to view this uneasiness as an *explanandum* and empirically to uncover its causes in an objectivising and scientific procedure; far more, it must be taken seriously for its content. Moral feelings may not be taken simply as personal idiosyncrasies, but as references to norms and values valid beyond the individual. Thus the ethicist – unlike the sociologist or the psychologist – cannot be content to assume the position of an uninvolved observer who analyses the empirical causes of the moral feelings reigning within a society and/or individual; his job is far more to pick up on these feelings and to use them as a starting point for his argument.

Feeling and objectivity

Of course, this does not mean that such feelings can *justify* moral judgments: often the former are not even uniform, which is reason enough. Uneasiness regarding reproduction technology is often countered by a no less strong fascination at the enormous progress being made by science, and repugnance at technological manipulation of human reproduction countered by enthusiasm at the possible therapies being made available. Contradicting empirical perceptions usually provokes even more intense research in order to decide which of the two perceptions is the more adequate, previously accepted 'facts' having to be corrected in the light of such research when they turn out – think of the geocentric perception of the Earth – to be the result of specific perceptive conditions or of an optical illusion, and moral feelings should not be immunised against correction and revision either. Everybody may and must have an undisputed right to his/her feelings; anyone experiencing uneasiness in the face of gene and reproduction technology thus has a right that this be respected, as long as it is clearly an expression of his/her personal attitude. Such expression does not, however, usually stop at announcing personal displeasure. Moral feelings are two-sided: on the one hand, they share with all other feelings a spontaneous origin and an emotional effect on the subject in question; at the same time, they differ from other feelings in that they are not usually expressed as purely 'private' emotions. This being so, they often lead to moral judgments, announced publicly, and linked with a claim to validity beyond the individual. As soon as a feeling is understood as being actually moral, it loses its private character; it becomes the motivation for a normative expectation upon all the members of the society in question. Only this claim to common validity renders a feeling – thus also an interest, a will, a judgment – specifically *moral* and distinguishes it from mere expressions of taste.

Our moral feelings are closely related to our tastes only at first sight. Whether I experience uneasiness over *in vitro* fertilisation or over the way a house is furnished, in both cases I may be emotionally moved by an object or process in a way I am powerless to control. Emotivism is based on this similarity, systematising it to a

concept, according to which moral judgments are no more than
expression of our attitudes towards or against particular phenomena. In actual fact, however, this confuses very important distinc-
tions. Whereas in mere matters of taste, reasons are neither
demanded, nor deemed necessary, or even possible, we connect
moral feelings and the judgments which result from them with a
need to justify them. Opposing tastes can exist alongside each
other without a problem, whereas opposing moral institutions usually provoke a debate based on, and aspiring to consensus. It is not
a problem if one speaker within a discussion prefers houses with
modern, practical furnishings and the other feels more at home in
cosy, antique surroundings; the case is different, however, when
one speaker expresses his deep uneasiness regarding the practice of
in vitro fertilisation and the other welcomes the introduction of
this procedure as progress. This kind of dissent is on a different
level, one which not only enables, but demands that a debate
aimed at its solution take place.

Clarity is seldom within biomedical discussion of this point.
During a debate in the German Ministry for Research and
Technology on the problem of 'spare' embryos, for example, a
leading German IVF specialist said:

> Edwards and his research group believe experimentation with these
> embryos to be ethically justifiable. Within other Anglo-Saxon coun-
> tries, this procedure is also more readily accepted than rejected. *We*
> categorically reject it. For *us*, the destruction of 'spare' embryos is also
> out of the question. Neither do *we* accept the donation of such
> embryos to women who could otherwise not become pregnant. *We*
> have always rejected heterologous insemination, and *we* shall therefore
> act accordingly with regard to female gametes and embryos.
>
> (Trotnow 1984, pp. 56–7, my italics)

Questioned more closely, Trotnow added: 'To make the point
quite clear, *we* have never experimented with embryos, and *we*
have no desire to do so' (p. 69). However honourable such an
explanation may be, it is not a *moral* opinion, but – as noted in the
Ministry debate – the formulation of a private attitude. The following consideration sheds some light on the difference between a
moral norm and a private attitude: we can say 'I personally would
never vote for the XYZ Party, but I consider it legitimate for
others to do so', but we *cannot* say 'I personally would never

deceive another person, but I consider it legitimate for others to do so'. The second statement appears almost absurd, and it would be difficult to take it seriously. The reason for this seems to be that any deception involves a violation of moral obligations; it cannot – apart from all the legal sanctions – be left to the whims of an individual. Thus moral norms must be able to be *generalised*;[1] they must be valid for every person, at every time, in every place and in all circumstances.

This kind of claim may be legitimately staked only when the moral norms and judgments involved are not dogmatically asserted but *justified*, in a way which anyone can understand. With regard to *in vitro* fertilisation, anyone who is content to stop at expressing his/her uneasiness or revulsion has a right to expect respect for these feelings; yet, as long as no reasons are given to justify these feelings, they will be regarded more as expression of a personal idiosyncrasy than as a moral feeling or verdict. Nobody is duty bound to justify publicly his/her private feelings; a sterile couple can at any time itself reject artificial insemination, *in vitro* fertilisation or any other therapy for sterility, without having to give reasons. *Moral* condemnation of these therapeutic interventions is totally different because it implies an expectation and a demand

---

[1] In more modern philosophical literature, this claim to trans-individual validity is made explicit through the *principle of universalisability*, which is, however, interpreted in different ways. Apart from a few diverging points of view, there seems to be agreement that moral norms, principles or values, have to be universal: neither implicitly nor explicitly may they be dependent upon time, space or other marginal conditions. This principle has a special importance in the ethical approaches which more or less attempt to bring moral validity into line with empirical truth; it then acquires a similar role for morality as the principle of induction has for the empirical sciences. Taking up the basic idea behind Kant's categorical imperative, which states that one may act only according to rules which one would welcome as a 'general law' (1949), these 'cognitivistic' ethicists formulate the principle of universalisation as *the* moral criterion.

It is not possible here to discuss whether the hopes which are linked with the cognitivistic approach are justified, i.e. whether it is possible to prove objectivity for moral claims to validity with the aid of the principle of universalisation. Yet it should be mentioned that this hope is questioned or doubted by many. For the deliberations which follow, it is sufficient to establish universalisability as a *necessary* premise for moral validity; it is unimportant for now whether it is, in addition, a *sufficient* premise. This principle is intended to prevent moral convictions from becoming too closely connected with personal taste, as suggested by Jean-Paul Sartre's statement that: 'the moral choice is comparable to the construction of a work of art' (1973, p. 48).

that all other people go along with this condemnation. Here we have the decisive reason behind claims to objectivity and the demand that moral norms be substantiated: they arise from the circumstance

> that we are subjected to these norms and sanctions, whether we like it or not, and that we in turn demand the same restriction of others (our children, for example). It is this restriction of our own actions, as well as the requirement that others restrict their actions in the same way, which has to be justified.
>
> (Tugendhat 1984b, p. 84)

If, in disapproving *in vitro* fertilisation or any other technology, we wish to express not merely a personal, more or less aesthetic opinion of taste but a moral verdict, then this disapproval must be able to be substantiated and generally understood; plausible arguments must be put forward to justify it.

Critical arguments

Reasons obviously become far more significant when contradictory moral feelings and verdicts about a particular phenomenon exist. This is where philosophical reflection comes in, making explicit the reasons put forward by each party, analysing them and weighing them up against each other; ideally, this process of reflection and discussion ends in consensus which, in turn, ends the conflict (cf. Bayertz 1994). For the participants in these ethical debates, this means not just being content to formulate their own positions, but – if they want to be taken seriously – developing and putting forward arguments to support their own positions and/or weaken those of the opposition.

This is what the critics of gene and reproduction technology have done; just as the advocates have not stopped at heralding their fascination, preferring to bring forward reasons and arguments to make their position more secure. The following overview presents the most important arguments *against* gene and reproduction technology. In the main related and connected, there is usually not much difference made between these arguments. Until now they have also been proclaimed as an inseparable unity, in the interests of viewing the object with a 'uniform' method. Since this kind of emphasised unity makes the debate more difficult, however, I have taken pains in the following reformulation to differentiate as precisely as possible between the various arguments, and to classify them in clearly distinguishable groups. Two main groups of critical arguments crystallised, each made up of three sub-groups.

1. *Technological* doubts usually refer to the problems of risk and safety. Interventions in human reproduction differ from other technological manipulations in that the risks involved always directly affect human individuals. Whereas an unsuccessful, functioning machine may be repaired or taken to pieces, any mistake in an instance of *in vitro* fertilisation or gene manipulation would be irreparable. Future projects for improving the human race involve, in addition, the difficulty of determining the aims of the project; preparing future human beings to cope better with the constantly increasing demands of a scientific and technological civilisation calls for a prognosis of those characteristics which the generations of tomorrow will require. A look at the sometimes grotesquely false prognoses of the visionaries shows how great the probability of making mistakes in such an undertaking could be.

2. *Political and social* doubts are mainly directed at the possibility of authoritarian political systems abusing the new technologies; Aldous Huxley's *Brave New World* is the literary paradigm of such a system. The 'racial hygiene' practised during the Nazi regime should also remind us of the dangers involved in instrumentalising gene and reproduction technology. There is also the possibility of these technologies being individually abused; ambitious parents, for example, could have their children programmed as highly specialised – and just as highly inconsiderate – freaks in a particular subject. Less Utopian is a commercialisation of the reproduction business via 'quality sperm' and/or surrogate mothers.

3. *Psycho-social* doubts result from the observation that an urgent desire to have children, although infertile, often stems from a neurotic compensatory strategy; satisfying it with new technology does not solve the actual problem: on the contrary, it creates additional ones. On top of this, there is the danger that a wide-

spread technologisation of the reproduction process, especially artificial procreation, will undermine the parent–child relationship. Emotional security within the family, fundamental to the social life and mental balance of every individual, could thus become endangered.

It is easy to see that this first group – however much its individual doubts and arguments may vary – forms a uniform category in the way that all the arguments refer to the *consequences* of applied gene and reproduction technology. It is impossible to overestimate the importance of this kind of anticipatory observation and evaluation; the introduction of new technologies has led to unwanted, even catastrophic, consequences far too often in the past for anyone to doubt seriously the necessity of technology assessment. Nevertheless, the considerations within this book do not deal primarily with such matters; they concentrate far more on the problems raised by a second group of critical arguments. This group aims less at the consequences of applied gene and reproduction technology, training its sights on the technologies themselves. It is conceivable that precautions could be taken to exclude all of the undesirable and dangerous consequences. Strict tests could go a long way in eliminating the safety risks, democratic political institutions and shrewd laws could prevent both State and individual abuse of the technologies, and appropriate application limitations could prevent the feared psycho-social consequences. Even if we assume all of this, the question still remains of whether we are allowed to make test tube babies and clones, improve the species and steer the autoevolutive process in the direction of gaseous or crystalline 'human beings'. The assumption just mentioned really does nothing to alter the three arguments belonging to the second group.

4. The *naturalness* argument states that interventions in human reproduction imply illegitimate manipulation of natural processes and lead to the creation of unnatural products. Yet especially human nature must be respected as holy.

5. The *technologisation* argument criticises science and technology for forcing its way into the business of reproduction; intimate processes are dragged under harsh laboratory lights, and secrets are destroyed. Gene and reproduction technology grants human beings access to the early stages of human life, procreation loses its

character of human 'becoming' and turns instead into the 'making' of human beings.

6. The *hybrism* argument refers to the attitude underlying the development and application of such technologies: by 'making' or 'manufacturing' its own kind, the human being assumes a heavenly rôle as creator. This assumption is most obvious in the project to reconstruct or improve the genus. But it is also behind technologies such as *in vitro* fertilisation; for here too, the human being is trying to manipulate its fate and break through natural barriers.

Holy war against human nature

If we compare these last arguments with the first three, it is obvious that the former belong to a different type of moral argumentation: they fall under a *deontological* concept of morality, thus substantiating a much more rigorous rejection of all forms of manipulating human reproduction. What makes them philosophically the most interesting is that they raise a series of fundamental philosophical problems connected with the concept of 'human nature'. Since the uneasiness mentioned is without doubt rooted in a feeling that technological intervention in human reproduction is unnatural, the last three arguments may be taken as its philosophical expression. In the debates about the moral legitimacy of these technologies, violation or disdain of human nature is a key argument. In his essay on *New Beginnings in Life*, published in 1972 and much quoted thereafter, Leon Kass centred his argumentation around this point; technological intervention in human reproduction for him implies morally illegitimate intervention in human nature. *In vitro* fertilisation turns the process of reproduction into an artificial procedure:

> What has been violated, even if only slightly, is the distinction between the natural and the artificial, and, at its very root, the nature of man himself. For man is the watershed which divides the world into those things that belong to nature and those that are made by men. To lay one's hands on human generation is to take a major step toward making man himself simply another of the manmade things.
>
> (Kass 1972, p. 54)

According to Kass, with gene and reproduction technology we have started a 'new holy war against human nature' (p. 20).

From this point of view, rejection of the Utopian projects which are not content to control the process, but which want to alter its product, must appear even stronger. Eugenic improvement of individual human characteristics, or even a complete gene technological reconstruction of the human being, as presented in its most extreme form by Stanislaw Lem in his concept of autoevolution, are aimed in a singularly radical manner at dissolving the natural in and about human beings through the artificial. Lem himself was of the opinion

> that autoevolution, the act in which the human being takes control over its own biology, is bound to provoke the heftiest conflicts between faith and empiricism ever known in history.
>
> (Lem 1980, p. 230)

It is irrelevant for now whether they really will be the heftiest in history; conflicts about the problem of human nature are certainly well under way. *Ethical* and *moral* problems seem to begin long before autoevolution; they are thus dependent less on the state of progress of technological options, and more on the normative significance of the object of these options. The problem of human nature and its moral dimension does not suddenly arise with the reconstruction of human beings; it is already present with contraception or *in vitro* fertilisation. For this reason, the science-fiction objection circumvents the philosophical problem. From a *philosophical* and *ethical* point of view, the question of when something may be realised – and even the possibility of realisation at all – is not all-important; even fantastic projects, by bringing an object or an action into the harsh light of futuristic visions, may reveal a moral dimension and provide access for ethical analysis. It is thus appropriate for Hans Jonas to speak of 'heuristic casuistry that is to help in the spotting of ethical principles' (Jonas 1984, p. 29). It is not the steadfastness of a prognosis which is important, but its content, because it allows moral principles, never needed before and thus implicit, to become visible.

> What is here contemplated, therefore, is a casuistry of the imagination which, unlike the customary casuistries of law and morality that serve the trying out of principles already known, assists in the tracking and

discovering of principles still unknown. The serious side of science fiction lies precisely in its performing such well-informed thought experiments, whose vivid imaginary results may assume the heuristic function here proposed.

(ibid., p. 30)

Part II
The destruction of
human substance

6

Human nature

Thus there is no human nature,
because there is no God
to have a conception of it.
Jean-Paul Sartre

The term 'human nature' epitomises everything which, regardless
of will, merits or society, the human being is *by Nature*. Like every
other form of life, the human being has a biological constitution
which determines certain essential features of its corporeal organisation and its behaviour. Thus this 'nature': (1) is common, since
it is shared by all members of the human race; (2) is not created
by ourselves, or by any other human individual, but is given; (3) is
the natural basis for individual existence and unfolding; (4) yet it
also limits these, since it is inaccessible and unalterable. Since we
all have an intuitive picture of what constitutes the human being, a
definition of human nature should not pose much of a problem.
The popularity of the term in many different contexts is therefore
no surprise; it always surfaces in discussions on the fundamental
aspects of anthropology or psychology, ethics or political philosophy. Yet a brief glance at the way it has been employed in philosophical discussion since Ancient times is sufficient to confuse the
picture: its meaning has usually remained implicit, precise definitions are hardly ever given, and every attempt to reconstruct one is
plagued by a multitude of competing modifiers. The 'strategic'
function of the term seemingly corresponds to insurmountable
ambiguity.

Body and spirit

The first manifestation of human nature is an organism comprising a particular structure. We can recognise from the external form of a living creature whether or not it is a human being, without becoming more closely acquainted with it in any way. In the Ancient world, the human being's characteristic upright gait and free hands were already being used to distinguish it physically from the animal kingdom; modern anthropological research also considers these characteristics to be biological prerequisites for anthropogenesis:

> Upright gait, a short face, hands which remain free during movement, and the possession of mobile tools, these are the fundamental characteristics of humanity.
>
> (Leroi-Gourhan 1980, p. 36)

Consequently, we cannot separate the 'humanness' of the human being from its existence as a natural – and, above all, that means corporeally organised – being. Insight had been gained into the natural and biological basis of *Homo sapiens* long before its origins were proved by Darwin. Not even the tendency to devaluate the bodily existence, beginning in Ancient times and especially prevalent during the Christian Middle Ages, has principally denied this. Even the conviction that the soul has to leave the flesh in order to regain itself or regain God concedes that the body is an essential part of the human being. The human self-consciousness which had been growing stronger ever since the Renaissance was not satisfied with this; the 'rehabilitation of sensuality' (Kondylis 1981), which resulted during the Modern Age period of Enlightenment led to a radical increase in the value of the human body. Materialist philosophers of the 18th century – for example, LaMettrie and d'Holbach – defined the human being as a machine. Opposing overemphasis of human spirituality, and especially rejecting Christian contempt for 'the flesh', human corporeality was accentuated to such an extent that the human being appeared as an exclusively material being, as an organised whole, made up of various matter, subject, like all of Nature's products, to her laws. Not even the human being's intellectual capabilities fundamentally distinguished it from other natural beings, since these capabilities were no more than modifications to its corporeal organisation, belonging to the human being alone, its bodily structure, the particular links between the matter joined within it. Even though this was extreme, and in no way representative, not even the idealistic countercurrent is blind to the insight that the human being is, and can only be, alive as an individual person in the form of an organic body. Although this philosophy attributes a status of decisive weight to the spiritual dimension, and although Hegel, for example, assumes that the human body is 'not in conformity with the mind' (Hegel *PhR*, §48), Hegel nevertheless emphasises that, at the same time, this body 'is the real pre-condition of every further determined mode of existence' (Hegel *PhR*, §47).

This implies that human nature is more than just the human body, including typical human capabilities and types of human behaviour. The animal also has a body, and if one does not share the materialists' opinion that human beings and animals are separated by a mere gradient, the question of what the specifically human characteristics are becomes even more acute. Mainstream philosophical thinking has therefore always assumed that an adequate definition of the term 'human being' must be more than merely a reference to its corporeal organisation. The human being *is* a natural being, but is not *just* a natural being. Since Ancient times, the question of what may be considered human has therefore been pondered not only with regard to the biological peculiarities of the species, but also to the characteristics which extend beyond the natural and the biological. For Aristotle, the human being distinguishes itself from the animal primarily in its cognitive faculty, its spirit, its reason – characteristics directly granting it a place next to God (*Eth. Nic.*, 1177b). The human being may be *animal* – but animal *rationale*. With regard to morality, Aristotle also maintains that the human being has an intermediate position of its own: the human being distinguishes itself from the animal in its moral faculty; its need for morality separates it from God (ibid., 1145). If Nature merely endows the human being with its moral faculty, the actual cultivation of this faculty emerging with habituation (ibid.. 1103a), then this reinforces the human being's affiliation to Nature, but lowers its status to that of a mere pre-requisite, on the basis of which the 'specifically human' is then to be created. Regardless of how the 'specifically human' was to be defined in the centuries which followed, whether as reason, spirit, morality, autonomy, freedom of will, perfectibility, etc., it was always considered as something more than just Nature, something projecting from her. This is the case, for example, when Descartes (1953), in his *Discours de la méthode*, localises the *differentia specifica* between the human being and the animal in language and reason, insisting that they cannot be derived from the moving forces of matter, being totally independent of the body. We are thus confronted with the human being as a double being, belonging to Nature through its body, but exceeding beyond her through its intellectual capabilities: *res cogitans* and *res extensa* simultaneously.

This dualism gave rise to the question of unity between the two substances within the – undivided – human being. Descartes certainly recognised this problem; yet he was not capable of drawing any conclusions regarding a conceptual unification of the two sides from his insight that the human spirit and the human body form a unity and are thus closely correlated. In this way the dualism continued to exist, although heavily under fire: in the attempt to dissolve the *res cogitans* in the *res extensa* and to found a materialistic monism; or in replacing reason with other criteria to distinguish between human beings and animals. Jean-Jacques Rousseau's idea of human *perfectibility* proved to be particularly influential. According to Rousseau, there is only a gradual difference between the intellectual faculties of human beings and animals:

> Thus it is not his understanding which constitutes the specific distinction of man among all other animals, but his capacity as a free agent. Nature commands all animals, and the beast obeys. Man receives the same impulsion, but he recognizes himself as being free to acquiesce or resist.
>
> (1984, p. 88)

For Rousseau, the real difference is 'one further distinguishing characteristic' of the human being, about which there can be no dispute:

> the *faculty of self-improvement* – a faculty which, with the help of circumstance, progressively develops all our other faculties, and which in man is inherent in the species as much as in the individual. On the other hand an animal at the end of several months is already what it

will remain for the rest of its life and its species will still be at the end of a thousand years what it was in the first of those thousand years.

(p. 88)

Human nature appears here not as a set of fixed characteristics and features, but as the basis and foundation of a developmental process in which the human being redefines itself constantly throughout history. The concept of perfectibility brings historical dynamics into the definition of humanity. The human being is no longer considered as what it is by Nature, but as what it makes of itself during the course of history: 'human nature' and 'human being'[1] drift apart.

Open relationship to Nature, decay of order

This implication is strengthened by the second perspective, which attempts to extract a philosophical concept of human nature from its relationship to (non-human) Nature. A direct consequence of *Homo sapiens* being a natural being is that it is a needy being. Its organism is maintained through continual metabolism, absorbing energy from the environment. In contrast to all the other biological species, the human being is not restricted to one type of behaviour towards its natural surroundings; it can satisfy its metabolic needs with the environment in very different ways and is even capable, beyond the mere acquisition of necessities, of consciously controlling and deliberately changing the natural conditions governing its life. As early as Ancient Greece (Plato, Protagorus), this was traced back to an 'unfitness' with regard to external living conditions, specific to the human race. The human being does not possess any specialised organs for the finding of food, nor natural protection against the rigours of the weather, nor natural weapons against its enemies: it does not possess a particular 'ecological niche'. The human being does not simply adapt to its environment: it adapts to its environment with the aid of technology. Originally just a product of Nature, the human being has become

---

[1] *Translator's note*: in this context the German 'menschliches Wesen' may be equally interpreted as 'human being' and 'human essence'.

'the creator and subject of its natural state' (Moscovici 1982, p. 27). Technological development and the relationship it constitutes between the human being and Nature was the start of a special dialectic: as a living creature not restricted to one specific relationship with Nature, the human being is capable of changing this relationship all the time, yet with each transformation, the human being also changes itself.

> It is impossible to make a strict division between human nature and *natura rerum*, the nature of things, and there is no way of pinpointing them to a fixed and ultimate stage [for their relationship].
>
> (p. 28)

Human plasticity and the openness of the human being's relationship to Nature did not become obvious until more recent times. With constant expansion and radical change in its metabolism with Nature, the human being is not simply granted its continued existence. Continued existence is guaranteed neither by Nature itself – by appropriate, instinctively guided behaviour, for example – nor by heavenly care. Instead, it is something which the human being has to achieve all on its own, time and again. The beginning of the Modern Age thus saw the term *self-preservation* becoming a central issue of philosophical perception of the world in general, and human self-understanding in particular. This term evolved in the context of a transformation of the entire perception of the world, beginning with the removal of God from the empirical world, dating back to the late scholastic theologians. In perceiving God as a sovereign facing Nature, free to create the world as He deemed fit, Nature became – theologically speaking – increasingly neutral. The structure of creation could no longer be traced back to reasons which could be rationally reconstructed by human beings; with the world's origins embedded in an act of God's free will, the human being can do no more than factually accept the world as it is. This neutralisation leads to a metaphysic excluding the notion of a teleological ordering of Nature. Whereas in Ancient times and the Middle Ages, the cosmos was observed as a hierarchy of purposes, in which every object had its natural place and every process its goal, Modern philosophy perceives the universe as a totality of material things and their natural relationships. A trenchant consequence of this deteologisation of the world is its demoralisation. A teleologically ordered cosmos always has a moral dimension; its structure of being coincides with a hierarchy of values, purposes and goals. At the beginning of the Modern Age, this notion was replaced by a picture of the world stripped of all its inherent moral qualities, like perfection, harmony, meaning, purpose; there ultimately remains 'the utter devalorization of being, the divorce of the world of value and the world of facts' (Koyré 1970, p. 2).

For modern humanity, the security offered by a meaningfully ordered cosmos is replaced by a 'plunge' into an unknown universe, governed by Nature's blind laws; the modern human being is not given a destiny in the world, but has to define its own. The 'decay of order' emerging with the decay of teleological ontology strips from the human being the possibility of being carried along by a purposeful ordering of the world or a heavenly plan for the world's salvation, and forcibly bestows upon it an existence which requires self-assertion and self-preservation. The specifically modern concept of subjectivity is thus constituted in connection with an altered view of the essence of Nature and of the human being's relationship to Nature: a *natural* world of matter and necessity, objectivity and quantity opposes a *human* world of reason and freedom, subjectivity and quality. The inner dualism of natural and non-natural finds support here in the *ontological*. Although in existence long before the Modern Age, this dualism becomes acute with the neutralisation of Nature and the emergence of the concept of subjectivity, ultimately conceptually cemented in Descartes' distinction between *res cogitans* and *res extensa*. This dualism carries on into Kant's interpretation of the human being as a citizen of two worlds – as a natural being living in a 'world of senses' and subjected to its determinism, and as a spiritual being belonging to an 'intelligible world' and free.

Subjectivity and insubstantiality

Nevertheless, Kant made efforts to bring the two worlds together and view them as a unity, at least in their origins. We could summarise this by saying that the human being is, according to its nature, *subject*. Human biology specifically prevents the human being from having a set, unchanging relationship with its natural surroundings, forcing upon it openness and freedom. Kant provides us with impressive argumentation along these lines, also serving as a summary of essential motives for the anthropological discussion earlier on:

> Since Nature gave Man his Reason and Free Will, this was a clear indication that he was to be guided neither by instinct nor inborn knowledge.
>
> For his food, clothing, external security, and defence, she gave him neither the horns of the bull nor the claws of the lion nor the teeth of the dog. Everything, including his entertainment, his insight and intelligence, even the goodness of his Will, were to be entirely his own accomplishment. But Nature's objective is not that he should live well and in comfort: a host of hardships attack him and make him acquire a rational esteem.
>
> Something is very odd in all this. Earlier generations have gone about their troublesome business only to prepare a foundation for the structure which Nature has in mind, yet only the last generations will have the good fortune to live in the building.
>
> (Kant 1963b, p. 135)

There are three closely interwoven arguments formulated here, together forming the basis for a theory on humanity. First of all (1), Kant takes up the matters of biological helplessness, unfitness, deficiency of instinct, etc., all specific to the human race and distinguishing it from other forms of life, reformulates them and thus lays the foundations for a tradition of defining the meaning of human nature, later to be taken up by Herder and pushed, especially by Arnold Gehlen, to the centre of 20th century philosophical anthropology. (2) Because of this 'sparingness' in its natural equipment, the human being is to be understood not on the grounds of its biological substratum, but only on the grounds of its enforced self-alteration and self-completion abilities. Its essence is not established, but consists in its continually growing powers. Finally (3), the realisation of this perfection process is comprehended as a process for which the human being itself is responsible; its nature does not guarantee perfection, but it facilitates perfectibility; the human being is not given its essence: its essence is its responsibility.

However, with regard to the concept of 'human nature', this attempt to present human subjectivity as having emerged from the biological nature of the human being is somewhat dissatisfying. The connection between human nature and human subjectivity remains genetic; it refers exclusively to the *emergence* of subjectivity from its natural basis. Once it has acquired an existence as subject, this basis seems to evaporate into insignificance – as subject, the human being remains curiously 'without substance'. The central dilemma involved in a definition of human nature remains unsolved: either we assume a clearly defined set of natural human characteristics and qualities; then we are forced to arrive at a substantialist image of humanity which cannot do justice to the manifold forms of human existence and their historic capacity for alteration. Or we focus on this plurality of existences and their historicity; then 'human nature' dissolves in a stream of changeable definitions.

Nothing alters in post-Kantian philosophy in this respect either. After Feuerbach had, at the beginning of the 19th century, once more made the concrete bodily nature of the human being a central problem of his philosophy, a process of historising the image of humanity began, beginning with Marx, to gain in strength, gradually to dissolve all of the anthropological constants into history. In *The German Ideology* – in indirect polemic against the idealist philosophy of the time – the 'physical organisation' of the human being is particularly emphasised as a 'premise of all human history', yet this natural foundation does not become a systematic part of the philosophy of Historical Materialism:

> The first premise of all human history is, of course, the existence of living human individuals. Thus the first fact to be established is the physical organisation of these individuals and their consequent relation to the rest of nature. Of course, we cannot here go either into the actual physical nature of man, or into the natural condtions in which man finds himself – geological, orohydrographical, climatic and so on. The writing of history must always set out from these natural bases and their modification in the course of history through the action of men.
>
> (Marx & Engels 1965, p. 31)

In actual fact, these 'natural foundations' are hardly ever mentioned by Marx or Engels in their theoretical works on history and society; not because they were forgotten, but because they were only *foundations*. What is really interesting is what takes place on top of these foundations: the social self-definition and historical self-alteration of the human being as 'the ensemble of the social relations' (ibid., p. 652).

Human nature fared no better within other 19th century philosophical movements. As Helmuth Plessner writes, for example, in Ernst Cassirer's Neo-Kantianism:

> human nature can only be defined functionally, and not substantially. There is no inherent principle or *vinculum substantiale*, as the scholastics believed, no specific ability which could be taken as a definition for the human being. There is only one characteristic, and that is its achievements: language, myth, religion, art, science, history . . . Cassirer knows that the human being is a living creature, but he makes no philosophical use of this information.
>
> (Plessner 1983c, pp. 242–3)

This way of viewing things fails to deliver an insight into:

> the obvious interlocking of the human manner of being and the human organism . . . In the tradition of Kant, the philosophy of identity and Neo-Kantianism, Nature is the Other, which is constituted, the product of creative functioning, and, even as a spirit, is in its otherness a mere interlude on the journey back to origin.
>
> (ibid., pp. 244–5)

This point has been taken up within our century by the philosophical anthropology represented by Max Scheler, Helmuth Plessner and Arnold Gehlen, attempting on the empirical basis of modern biological theories to produce a philosophical understanding of human nature which takes its naturalness seriously, without reverting to rash biologism or naturalism. The historicity of the human race and its plasticity in various natural and social living conditions are neither disputed nor trivialised. Plessner prefers to see the experience of history precisely as the basis for questioning human nature. It is this experience which enables clear vision of:

> what always asserts itself, in all forms of human appearance, in forever differing ways, as the same: *semper aliter, semper idem* . . . Not much philosophising is necessary in order to comprehend that the experience of variety and change within the human race and human fates is only possible against the simple and constant background of the

human genus. Variability involves constancy. The richer and more disparate our historical experience becomes, the more urgent the need for unity becomes. This need cannot, however, be stilled with a generalising synthesis, but only by resorting to the conditions of the possibility of confusing variety.

(Plessner 1983b, pp. 139–40)

Yet even this line of argumentation demonstrates the common problem of attempting to define human nature in general terms, since any such definition is only possible abstractively, by disregarding the concrete appearances of human beings throughout the course of history. For, regardless of which concrete human beings we are confronted with, their characteristics and methods of behaviour are always socially and historically conditioned, and the concept of 'human nature' can be constructed only if we disregard these visible social and historical phenomena. If we do this empirically, we are ultimately left with just a few non-committal platitudes about 'the' human being; if we do so theoretically, we may be able to arrive at definitions with some content, yet they will be extremely abstract. Plessner's own term 'eccentric positionality', which he employs in *Die Stufen des Organischen und der Mensch* (Organic Stages and the Human Being: Plessner 1981, pp. 360–5) to characterise the fundamental feature of the manner in which human beings exist, is one example of this. It refers to the circumstance that the human being not only *is* its being, but behaves actively and consciously towards it. The human being is thus forced 'to make itself what it already is, to lead the life it lives' (ibid., p. 384). Plessner's choice of tracing the manner in which human beings exist back to their natural circumstances thus no longer serves to deliver a precise definition of 'human nature' – the term does not play a systematic rôle in *Stufen des Organischen* – but rather the exact opposite: 'eccentric positionality' defines precisely the reason why, in the case of the human being, there can be no fixed set of unalterable, natural definitions.

Because the human being is forced, as a result of its manner of existence, to lead the life it lives, i.e. to make itself what it is – since the human being only is when it executes, it needs a a non-natural, nongrown complement. It is therefore by Nature, due to its form of existence, *artificial*. As an eccentric being, without equilibrium, without time or place, nowhere, constitutively homeless, the human being has to 'become something' and – thus create its equilibrium . . . An eccentric form of life and a requirement for supplementation amount to the very same thing. Requirement is not to be understood here in a subjective, psychological sense. It is precedent to all human needs, to each compulsion, each drive, each tendency, each human will. In this requirement or nakedness lies the drive behind each specifically human activity, i.e. each activity geared towards the unreal and involving artificial means, the ultimate reason behind the *tool* and behind what the tool serves: *culture*.

(ibid., pp. 384–5).

The result appears to be paradoxical: the human being's nature is its culture, and its natural definition is to define itself. With the findings of philosophical anthropology, the notion of human nature in the sense of a fixable substance which is unalterable, and which places limits on thoughts and actions, proves to be an illusion. Not much more is required to reject this notion totally. Taking up on existentialist 'belief that existence comes before essence' (1973, p. 26), Jean-Paul Sartre drew the radical conclusion that there is no such thing as human nature (p. 28). In *Being and Nothingness*, Sartre had already defined and emphasised freedom as the fundamental characteristic of human existence (1958). Instead of being committed through natural preconditions in any way, the human being can and must design itself. Sartre's existentialism assumes individual subjectivity to be absolute. Plessner – and Kant before him – had already emphasised that the human being is not committed by its biological constitution, that the latter rather enables and forces the human being to lead its own life and actively shape its own history. Sartre radicalises these thoughts by additionally rejecting the genetic connection between human nature and human subjectivity, philosophically speaking.

Normativity

The ease with which the term 'human nature' is employed is curiously disproportional to the difficulty experienced in assigning a precise definition to it. This is due to the fact that a large, maybe even major proportion of the ways in which 'human nature' is employed is not usually aimed at describing an object as exactly as possible, but is an attempt to label *normatively* a but vaguely defined image of the human being. The term 'human nature' shares this normativity with the general concept of Nature, which, as John Stuart Mill has shown, holds two major meanings: (1) it means the total number of forces in the world, including everything occurring due to these forces; (2) it refers to everything which occurs spontaneously, without deliberate and intentional human interference (1969b, p. 375). In addition, there is a third employment of the term which refers to 'nature' as a criterion by which to measure human thoughts, feelings and actions. From the Ancient Stoics via modern Natural Law to the present day, the *naturam sequi* has always been regarded as a fundamental ethical principle, and social institutions, human behaviours and moral norms have always been justified as (or criticised for) being (or not being) in accordance with Nature. Not only in some philosophical teachings, but also in the everyday consciousness of many human beings, the equation dictates that everything which is 'natural' is 'good'.

> That any mode of thinking, feeling, or acting, is 'according to nature' is usually accepted as a strong argument for its goodness. If it can be said with any plausibility that 'nature enjoins' anything, the propriety of obeying the injunction is by most people considered to be made out: and conversely, the imputation of being contrary to nature, is thought to bar the door against any pretension on the part of the thing so designated, to be tolerated or excused; and the word unnatural has not ceased to be one of the most vituperative epithets in the language.
>
> (ibid., p. 377)

Thus this third employment of the term 'Nature' does not constitute a third meaning, a third definition of what is to be understood by 'Nature'; it is much more the establishment of a norm. The normative dimension of the term 'Nature' is not a third definition alongside the first two mentioned, but hovers, as it were, above them, penetrating them in numerous contexts of use.

> Those who say that we ought to act according to Nature do not mean the mere identical proposition that we ought to do what we ought to do. They think that the word Nature affords some external criterion of what we should do; and if they lay down as a rule for what ought to be, a word which in its proper signification denotes what is, they do

so because they have a notion, either clearly or confusedly, that what is, constitutes the rule and standard of what ought to be.

(ibid., p. 377)

The problem with this kind of interpretation of Nature as normative is that, before Nature may be attributed with having a normative content, that same normative content has to have been placed there. One has to *view* Nature as morally relevant in order to use her as a point of moral orientation. Yet this in turn requires 'special religious or metaphysical premises not open to a general secular defence'.

> In order for the character of reality to serve as a criterion for resolving moral disputes, it must be shown to be morally normative. One must be able to show that the general tendencies of nature were established by God, not to test the abilities of humans to redirect them, but to guide humans to their proper goals. To establish such a proposition would require special religious or metaphysical premises not open to a general secular defence. In order to know whether the general tendencies of nature or the structures of reality are to be acknowledged as morally instructive rather than confronted as challenges to human manipulative capacities, one must have standards by which to judge states of affairs or structures of nature or reality to be good or bad, as being that to which one ought to submit or that which one ought to set aside. But the availability of such standards is what is at issue.

(ibid., p. 377)

The situation is similar with 'human nature'. Nearly every non-trivial philosophical definition of 'human nature' is already influenced by normative prerequisites and/or directly leads to normative consequences. This link is particularly significant within political philosophy: whether the human being is regarded as naturally bad (cf. Hobbes) or naturally good (cf. Rousseau), both cases result in – differing – political consequences. In the first case, it will be deemed unavoidable to curb in an authoritarian manner the anti-social drives of individuals[2] – for example through a 'strong'

---

[2] Sigmund Freud, emphasising an inherent human tendency towards aggression, offers a more modern theoretical example of the *necessary* suppressive function of social institutions. 'The existence of this inclination to aggression, which we can detect in ourselves and justly assume to be present in others, is the factor which disturbs our relations with our neighbour and which forces civilization into such a high expenditure [of energy]. In consequence of this primary mutual hostility of human beings,

State; in the second case, one can only expect a depravation of virtue from such a State. Turned around, the various interpretations of human nature can serve to legitimise the different political positions held in each case, and since Ancient times hardly any other term has been employed as frequently by very different parties for purposes of legitimation. – In other areas, views as to what is 'human' or 'humane', and thus morally good, usually involve particular interpretations of human nature. Critical statements about gene and reproduction technology from Leon Kass, quoted above, have already demonstrated that scientific and technological developments are also subject to being judged according to criteria of 'naturalness'.

Our century has not been wanting in technological innovations and breakthroughs in previously unavailable practical experiences and options. And, since all of these innovations come into conflict with traditional forms of life within society, as well as the values associated with these forms of life, all of them give rise to social and moral problems in one way or another. Even if they do not cause any grave shake-up in our system of values, they repeatedly pose the question of whether the loss in familiarity with our surroundings, which we experience with each trenchant technological innovation, is not too high a price for the blessings they bring. It is thus no surprise that criticism of progress and civilisation – a constant within modern Western history – has been raging more than ever recently. Yet the tenor of this criticism is not the same everywhere. Uneasiness and criticism are usually directed at the *consequences* of technology: the destruction of the countryside, the extinction of certain species or the looming extermination of the human race. The 'naturalness' argument usually plays a minor rôle. Criticism of the hydrogen bomb as 'unnatural' would be regarded bizarre, and an atomic power plant is disturbing for its

civilized society is perpetually threatened with disintegration. The interest of work in common would not hold it together; instinctual passions are stronger than reasonable interests. Civilization has to use its utmost efforts in order to set limits to man's aggressive instincts and to hold the manifestations of them in check by physical reaction-formations. Hence, therefore, the use of methods intended to incite people into identifications and aim-inhibited relationships of love, hence the restriction upon sexual life, and hence too the ideal's commandment to love one's neighbour as oneself – a commandment which is really justified by the fact that nothing else runs so strongly counter to the original nature of man' (Freud 1969, p. 49).

potential danger and not its 'unnaturalness'. In the debate on gene
and reproduction technology, however, 'naturalness' is the central
problem; its provocation is based on a collision with deeply rooted
views on human nature. This becomes clearer if we compare
'intranautic' venturing into the reproductive process with astro-
nautic venturing into space.

Venture into space

Space technology has led the human being to cross one of the
boundaries fundamental to its existence – at least until two
decades ago: that of the planet where the human being was created
and lives. Space travel could thus serve as the paradigm of a technological breakthrough. There has certainly been no lack of voices
eager to proclaim the progress of space technology as a turning
point in human history.

> Having succeeded in populating the entire planet, the only living
> creature to do so, the human being prepares to become a species capa-
> ble of existing at the solar system level, begins to unify its geography
> and astronomy. The employment of space rockets suggests more than
> just the mere discovery of a new means of transport and communica-
> tion; it suggests that at some stage the human race will discover and
> occupy worlds of a different physical quality. For hundreds of years,
> sceptics were angry or amused at the idea of venturing into extrater-
> restrial territory, a topic passionately cultivated by its pioneers. Today
> we return to it, equipped with the teachings of the 19th century and
> eager to explore the extent of such an extraordinary and radical revo-
> lution. What used to be Utopian, an exaggeration of innocent imagi-
> nation, has now become part of our *expanding* natural order.
> Everything which has been thought of and tried out on our planet
> now has to be revised. We already have the preliminaries, which are
> to be taken as hints. A strengthening of our links to material powers,
> an expansion of our possibilities in life beyond the surface of the
> Earth, a corresponding revolution of our intelligence and our instru-
> ments: these are the components of our visible, immediate reality.
>
>   (Moscovici 1982, pp. 15–16)

However dramatic these words may be, it is impossible to hide
the fact that they are far removed from reality. Satellite technology,

flying to the moon and investigating far-off planets with space probes are all, of course, impressive technological achievements. Why a revision of everything conceived and tested on Earth should be necessary, however, remains incomprehensible. Not only has such a revision not taken place: there is hardly any reason why one should – hardly any reason why an astronaut walking on the moon should be viewed as a more trenchant event than the first hot air balloon trip or the maiden voyage of the first submarine. With space travel, we have exceeded the boundary separating our earthly atmosphere from extra-terrestrial space; yet was this really fundamentally different from overcoming the limits to human mobility posed by conventional transportation methods? Space technology has forced open the door to a part of Nature which differs from the Nature familiar to us on Earth only in its emptiness and immeasurable extent, but not in its moral quality. The Modern scientific revolution has done away with Ancient and Mediaeval differentiation between the cosmic spheres, thus destroying the hierarchy of values connected with that differentiation. We no longer distinguish between an imperfect sublunar sphere and the supralunar spheres which are gradually more perfect. Considering a world view

> in which the hierarchy of value determined the hierarchy and structure of being, rising from the dark, heavy and imperfect earth to the higher and higher perfection of the stars and heavenly spheres
>
> (Koyré 1970, p. 2)

the venture into space would have included a violation of the valuable ordering within the world. For us, on the other hand, viewing the universe as an homogenous space, with no difference between the inherent moral qualities of its various regions, the flight of a rocket merely appears as the bridging of a quantitatively measurable distance. Even if we would like to be impressed or moved by the sight of a starry sky above us, the 'awe' that we experience is no longer moral, but merely psychological. We no longer view the sky as the home of the Gods, and certainly not as the blackboard upon which all the moral laws are written. In this sense, it is not a moral feeling which is involved in awesome amazement at the eternity of the universe:

> A little interrogation of our own consciousness will suffice to convince us, that what makes these phenomena so impressive is simply their

vastness. The enormous extension in space and time, or the enormous power they exemplify, constitutes their sublimity; a feeling in all cases, more allied to terror than to any moral emotion. And though the vast scale of these phenomena may well excite wonder, and sets at defiance all ideas of rivalry, the feeling it inspires is of a totally different character from admiration of excellence. Those in whom awe produces admiration may be aesthetically developed, but they are morally uncultivated.

(Mill 1969b, p. 384)

Holiness

In this respect, interventions in human nature are fundamentally different from interventions in non-human Nature. Human nature is not morally neutral and valueless for us in the same sense as Nature is. The demoralisation of matter, which took place at the beginning of the Modern Age as an ontological correlate for the development of modern consciousness of subjectivity, omitted the human body. Human nature has retained the inherent value which Nature also possessed before the scientific revolution: it is 'holy' to us as, in a similar way, the starry night sky must have been to those who lived in the Ancient and Middle Ages. Just as, in the past, travelling heavenly bodies were observed not as planetary and stellar movements which obey the law of gravity and which may be calculated according to it, but as the manifestation of a reasonable order inherent to the cosmos, so the human body appears not merely as an apparatus obeying physical and chemical laws, but as the natural basis for the person in question. In his letters *Über die aesthetische Erziehung des Menschen* (On the Aesthetical Education of Man), Friedrich Schiller lends expression to the opposition between Nature's freedom from value and the inherent value of the human sphere – albeit in a different context, and with reference not to biological and medical, but to pedagogical and political practice.

When the artist dealing with the mechanical lays his hands on a shapeless mass in order to give it the form he intends, he has no scruples about treating it roughly. The Nature with which he works does not deserve respect in itself, and he is not concerned with the whole for the sake of its components, but with its components for the sake of the whole. When the artist dealing with the beautiful lays his hands on the same mass, he has just as few scruples about treating it roughly, but he avoids letting this show. He does not respect the matter with which he is working any more than the artist dealing with the mechanical, but he will attempt to deceive the eye which defends the freedom of this matter by seeming to treat it with compliance. The artist dealing with the pedagogical and political is altogether different, for he views the human being as both his matter and his task. The purpose returns to the matter, and only because the whole serves its components may the components bow to the whole. The artist dealing with the political has to approach his material with a totally different respect than that feigned by the artist dealing with the beautiful. He has to care for its uniqueness and personality, not subjectively and for show, but objectively and for the inner essence.

(Schiller 1967, p. 578)

This feeling of holiness with regard to human nature, and the moral postulate deeming it to be cared for and respected, have their origins in Western religion. According to Christian tradition, the human being is as much one of God's creatures as any other living being; yet the fact that the human being has a soul and was created in God's image gives it a special place amongst other creatures.

And God said, Let us make man in our image, after our likeness; and let them have dominion over the fish of the sea, and over the fowl of the air, and over the cattle, and over all the earth, and over every creeping thing that creepeth upon the earth. So God created man in his *own* image, in the image of God created he him; male and female created he them.

(Genesis 1: 26–27)

This similarity in image to God is expressively reinforced in the New Testament with the words:

But we all, with open face beholding as in a glass the glory of the Lord, are changed into the same image from glory to glory, *even* as by the spirit of the Lord.

(II Corinthians 3: 18; cf. Benz 1961, p. 32)

There is no need to go into the depth with which Christian beliefs have characterised Western thinking – and still do. Views regarding human nature are no exception. Even if, within this tradition, the body was attributed a lesser value than the spirit and soul, it was never considered merely as matter, and research into the human body at the beginning of the Modern Age could therefore still be justified with the theological argument that anatomy 'leads us directly to our creator, just as the effect leads us directly to the cause' (quoted from Jacob 1983, p. 43). Theological neutralisation of Nature did not directly exclude human nature; yet the latter was considered to be in the image of God, and thus demanded reverence and respect. Besides religious convictions, there were also philosophical arguments opposing a complete demoralisation of the human body. That is, despite the fact that – apart from the materialist thinkers – there is consensus that the essence of the human being is more than its nature, even the most consequent of idealists could hardly deny that human nature is at the same time the basis of non-natural human characteristics. Hegel, in his *Philosophy of Right* (§48), categorically denies the attempt to separate the person from the body:

> It is only because I am alive as a free entity in my body that this living existent ought not to be misused by being made a beast of burden. While I am alive, my soul (the concept and, to use a higher term, the free entity) and my body are not separated; my body is the embodiment of my freedom and it is with my body that I feel. It is therefore only abstract sophistical reasoning which can so distinguish body and soul as to hold that the 'thing-in-itself', the soul, is not touched or attacked if the body is maltreated and the existent embodiment of personality is subjected to the power of another . . . If another does violence to my body, he does violence to me.

Also enlightening are Hegel's considerations in his *Ästhetik*. Talk of the human *Gestalt* belonging to Nature is criticised here as 'a very vague expression' (II, p. 98) for the way it disregards the fact that the spirit is manifested in this *Gestalt* as well, and that the spirit lends the *Gestalt* sensual expression:

> The expression in the human face, its eyes, its stance and gesture may be material and not spiritual; yet within this corporeality, the human exterior is not only vital and natural in the way of an animal, but an incarnation, a reflection of the spirit within. Through a man's eyes one sees his soul, just as his entire form expresses his spiritual character. If the incarnation is part of the spirit, *its* representation, then it follows that the spirit is also the inner part of the body, and not an

inwardness which is foreign to the external *Gestalt*. The materialness of the body therefore neither infers nor implies a different meaning. It is true that the human *Gestalt* has much in common with that of the animal, but the difference between the human body and the animal body is that the human body proves to be the domain, the only true, natural representation of the spirit.

(I, p. 419)

In contrast to the rest of Nature, the human body is not value-free matter, but bespirited, and thus in possession of an inherent value. It may not *be* what is specifically human, but it is its 'domain'.

The valuable dimension of the human body, based on its identity with the spirit, is manifested, on the one hand, in the body's beauty. It is no coincidence that, for Hegel, the most complete realisation of art's ideal – mutual adequacy of content and form – is the human *Gestalt*, 'because only the human exterior is capable of sensually disclosing the spiritual' (ibid., p. 419). On the other hand, in ceasing to be mere facts of Nature, the features constituting the human *physis* become symbols of humanity. This is especially true of the upright gait differentiating human beings from all other animals, and therefore regarded from time immemorial to be as much the foundation as the symbol of human peculiarity.

Look up to Heaven, O human, and take pleasure in your great advantage, linked by the creator of the world to such a simple principle, your upright gait! If you were to walk on all fours like an animal, your head would be shaped in the gluttonous manner favouring mouth and nose, and the rest of your body would be structured accordingly: what would become of your higher level of intelligence, the image of God, invisible within you? ... Through the structuring of your limbs to suit an upright gait, however, your head received a handsome position and direction; the brain, that tender, ethereal, heavenly growth, gained enough space to spread itself out and branch downwards. Full of thoughts, the forehead domed, the animal organs retreated, the human being was formed.

(Herder 1965, I, p. 128)

Even in the 20th century, upright gait has lost none of its significance. This is shown, for example, in the following line from Ernst Bloch: 'For every thousand wars there are not even ten revolutions; such are the difficulties of upright gait' (Bloch 1959, p. 551).

Monsters

If the holiness and value inherent within human nature is embodied in the aesthetic and symbolic dimension of the human *Gestalt*, then it is easy to comprehend why artificial people in literature so often appear as ugly, vile monsters. We only have to think of Victor Frankenstein's horror, as already quoted. It would be too superficial to attribute the ugliness of this nameless creature to its creator's lack of craftmanship or – Mary Shelley's novel appeared in 1816 – to the underdeveloped state of science and technology at the time. Far more, the monstrosity is literary expression of the illegitimacy of manipulating human nature. Up until now, the manipulation of non-human creatures has aroused as much uneasiness, even with regard to genetically manipulated bacteria:

> If Dr. Frankenstein must go on producing his little biological monsters – and I deny the urgency and even the compulsion – why pick *E. coli* as the womb?
>
> (Chargaff 1976, p. 938)

Monsters are not as far removed from our theme as it might at first appear, as illustrated by the debate on the permissibility of human/animal hybrids. Whilst Joseph Fletcher considers the creation of such beings permissible (1974, p. 171–3), others remind us of the 'Minotaur' in Greek mythology, a bull/human hybrid which had to be locked up in that famous labyrinth because of its ugliness and awfulness (Walters 1982, p. 117). In Lederberg's considerations, the external form of the beings to be created, the attractiveness of their appearance, also plays a particular rôle. In answer to the question of how the human being is, in future, to dissociate itself from isolated or scattered tissue and organs, on the one hand, and experimental, karyotype hybrids, on the other, he offers the following as a pragmatic criterion: human legal privileges will be granted to those 'objects' which are similar enough to human beings in appearance to move human conscience, and which are not too expensive to keep (Lederburg 1966, p. 11). Moreover, Lederberg assumes that public acceptance concerning trenchant manipulations of human beings will partly be influenced by 'the handsomeness of a parahuman progeny' (ibid.). However, he does not consider this to be a well-reflected criterion, but to be unreliable.

Nature and sexuality

Thus the uneasiness aroused by developments in gene and repro-duction technology stems from the fact that the interventions which this technology makes possible concern not just any neutral matter, but human nature, as holy as ever and – morally and aes-thetically – valuable in its own right. This is especially the case as the new technologies invade an area of human nature which is par-ticularly 'sensitive': sexuality and reproduction. Not surprisingly, all the types of behaviour closely or loosely connected with sexual-ity and reproduction are usually attributed to human nature. There is no need to go into the biological significance of these processes and there can be no doubt that the driving forces behind our reproductive behaviour are deeply anchored in our biological constitution. Clifford Grobstein attempted to identify specifically human reproductive behaviour as a unity of five moments ('basic human pentad') which include the biological, the human behav-ioural and the sociological fields, as well as forming a kind of gra-dient from the animal to the human, along which our species has evolutionarily developed, and is developing further, from genera-tion to generation (1981, pp. 60–1). Central to this complex is the biological phenomenon of internal fertilisation and pregnancy. According to Grobstein, this manner of reproduction is much older than human culture; it conditions the sexual intercourse strongly influencing our experiences, dreams, individual lives and social behaviour. Five elements orbit internal fertilisation and pregnancy as a biological fact: (1) the roles of the sexes and sexual behaviour, (2) marital love, (3) the institution of marriage, (4) the conception of and care for children, (5) the family institution. In actual fact, the key biological and social significance of sexuality and reproduction may be found in all the societies we are aware of, in the institutionalisation of their control, and in the manifold rit-uals and symbols connected with sexual procedures – typically enough, even in the industrial societies characterised by a strong trend away from rituals, a 'minimum of social aestheticism' (Leroi-Gourhan 1980, p. 441) has been preserved precisely in connection with sexual maturity.

Here we again have the fundamental problem involved in any conditioning of human nature: the transition from the *biological* fact of internal procreation and pregnancy to the *social* facts of marriage, family and ritualisation clearly shows how difficult it is to separate a human characteristic or behaviour from its – no longer natural – manifestation. More importantly, the biological and social 'nature' of sexuality and reproduction is not merely regarded as an historical fact, but – in the manner already mentioned – is attributed with normative significance. In hardly any other area of life does the term 'naturalness' have such a strong and duty-binding effect or, *vice versa*, the term 'unnaturalness' produce such a spontaneous and deep feeling of repugnance. Even if, with an historical perspective and in an intercultural comparison, this pair of opposites, naturalness and unnaturalness, proves to be an antinomy between the socially allowed and the socially not allowed, this still does nothing to change the fact that there is a strong normative bond between this pair of opposites. It is significant here that the concept of naturalness not only excludes sexual practices which deviate from accepted social norms, but also renders 'unnatural' technological manipulation of the normal procedure, with violation of a strongly symbolic and normative field moving us much more deeply emotionally than any other form of manipulation.

Based on his concept of the 'basic human pentad', Clifford Grobstein also drew attention to this circumstance with regard to *in vitro* fertilisation:

> In no way, therefore, can the sudden displacement of so primordial a process be treated as such a simple translocation in space from internal to external. The wrench is epic in human history. However cleverly biological consequences may be technically minimized, the translocation cannot fail eventually to generate profound emotional, cultural and social reverberations.
>
> (1981, p. 61)

Technological intervention in the process of sexuality and reproduction provoked this kind of emotional, cultural and social reaction long before the most recent scientific developments. And the dichotomy of 'naturalness' and 'unnaturalness' has always served as the basis for condemning these interventions. In his critical analysis of human society and culture, Jean-Jacques Rousseau (1984, p. 150) mentions this kind of manipulation together with war, piracy, shipwreck, murder, intoxication and robbery, all sources of loss for the human species which necessarily result from civilisation turning its back on Nature.

> How many shameful methods there are to prevent the birth of man and deceive nature; whether by those brutish and depraved tastes which insult her most charming work, tastes that neither savages nor animals have ever known, and which are born in civilised countries only from corrupt imaginations; whether by secret abortions, worthy fruits of debauchery and vicious honour; whether by the exposure and murder of a multitude of infants, victims of the poverty of their parents or the barbarous shame of their mothers, finally, by the mutilation of those unfortunates, in whom a part of their existence and all their posterity are sacrificed for the sake of some worthless songs, or worse still sacrificed to the brutal jealousy of a few men; a mutilation which, in the last case, doubly outrages nature, both in the treatment received by the victims and the use to which they are destined.[3]

Even today, the naturalness argument plays a key rôle in the Catholic condemnation of contraception, artificial insemination and *in vitro* fertilisation. The justified desire to have a child may never – according to Pius XII in the speech quoted earlier (from Gründel 1983, p. 255) – be satisfied by way of 'anti-natural actions'.

[3] There are three points to be noted with regard to this passage. (1) As we have already seen, it is not true that the 'savages' were unaware of contraception and abortion (cf. Himes 1970; Devereux 1976); thus the latter cannot be traced back to a 'corrupt imagination' as a result of civilisation. (2) This allusion to the abandonment and murder of children confirms more recent beliefs (McKeown 1976) regarding widespread infanticide within Europe until into the 19th century. (3) With 'mutilation', Rousseau is referring to the castration of oriental harem guards, and of young choristers who were put in – mainly church – choirs as eunuch sopranos. In the Pope's chapel this took place until the year 1900.

7

Substantialism and its difficulties

*. . . the word 'unnatural' has not ceased
to be one of the most vituperative epithets
in the language*
John Stuart Mill

Until recently, there was very little chance of controlling or directly intervening in human reproduction. The latest achievements within the field of reproduction technology have changed all this; with *in vitro* fertilisation, for example, procreation – if not the human being itself – has become a technological process. Each new breakthrough in this field represents a further step towards a technological control over human nature. With gene and reproduction technology – as critics have repeatedly emphasised – it is no less than human nature which is at stake and, with it, all that is human, *humanum* itself. In connection with the problem of surrogate motherhood, Ernst Benda proposed that an affliction of human dignity occurs when

> the human being's natural moulding is fundamentally violated. The mother–child relationship is the most natural conceivable relationship between two human beings. It is inhuman to hinder or divide this relationship through technological manipulation.
>
> (Benda 1985, p. 147)

Yet what does this character, with which Nature has endowed the human being, actually consist of? If the term 'human nature' is to have more than a declamatory function, if it is to provide effective moral orientation as a key GenEthical term, then light must be shed on its scope and its content.

Practical dualism

As we have seen, there is a dualism characterising Western anthropology. On the one hand, the human being is viewed as a natural being; modern philosophy has placed the human being in the midst of Nature, considers it Nature's product and part of her. The empirical sciences have substantiated this theory, as well as adding an important dimension to it: naturalisation does not stop at making the human race theoretically a member of Nature's extensive household, it also renders the human race open to technological manipulation. Technological control over human nature, as we notice today with shock, is proving to be a true consequence of scientific enterprise; it is stage two of the naturalisation of humanity. First of all, science stripped the human being theoretically of its supernatural attributes, comparing it with other natural, organic beings; now it begins to make the human being a 'natural object' in practice, bringing it into line with technologically manipulable objects.

On the other hand, anthropological philosophy – apart from radical movements, such as the materialism in France or the behaviourism in our century – has always believed in the specificity, the particularity of the human race. Not even Darwin's erasure of the principal difference between the human being and the animal cast doubt on the special position held by the *Homo sapiens* at the top of the evolutionary tree. On the contrary, parallel to the process of human naturalisation, a process of human subjectivisation took place, which was no less significant. Creation of the modern human self-consciousness as an autonomous subject is very recent and, with it, the conviction that each human individual possesses its own unique value. Especially in moral and political philosophy, autonomy and subjectivity have become fundamental categories, making their impression and finding their institutional anchor in the concepts of human rights and democracy. Seen this way, the human being does *not* appear as just any 'natural object': moral qualities are also attributed to its *physis*. The rights to personal freedom guaranteed in the German Constitution (Article 2) thus include not only the right to unfold one's personality freely (Para 1), but also the rights to life and to freedom from bodily injury (Para 2); the personality is obviously dependent upon life and the freedom of 'its' body from injury.

With this in mind, the uneasiness felt in connection with gene and reproduction technology may be regarded as expression of a collision between these two basic Modern Age tendencies. On the one hand, technological intervention in human reproduction is represented as a continuation of the naturalisation trend; there are even good reasons to interpret it as modern confirmation of human subjectivity, bestowing a new quality upon the understanding of and control over Nature. On the other hand, this technology takes control over *human* nature, which we have just as many good reasons to believe the natural basis of the personality and subjectivity. Thus the advance of scientific and technological progress into this non-demoralised part of nature represents a moral problem of a particular kind: it supports human subjectivity *and* threatens it. With the control over human nature which gene and reproduction technology has provided, the central dualism existing within the Western image of humanity begins to acquire concrete form. The opposition between human nature and human subjectivity may be seen to exceed the realms of human self-interpretation and become a practical problem.

What is substantialism?

There are two ways in which one can attempt to solve this conflict. One may adhere to subjectivity as the actual fate of the human race, and accept further naturalisation of humanity as an unstoppable destiny. The technologisation of human reproduction then no longer appears as a threat to the very essence of the human being, but as its unfolding. As a *subject*, the human being would not even be endangered by the transition to an autoevolutional alteration of the natural historical human organism, as

Helmuth Plessner emphasised more than half a century ago –
albeit without a thought for gene manipulation and the like:

> If the animal becomes human through the characteristic of being out-
> side of itself, then it is clear that – because no new organisational
> structure is possible through eccentricity – the human being has to
> remain bodily an animal. The physical characteristics of human nature
> thus have a purely empirical value. Being human is not bound to one
> particular *Gestalt* and one could thus . . . be human within various
> *Gestalten* other than the one with which we are familiar.
>
> (Plessner 1981, p. 365)

The second way is to oppose this kind of emphasis upon human
subjectivity and insubstantiality and insist upon a direct connection between human personality and human nature.

This alternative point of view sees human nature not merely as
an empirical fact, but as a morally relevant fact. It may and must –
secularly – be viewed as 'holy', as an area removed from the merely
profane, its boundaries also constituting the boundaries of morally
legitimate human action. If it is correct that human personality, subjectivity, dignity, etc. are not freely existing entities, but characteristics of an organism, then, with technological access to this organism,
these characteristics are also threatened. Anyone prepared to dispose
of human nature is prepared to dispose of not only a whole series of
physiological characteristics of the species *Homo sapiens*, but *human
substance* itself: the unity of body and spirit, of nature and dignity,
of biological substratum and human personality. A GenEthics
claiming to be philosophical expression of the uneasiness surrounding a technologisation of human reproduction, as described above,
must be concerned with protecting, maintaining and securing this
human substance, where substance may be described in religious
terms – for example as 'bearing the image of the Creator'
(Instruction 1987, p. 11) – or in terms of constitutional law:

> A technological alteration of human nature affects the image of the
> human being assumed within constitutional law. Article 1 of the
> German Constitution desires to protect the 'intrinsic value' or 'dig-
> nity' of the human being, in other words, to protect everything which
> forms an essential part of the human being's physical, psychological
> and spiritual existence. This does not refer to casual acts, but to
> processes which affect the very core of the human *being* .
>
> (Benda 1985, p. 130)

Internal differentiations aside, substantialism within GenEthics may be characterised with the help of two assertions. (1) There exists a *human substance* which must be regarded as the epitome of the psycho-physical unity of the human being, and which may be expressed in a more or less sharply defined view of humanity. This view of humanity is the basis for a moral evaluation of gene and reproduction technology. In the light of the growing likelihood that alterations be made deliberately to the human biological constitution, Hans Jonas calls for 'a reflection on what is humanly desirable... and on the image of man' (Jonas 1979, p. 41). (2) As a fundamental element of this substance, *human nature* cannot simply be diminished to a biological fact; it acquires particular significance with a view to GenEthics because it represents the starting point for technological erosion of human substance, and thus of *humanum* itself. For this reason, human nature must be respected as holy.

Non-inviolability

At this point it should be noted that the holiness of human nature is not to be understood in the sense of an inviolability which is absolute and without exception – and the substantialists do not understand it this way. From the very beginning, human beings have attempted to manipulate not only Nature, but also their own nature. In all human cultures of which we are aware, there has been, and still is, a strong desire within the scope of medical practice to hinder unwanted external influences on the human body, or even unwanted processes within it, at the very least to restrict the latter's consequences. In its attempts to heal wounds, fight diseases, reduce pain, etc., the field of medicine amounts to an effort to control human nature. Drastic and far-reaching interventions are not only found within the realms of modern 'apparatus medicine'; operations and amputations alter the physical structure of the human organism, herbal remedies and medicines alter its chemical structure. If the holiness of human nature were to be interpreted as strictly inviolable, then medical control over human nature would have to be rejected as immoral.

The principal holiness of human nature has never been regarded – other than by a few religious sects – as prohibiting the medical treatment of diseases, injuries, etc. On the contrary, it seems appropriate to derive from the holiness of human nature a duty to protect it, care for it and maintain it, leading in turn to the legitimacy of certain kinds of technological intervention and manipulation: namely, those which are aimed at protection, care and maintenance. Control over human nature is therefore usually regarded as legitimate insofar as it is orientated towards medical tasks, and thus the goal of health. A physician is justified in amputating a leg if, in so doing, he is able to save the life of the patient; but the amputation is not justified if there is no such therapeutic goal – not even if the patient, for whatever reason, desires the operation. We thus view the holiness of human nature not as a restricting taboo, but in the sense of a fundamental respect, making it our duty to come up with good reasons to justify each intervention. Generally speaking, the therapeutic goal behind an intervention, such as the healing of a disease, the reduction of pain or even the compensation of a physical defect, is always a good enough reason.

This is also true of interventions in reproduction. We have already seen (in Chapter 2) that human reproduction has been subject to numerous technological interventions with varying purposes from time immemorial. However they might be evaluated morally, there can be no doubt as to the legitimacy of at least some of these interventions. This is especially true of the interventions concerned with the final phase of the reproductive process. Progress in the fields of gynaecology, prenatal surgery and embryology over the past hundred years has led to efficient perinatal medicine: premature babies which never could have survived just a few decades ago can now be saved without incurring permanent damage; in difficult cases, a Caesarean section often permits a safe birth. The consequently reduced number of deaths in infants and mothers indubitably represents a far-reaching technological intervention in human reproduction, yet without giving rise to the uneasiness and criticism confronting more modern reproduction technology. This observation should in no way be taken for granted; it is not all that long ago that medical obstetrics faced severe opposition: reducing the number of deaths in infants and mothers would lead to a watering down of the natural selection process, and thus ultimately to a biological degeneration of civilised humanity.

> The success of medicine and hygiene, together with better living conditions for the masses, in combatting *infant mortality* is another way in which culture is removing one of the selective factors which produced the quality of our race. As a result of better infant care and more digestible baby food, children of a weak disposition who in the past would have perished are now being kept alive.
>
> (Schallmayer 1903, p. 150)

If this kind of argumentation is rejected today, then this is because we do not regard the natural course of human reproduction as an inviolable, holy process, rather considering it our moral duty to alleviate the cruelty of natural selection. The Social Darwinists and eugenicists who insist upon the inviolability of natural selection seem to do so, in our eyes, not as an expression of respect for the holiness of Nature, but out of moral cynicism.

In addition to interventions within the scope of perinatal medicine, surgical measures to counter infertility often escape scepticism, too, and are even welcomed as progress. Even the most severe critics of the latest reproduction technologies now refer to these surgical measures as an acceptable alternative to, for example, *in vitro* fertilisation: instead of 'artificial' procreation in a glass dish, infertile women could be helped by an operation to the Fallopian tubes; should this not prove practicable at the present time, then research must be carried out in order to provide the conditions necessary for it to become practicable. Yet there can be no doubt that a Fallopian tube operation also represents a grave intervention in human nature, nor that the raising of a five-month-old embryo in totally artificial surroundings implies a comprehensive technologisation of vital processes.

Accordingly, a strict reformulation of the holiness principle, forbidding *every* intervention in human nature in general, and every intervention in human reproduction in particular, would have no hope of surviving. A GenEthics adhering to the principal holiness of human nature, yet wishing to maintain a minimum of argumentative consistency, is faced with the following alternatives: either to expand its rejection of technological interventions in human nature to cover the entire field of medical manipulations; or – in order to avoid this obviously inacceptable conclusion – to withdraw its rejection of reproduction technology. The only chance of avoiding this second conclusion is to define more precisely the 'substance' of human reproduction rendering it a specifically human process. From such a definition, criteria could then be derived to help distinguish between morally legitimate interventions in human nature or reproduction – e.g. Fallopian tube operations and obstetrics – and other, morally illegitimate interventions – e.g. artificial insemination or *in vitro* fertilisation. One such definition of the human substance behind the human reproductive process is put forward in an 'Instruction' by the Vatican *Sacred Congregation for the Doctrine of the Faith* on the problems raised by reproduction technology:

> The fundamental values connected with the techniques of artificial human procreation are two: the life of the human being called into existence and the special nature of the transmission of human life in marriage. The moral judgment on such methods of artificial procreation must therefore be formulated in reference to these values.
>
> (Instruction 1987, pp. 9–10)

This definition may be considered representative in that the two points it mentions are actually the ones which play a key rôle in the various approaches of substantialist GenEthics: (1) the moral status of the embryo, and (2) the unity of sexuality and reproduction.

Unity of sexuality and reproduction

Due to the biological fact that mammalian fertilisation and pregnancy take place within the body of the female, human reproduction is possible only as the consequence of a physical union between a male and a female partner. Thus throughout human history to date, the sexual act has been a prerequisite for human reproduction. Artificial insemination made it possible for the first time to separate fertilisation and pregnancy from the sexual act; going further, *in vitro* fertilisation removed the fertilisation process to extracorporeal vessels. Through these technologies, the unity existing for hundreds of thousands of years between sexuality – in terms of the sexual act – and reproduction has, for the first time ever, been destroyed. In the eyes of numerous bioethicists, this means the destruction not only of a factually existing link, but also of a morally relevant unity. One of the first people to make the violation of this morally relevant unity a key argument against reproduction technology was Paul Ramsey, who, in his book *Fabricated Man* (1970) focuses on the question of: 'whether sexual intercourse as an act of love should ever be separated from sexual intercourse as a procreative act'. It has to be asked: 'Ought men and women ever to put entirely asunder what God joined together in the covenant of the generating generations of mankind?' And the answer reads:

> I will state as a premise of the following discussion that an ethics (whether proposed by nominal Christians or not) that *in principle* sunders these two goods – regarding procreation as an aspect of biological nature to be subjected merely to the requirements of *technological* control while saying that the unitive purpose is the free, human, personal end of the matter – pays disrespect to the nature of parenthood.
>
> (p. 33)

For Ramsey – and the majority of Christian sexual ethicists – the unity of sexuality and reproduction is not only a biological fact, but a moral postulate, a norm which may not be violated by modern reproduction technology.

It is not possible here to go into the specifically theological prerequisites and implications of this postulate. Inasmuch as it may claim universal validity as a *moral* postulate, it must also be justifiable independently of theological prerequisites. We can start by excluding *per se* any interpretation based on natural fact with an obliging character. This kind of interpretation would imply the derivation of an 'is' from an 'ought', making it subject to the 'naturalistic fallacy'[1] accusation. Independent of the naturalism

---

[1] The assumption that concluding an 'ought' from an 'is' is a 'fallacy' is not as self-explanatory as the moral philosophical *communis opinio* would have us believe since the writings of David Hume and G. E. Moore. Apart from the fact that Moore has been unable to come up with a satisfactory and precise characterisation of this fallacy (cf. Frankena 1973), the term 'fallacy' suggests that a formal mistake is meant, a violation of logical laws, all of which throws a veil over the metaphysical prerequisites of the problem. Prohibiting the deduction of normative statements from descriptive ones is only plausible within the framework of an ontology which removes all normative contents from reality, which declares 'ought' to be a strictly separate entity from 'is', and which believes the origin of all values to lie in the subject.

problem, which shall be returned to later, this kind of interpretation must be disregarded just on empirical grounds. Firstly, it is a well-known fact that fertilisation in humans – as in all of the advanced mammals – is possible only on certain days of the female cycle; this renders the unity of sexuality and reproduction only partial, destroying the factual basis of the unity postulate: the naturalness argument cannot turn something which is not even universally present in Nature into a binding norm for the human race. We should also remember that the questionable unity of sexuality and reproduction, inasmuch as it exists at all, definitely comes to an end with the female menopause. Secondly, and more importantly, this unity does not exist *per definitionem* for all the couples who are unable to have a child naturally, and who for this reason view artificial insemination or *in vitro* fertilisation as the last chance to fulfil their desire to have children; a unity which obviously does not exist cannot be destroyed by technological intervention.

Instead of presuming a 'naturalistically' given unity of sexuality and reproduction, which *eo ipso* involves a moral obligation, it seems more sensible to interpret the loving union of the sexual act as a realisation of personal care and affection between the partners involved, anticipating their relationship later on to the child thus created. Accordingly, the tender embrace of the couple would be viewed as a symbolic anticipation of the affection which this couple is to show its future child. This – a symbolic anticipation of a moral relationship, and not merely a natural fact – lends the unity of sexuality and reproduction a dimension of normative obligation. This kind of symbolic anticipation also affects artificial procreation in the laboratory, with the essential difference that here the procreation takes place in a totally objectified environment, in line with the criterion of scientific and technological rationality and controlled by an extensive apparatus, anticipating a relationship between parents and child which is just as objectified and depersonalised. There are many reasons to believe that these or similar ideas are behind the criticism of reproduction technology.

> The unity of love and life within marriage is said to represent God's love of the human race. Accordingly, all emergence of new life as part of the love of man and woman counts as a cooperation with God's loving creation. This creation has nothing to do with *a desire to have and possess*, and thus nothing to do with 'a desire to manufacture' chil-

dren. It is far more a case of partners meeting in love, a meeting which is God's medium for creating the life which he then gives and entrusts to human beings. Thus in theological anthropological thinking, the liaison, indeed the *union of love and reproduction*, is an essential, constitutive moment, for it not only enables the unity and integration of spiritual life (in the act of love) and natural life (the sexual act, insemination), but also prevents the emergence of human life from becoming a 'making' of and then a control over life, prevents life from becoming a manufacturable, buyable and controllable possession like anything else.

(Eibach 1983, p. 150)

Leon Kass puts forward similar arguments, refraining, however, from theological references.

Human procreation is human partly because it is not simply an activity of our rational wills. Men and women are embodied as well as desiring and calculating creatures. It is for the gods to create in thought and by fiat ('Let the earth bring forth . . .'). And some future race of demigods (or demi-men) may obtain its successors from the local fertilization and decanting station. But *human* procreation is begetting. It is a more complete human activity precisely because it engages us bodily and spiritually as well as rationally. Is there possibly some wisdom in that mystery of nature which joins the pleasure of sex, the communication of love, and the desire for children in the very activity by which we continue the chain of human existence? Is biological parenthood a built-in 'device' selected to promote adequate caring for posterity? Before we embark on 'New Beginnings in Life' we should consider the meaning of the union between sex, love and procreation and the meaning and consequences of its cleavage.

(Kass 1972, pp. 53–4)

This symbolic interpretation has the advantage over the naturalistic interpretation of not merely being dependent upon a continual, factual existence of the unity, but of also having clear, moral content: it refers to the character and the 'quality' of human relationships. This signifies a change of direction within substantialist argumentation: a turn away from human nature as an obliging fact, towards human interests and needs. The symbolic interpretation of the unity postulate implicitly recognises that the decisive point of consideration cannot be the natural fact of internal fertilisation, but only the consequences for the living conditions of future offspring of replacing it technologically.

Four problems

However, this symbolic interpretation is not without its share of difficulties.

1. First of all, there is no reason at all to assume that the sexual relationship between the parents provides if not a guarantee, then at least a better basis for a loving relationship to their child. Historical family research has shown that the parent–child relationship is influenced by a great many social factors beyond the realms of the personal relationship between the parents. We also know that 'natural' parenthood does no more to prevent the frighteningly abundant cases of child abuse than 'artificial' parenthood – e.g. by adoption – does to hinder the establishment of a loving relationship. There is no empirical evidence to support the concern that conscious family planning could be expression of a reified relationship to human life or that it could lead to an objectification of the parent–child relationship. Often enough in the course of history, as well as nowadays, the opposite has proved to be the case: the unwanted, unplanned child is subject to the danger of being merely acknowledged, maybe even rejected, and of growing up in an environment devoid of love and affection. Judging by our experience throughout history, it is barely comprehensible how, of all things, the spontaneity and lack of planning behind procreation can be made into a moral value (cf. Eibach 1983, p. 146; Löw 1983, p. 39), as if the coincidence of their creation and the thoughtlessness of their parents could provide children with optimum chances for the future. Just as unjustified is the fear that the technological and rational character of laboratory procreation could affect the character of the parent–child relationship and lead the parents to a similarly technological, rationalised attitude towards the child. 'Acquiring' a child like a consumer article is much easier within the framework of unified sexuality and reproduction than beyond it; the procedures involved in 'artificial' procreation are so unedifying and burdensome that there is less reason here than anywhere to expect thoughtlessness and mere consumer behaviour. Rather than the fear that 'test-tube babies' may be emotionally at a disadvantage compared with other children, the exact opposite would seem more plausible: namely, that

children who are created 'as an unintentional side-effect' (Eibach 1983, p. 146) of their parents' sexual intercourse are more likely to be threatened with being unwanted and unloved than other children.

2. Talk of destroying the unity of sexuality and reproduction often seems to suggest that the aim behind introducing these technologies may be a *general replacement* of the normal process of procreation with artificial procedures. The tendency of reproduction technology towards 'unlimited application' is deplored by many: test-tube fertilisation could easily become an all-round cure, even the norm for human reproduction, totally separate from human sexuality. These visions are put forward by Utopian technocrats, prognosticating as the norm a complete division of reproduction and sexual intercourse:

> The quip heard in corner bars is quite soundly based: We first found out how to have sex without having babies, and now we are finding out how to have babies without having sex. No longer is human reproduction centered in the genitalia or even dependent on them. Even the gonads, testicles and ovaries are no longer necessary. In fact, we have bypassed in theory even the 'gametes' or germ cells (eggs and sperm) supplied by the gonads, since theoretically they can be artificially synthesized – that is, constructed chemically without the biological process of forming them.
>
> (Fletcher 1974, p. 10)

Yet these essentially compulsive notions of totally replacing the natural with the artificial are unrealistic. Just the high costs connected with such a replacement are a valid counter-argument, not to mention the fact that nobody can be seriously interested in such a replacement. Why should the majority of human beings subject themselves to a highly unpleasant procedure – after all, *in vitro* fertilisation does involve surgery – when the same goal may be attained not only more comfortably, but also involving more fun? Techniques such as artificial insemination and *in vitro* fertilisation only 'make sense' as therapeutic measures for the correction of infertility – and, in this function, they do *not* imply a destruction of the unity of sexuality and reproduction because, in cases of infertility, this unity does not exist.

3. It has already been hinted at that infertile couples are principally hindered in making their sexual relationship a symbolic

anticipation of their common affection for the desired child. They are not faced with choosing between the natural way and an artificial one, but between not having a child at all and creating one artificially. We may be forced to presume that a strong desire to have children is, in many cases, the result of a psychologically problematic motivational structure (Petersen 1985, pp. 52–3), and that fulfilling this desire, for example through *in vitro* fertilisation, does not always solve the actual problems in the lives of the couples in question. This gives rise to serious problems regarding the indication for such an intervention, yet a total rejection of such interventions would imply making decisions for those affected by unwanted childlessness, which would be neither morally justifiable nor politically feasible. Of course, it is also possible to recommend to unwantingly childless couples that they

> find in it an opportunity for sharing in a particular way in the Lord's Cross, the source of spiritual fruitfulness.
>
> (Instruction 1987, p. 34);

yet this kind of recommendation can hardly become a generally accepted moral rule.

4. This ultimately raises the matter of how relevant human needs and desires are to GenEthical considerations. If we have spent thousands of years trying, more or less successfully, to separate sexuality from reproduction with contraceptive means, then this must be regarded as indication that the unity of sexuality and reproduction is *not* in the interests of the human race. Yet if it is legitimate to separate sexuality from reproduction, why should it be reprehensible *in principle* to separate reproduction from sexuality? Individual Catholic theologians have developed a sophisticated line of argumentation regarding this point, based on the assumption that, because of the spontaneity of the fertilisation process, the partners involved in the sexual act do not have the opportunity

> to use fertilisation itself as expression of their personal inclination. This process is structured according to its own objective laws which have no direct effects on the personal dimension. They are objective, and are thus principally separable from those involved. They are not directly personal *per se*.
>
> (Fraling 1984, p. 67)

Just as today there are no objections to certain other biological processes being controlled with the help of technology, fertilisation is also a morally neutral process.

> The body has a concrete materialness which may simply be treated according to material laws, and this is why I believe that couples are not necessarily affronted in their personal dignity when this natural course of events is hindered by obstacles and – assuming that both partners are in favour – manipulations are carried out in order to remove these obstacles.
>
> (ibid., pp. 67–8)

The postulate of unified reproduction and sexuality proves to be all the more problematic when the needs of the partners in question are no longer viewed merely as sources of illegitimate requirements and intentions, but are taken seriously in moral terms.

> Nature is familiar with periods of infertility. What is wrong with the human being adopting such natural behaviour, especially considering that marriage no longer stands solely, or even essentially, for the creation of new life, but for the manifestation of wedded love and faithfulness? In other cases, and for similar reasons, it can sometimes be very reasonable, and thus morally justifiable, to intervene in Nature. This line of argumentation was used years ago to question the close connection between the act of love and reproduction. New developments within theological ethics, as well as the modern, integral perception of marriage, no longer tend to reject interventions in Nature on principle – in this case a separation of the act of love from reproduction –, but instead weigh up the pros and cons involved. This is true of contraception, of sterilisation, of homologous artificial insemination and of extracorporeal fertilisation.
>
> (Gründel 1983, p. 257)

The embryo as a person

The debate on the moral status of the embryo refers to whether the fertilised human egg cell (zygote) is to be regarded as a human *person*, with all the rights consequently due to it – especially the rights to life and freedom from injury. Individual authors have exaggerated the question to the point of implying its counterpart: is the fertilised egg cell to be counted as part of the human species, and does its life therefore deserve full protection, as guaranteed by the German Constitutional Court, ('from the *point* of fertilisation onwards'), or is this formation nothing more than a highly complex conglomerate of organic compound within an organic environment?

(Löw 1983, p. 40)

From a substantialist point of view, everything else depends upon the answer to this question. Whereas the latter alternative would lead to an abolition of ethics, the former justifies the 'categorical foundations' necessarily underlying a genuine GenEthics:

Sound ethical argumentation can only be successful if it is based on the premise that every member of the genus human being respects every other human being as having the same rights and an equal dignity.

(ibid., p. 42)

Each intervention in human reproduction then becomes an intervention in the autonomy and dignity of the embryo; it violates the

right of each human being to originate naturally, allowing it to stand up to everyone else as a being with the same rights, and not as a being originating from the mercy of sperm donors and genetic engineers.

(ibid., p. 43)

It is essentially to be regarded or evaluated as the manipulation of a person.

The strength of these 'categorical foundations' lies in their ability to give human actions a clear orientation and to set them definite limits. If the direct result of fertilisation is a human being, then the same standards must be set for interventions in reproduction as for any other technological manipulation or therapeutic procedure. This could be the safety of such manipulations and procedures. The development of any form of reproduction technology requires that numerous individual stages and ultimately the entire procedure be tested; this cannot be covered by animal experiments alone: human beings must be tested too. If the embryo is a complete human person, then these tests have to be disqualified as immoral human experiments; for it must be assumed that numerous embryos are needed for such experiments. In short, technological intervention in human reproduction is immoral just because the know-how needed in order to carry it out can only be attained immorally, through experiments on or with human beings (embryos). Paul Ramsey (1970, pp. 113, 134) was quick in making this consideration a key argument against the entire field of reproduction technology:

> Let us imagine that there can be developed an artificial placenta as good for the child as the womb – or better, because it abolishes the limits imposed by the human pelvis upon brain development, and makes the child accessible to 'the management's' improvement. Even so, such a technological development skips over the crucial ethical question. Prescinding from the 'good' ends in view, the decisive moral verdict must be that we cannot rightfully *get to know* how to do this without conducting unethical experiments upon the unborn who must be the 'mishaps' (the dead and retarded ones) through whom we learn how.

It is obvious that the weight of this argumentation depends on its premise. As the following statement by a human geneticist demonstrates, it should by no means be taken for granted that a fertilised egg cell has to be respected as a human person:

> I am amazed at all this talk of embryos. Literally, embryo means in moss, i.e. in *villi*. Yet at the point in time at stake there are no *villi* present. At this point in time, I can see no difference between what is under the microscope and the egg cell of any other mammal. This seems to me to be important when considering what constitutes a human being. More than 40% of all fertilised egg cells fail to survive. This means that if we create a child at all, we have a 40% chance of creating a doomed embryo. I do not really understand why it is considered so important to speak of a person at this stage, since it is not even possible to differentiate in the slightest between these cells and those which are later to become the central nervous system, for example.
>
> (Lenz 1984, pp. 69–70)

Löw uses his 'categorical foundations' against this type of naturalistic argumentation. Whether we are able to distinguish a human egg cell from another mammalian embryo under a microscope is totally irrelevant:

> The decision to view a fertilised human egg cell as a human life which has to be protected finds its orientation in the only indubitable criterion as to whether a human being is a human being or not: its biological membership of the species *Homo sapiens*. Were this not to be the case, a newborn child would have less right to protection than a fully grown Alsatian. In reaching this decision, the human being recognises

the cell as a teleologically constituted germ, from which an equally free person *should* emerge, if all goes well.

(Löw 1983, pp. 41–2)

Against naturalism

If we take a closer look at the theory of the 'teleologically constituted germ', the question arises of how this teleological constitution can be made compatible with the fact that numerous embryos die spontaneously, as mentioned by Lenz. A number of years ago, we discovered that actually about two-thirds of all fertilised egg cells die without any human intervention. Most of them die before nidation, i.e. within the first seven to nine days; most of the rest die before the tenth week pending fertilisation (Biggers 1983, pp. 46–7; Soupart 1983, pp. 79–80). With this in mind, talk of the fertilised egg cell as a 'teleologically constituted germ' loses its plausibility. If two-thirds die from natural causes, then Löw's afterthought, with its restrictive 'if all goes well', appears to refer to the norm; it seems to be death which is teleological in this process, and not the emergence of an 'equally free person'. Karl Rahner used this point to question the coincidence of fertilisation and the becoming of a human being:

> For several centuries Catholic moral theologians have been convinced that individual *human* life begins at the moment when the two germ cells unite. Will the moral theologian still have the courage to uphold this prerequisite for so many of his moral and theological beliefs if he is suddenly confronted with the fact that 50% of fertilised female egg cells never get as far as lodging in the womb? Will he be able to believe that 50% of all 'human beings' – true human beings with an 'immortal' soul and an eternal destiny – never get beyond this first stage of human existence?
>
> (Rahner 1967b, p. 287)

We could go a step further: if such a high percentage of human embryos dies without human interference anyway, why should technological interventions in reproduction – whether for therapeutic or experimental purposes – also leading to the death of embryos be deemed immoral? Yet this question obviously implies the derivation of an 'is' from an 'ought', already mentioned as constituting a 'naturalistic fallacy'. The problems which this derivation involves become clear if we examine the remark often made by the advocates of gene and reproduction technological manipulations, namely that Nature does just the same: if genes are exchanged spontaneously between different species by Nature, then it cannot be immoral for us to mingle human with bacterial genes; if Nature creates identical twins, then it cannot be immoral for us to split embryos and create several human individuals from one zygote, etc. Löw (1983, p. 39) inveighs against this type of naturalistic argumentation with an impressive comparison:

> Two pedestrians are hit by roof tiles, both fatally. In one case, the tile was dislodged by Nature – a storm, for example, – in the other, a man deliberately let it come crashing down. In Court, the man on the roof tells the judge his action was justified because Nature did just the same. This illustrates why arguing that 'Nature does just the same' destroys our concept of justification. Nature does not have to be justified, but human actions do, and precisely because they are *not* natural events. To put it bluntly: anyone who manipulates genes is *not* doing the same as Nature. Just the fact that he or she is *doing* something makes it different. The effect may be the same, as with the roof tiles; seen in the light of our concept of justication, however, there is a categorical distinction to be made between these two cases: the first is an event, the second an action.

It is fairly obvious that this line of argumentation does not only apply to the attempt to legitimise technological interventions in human reproduction with a reference to Nature, but that it also applies to the attempt to illegitimise such interventions with a reference to Nature. Just as a human action may not be justified using the fact that its result also occurs 'naturally', so an action may not be criticised with the argument that it or its result be 'unnatural', a contradiction of human nature. If an 'ought' cannot be derived from an 'is', then, with regard to the moral status of embryos, facts cannot justify norms either. The biological *fact* of belonging to the species is not sufficient cause to justify *moral* rights. According to the views of several moral philosophers, drawing a conclusion about the moral status of a being from its affiliation to the species *Homo sapiens* implies a naturalism related to racism – in its argumentative structure, and not its political or moral content: in the same way as the racist derives moral rights from the empirical fact of race membership, the 'speciesist' derives moral rights from the empirical fact of species membership. This ignores the fact, however, that moral rights can only stem from morally relevant characteristics, such as conscience, autonomy, rationality, endurance, etc., and not from natural characteristics such as membership of a race or species. With this in mind, it seems inconsistent to ascribe a *special* moral status to the human foetus:

> I have argued that the life of a fetus is of no greater value than the life of a non-human animal at a similar level of rationality, self-consciousness, awareness, capacity to feel, etc., and that since no fetus is a person no fetus has the same claim to life as a person.
>
> (Singer 1979, p. 122)

This line of argumentation does raise its own problems: the ability to feel and the ability to suffer, which play a key rôle here, are also empirical characteristics, and yet regarded as morally relevant. It is nevertheless acceptable insofar as biological facts *eo ipso* do not imply any moral rights; thus, in order for such rights to be acknowledged, facts are at least *insufficient*.

In the light of this difficulty, the substantialist has two differing, but not mutually exclusive, strategies. The aim of the first is to find at least one embryonic characteristic which is morally directly relevant. Since rationality, autonomy or endurance cannot apply to embryos, *individuality* is focused upon. In contrast to asexual reproduction, the biological 'purpose' behind sexual reproduction is the creation of genetic and, ultimately, phenotypical variety; when the parents' sex cells come together, there emerges not merely a new human life, but a genetically unique individual, not identical with its parents, nor with any other human being (apart from the special case of identical twins). The question is whether personal individuality may be directly deduced from genetic uniqueness. This conclusion is drawn in the document of the Sacred Congregation for the Doctrine of the Faith already cited; quoting its own previous explanation of the abortion problem, it states:

> From the time that the ovum is fertilised, a new life is begun which is neither that of the father nor of the mother; it is rather the life of a new human being with its own growth. It would never be made

human if it were not human already. To this perpetual evidence . . .
modern genetic science brings valuable confirmation. It has demonstrated that, from the first instant, the programme is fixed as to what
this living being will be: a man, this individual-man with his characteristic aspects already well-determined. Right from fertilisation is
begun the adventure of human life, and each of its great capacities
requires time . . . to find its place and to be in a position to act.

(Instruction 1987, p. 13)

If genetic uniqueness coincides with personal identity, then not
only is every abortion a murder, but also every manipulation of a
zygote manipulation of a person. This is why Löw rejects every
form of germ-line manipulation, including those with an exclusively therapeutic goal:

it is not an existing human being which is being healed, but the identity of a human being which is being manipulated.

(Löw 1983, p. 45)

Although Löw does not claim that genetic individuality coincides
with personal identity, the *moral* connection between the two is
rendered so close that every embryonic manipulation must be
rejected as illegitimate. This argument is especially common
against cloning: by creating a human being asexually, its genetic
individuality is denied, and with it the chance to develop a
personal identity.

Our children begin with a unique genetic independence of us, analogous to the personal independence that sooner or later will have to be
granted them or wrested from us.

(Ramsey 1970, p. 72)

The creation of genetic copies, with pre-determined genetic dispositions, would dramatically increase the difficulty of establishing
one's own identity, and is therefore immoral.

According to findings in the field of modern genetics, however,
the relationships between biological uniqueness and personal individuality are much more complex and far less obvious than suggested here. There can be no doubt that fertilisation results in a
genetically unique being; yet even if we are not yet sure about the
connections between the genetic constitution and the personality of
a human being, we do know that personal identity is not simply
established at the moment of fertilisation, instead forming gradually

in a lifelong process of interaction with the environment. An organism is on no account the mere realisation of a particular genotype; even during embryogenesis, numerous epigenetic and environmental determinants become part of the somatic expression of genetic information, so that the identity of the genetic constitution cannot even pass as guarantee for the identity of the somatic structure of an organism (Eisenberg 1976). The same rules which apply to organic characteristics obviously apply even more to the development of personality. Probably the best example of this is identical twins, which, for all their similarity, are neither somatically nor even physically identical. The fact that they have a common genotype obviously does not prevent them from developing their own individual identities – despite the added factor of usually growing up in very similar environments. Not even a clone can be biologically denied the chance of developing its own personal identity; its genetic constitution does not predestine it to the limited status of a 'copy'.

The fundamental difficulties surrounding even this attempt to trace the personal dignity of the embryo back to its genetic uniqueness lead us smoothly to the *second* argumentational strategy mentioned above. At least the reflecting philosophers amongst the substantialists do not maintain that membership of the species or genetic uniqueness could *per se* be the foundation of an embryo's personality. Far more, Löw states

> that here a *decision* is at stake. The living human being is free to see it this way or that. It is therefore an action subject to ethical categories, in other words, a matter of practice and not just of theory. In both cases, we have to consider the consequences very carefully.
>
> (Löw 1983, p. 40)

Löw thus evades the naturalism accusation which he himself makes against some of its advocates, yet he tangles himself in other justification difficulties. (1) If recognising the embryo as a person has to do with the result of a decision, then we have to ask ourselves whether this means a *pure* decision or a *justified* decision. It is obviously the latter which is meant, for we are challenged to think carefully about the consequences of the alternatives. This leads, however, to the doubly strange circumstance that Löw justifies the 'categorical foundations' of his GenEthics with consequentialist arguments. This is strange because, firstly, foundations are not usually capable of, nor do they require justification; secondly, 'categorical' – i.e. unconditioned – foundations are justified in a consequentialist procedure, in other words one dependent upon conditions. (2) If we take a closer look at this consequentialist justification, we find the following explication: if biological membership of the species *Homo sapiens* were not acknowledged as being a criterion for personality, then 'a newborn child would have less right to protection than a fully grown Alsatian'. Yet we want to know *why* an embryo or a newborn child should receive more protection than an animal. Instead of receiving justification for this unequal treatment, we are told what we already knew: if we deny the embryo the status of a person, it is no worthier of protection than any other mammal. Thus even if we accept the notion of justifying 'categorical foundations' with consequentialist arguments, this justification proves to be circular.

Motives and reasons

An important *motive* behind the substantialist search for a basis of the moral norms within human nature is addressed by Helmuth Plessner in his inaugural lecture in Groningen in 1936:

> With the decay of a heavenly authority which until the denominational conflicts was respected by humanity throughout Europe, with the emergence of the nations as independent, worldly States, and with the secularisation of science, one instance after another – instances which considered the human being and none other than the human being to be God's creation and image, and to which the human being could only appeal as a human being, i.e. according to the generic character *to which it was obliged* – has become questionable. Because it has become possible since the Enlightenment to question the existence of God, the truth of reason, the binding force of humanity, every supernatural, spiritual, moral basis which guaranteed uniformity for all things bearing a human face has been discontinued. Apart from the natural basis, all the elements from which and as what the human being, with respect to its generic character, has to understand itself have been undermined.
>
> (Plessner 1983a, pp. 41–2)

Where are the norms to come from, one could also ask with regard to a GenEthics, what is to be their foundation, if not such a 'natural basis'? Have we not experienced the gradual undermining and colonisation of our traditional social values by scientific and technological progress? – It is obviously the need for a moral orientation with stable foundations which makes human nature so attractive to a substantialist GenEthics. And yet this hope is doubtful. In Chapter 6 we witnessed the difficulties encountered by attempts to define human nature precisely and unambiguously. This 'natural basis' is obviously not capable of serving as the foundation for a moral orientation either, as Plessner emphasises directly after the passage already cited:

> Yet the natural basis only demonstrates what is human about the human being in an abstraction of the average type, whom we can artificially construct from all the different racial variations, if we wish to. Who or what, however, should induce us to do so, if not either faith in the human being as God's creation and God's image, or at least faith that reason, and with it a higher ranking amongst all real things, is only given to the human race, faith in the dignity of a spiritual and reasonable existence committed to the character of the human genus? If this faith no longer exists, then scientific interest in cleanly dividing the species *homo* from other anthropoids is merely problematic. The natural basis of existence, which ultimately remained in the course of a global history of suspicion towards every form of authority, does not have a committing character *per se*.
>
> (ibid., p. 42)[2]

---

[2] In this context it should be remembered that Plessner's anthropology also had a political and moral tendency. At the end of his lecture – the year is 1936 – he says: 'Kant wanted to limit knowledge in order to make room for faith. He wanted to put a stop to the theoretical presumptuousness of being able to prove something with respect to freedom, immortality and the existence of God, because he feared that, in the face of human weakness, this kind of metaphysics could have devastating consequences for basic moral convictions. Today we are also dealing with the necessity of rejecting theoretical presumptuousness. Yet this is not directed towards metaphysics, but towards the human race, and how it is putting its own head on the block with its immensely increased powers of control due to progress in science and technology. This is why we have to put a stop to the increasingly inconsiderate presumptuousness of politicians, economists and doctors in matters of sterilisation, eugenics, racial politics, human breeding, or the human ability to play with Fate. Human ability has rendered the human being a threat to its own future, since its ability can only be overcome by more ability and there is no guarantee that the human race will not fall behind in the process. This reveals the true philosophical purpose behind philosophical anthropology, namely to limit human ability by infinitely restricting human knowledge, thereby restricting its unfathomableness and uncertainty with regard to the future, thus coming closer to faith in mankind' (Plessner 1983a, pp. 50–1).

Yet this undermining of committedness is not, as Plessner's reference to the 'global history of suspicion towards every form of authority' seems to imply, merely a non–committing development due to the factual course of history. It is a *principal* undermining of committedness. The search for a moral orientation within human nature encounters two fundamental difficulties.

1. The first difficulty stems from the impossibility of making a clear distinction between the 'natural' and the 'artificial' about or in the human being. Even for non–human objects we have no universal and unambiguous criterion, as Jacques Monod has demonstrated (1972, p. 15), for distinguishing whether an object is natural or artificial; only knowledge about its origins makes such a decision possible. The borderline between the natural and the artificial is thus not determinable ontologically; in many cases, we can only *grade* objects according to their level of naturalness or artificiality, measured by the anthropogenic alterations which the object has undergone. This has the direct consequence that we cannot expect absolute naturalness from the human being itself, its characteristics and manners of behaviour. For which human characteristic or manner of behaviour has not in some way been affected, modified or transformed anthropogenically? Every search for a human nature which is, let's say, pure and natural, is thus doomed to fail. The human being is, as Plessner puts it, artificial by Nature.

2. Even if we managed to find a definite, natural, human feature, we would not be much further on. There can be no doubt that the necessity of internal fertilisation is one such feature; yet what gives us the right to sell this feature which is characteristic of all mammals as part of *human* nature? The fact that *Homo sapiens* has reproduced on the basis of internal fertilisation throughout its entire history to date can hardly justify regarding this process as a moral norm. The substantialist is constantly in danger of stylising and dogmatising the human traits familiar to us from history and our own experience as indisputable, essential human characteristics.

Concrete morality has often involved talk of a factual, but not at all essential, as yet stable human state, drawn into the altering situation of the self-guiding human being, for example: this or that is against a woman's 'nature', against the essence of the family, against the natural function of a biological organ, etc., whereas what is really at stake is a changeable, only relatively fixed parameter within a constant being.

(Rahner 1967a, p. 274)

We obviously need a *criterion* to help us decide which factually ascertainable characteristics of one or all human beings are part of human nature – and must thus remain untouchable, and which characteristics are contingent – and may thus legitimately be manipulated. The problem of where to draw the line is not limited to the ideological danger, which should not be forgotten, that the established grade of human 'artificiality' at any one time in history could be declared as human nature. Philosophically important is something else, namely that every attempt to anchor the basis of justification for the morality of action in Nature itself tends – as formulated by Kant –

inevitably to move in a circle and cannot avoid tacitly presupposing the morality which it ought to explain.

(Kant 1949, p. 99)

Human nature must also be regarded and interpreted normatively, in order to identify the norms which at some stage have been interpreted into it. This circle can be broken only by the naming of a *criterion* or of *reasons*, independent of natural facts, for the selection of particular features of the human biological constitution to a normatively binding 'human substance'.

There are three types of reason put forward by the substantial-ists, starting with the *theological*, for example when Ramsey asks rhetorically whether men and women may ever put asunder what God has joined in the bond of procreative human generations. Secondly, *decisionistic* reasons, for example when Löw declares the acknowledgement of the embryo as a person to be the result of a decision. Since the first group cannot claim to be universally valid, and the second group cannot really, at least on its own, pass as 'reasons', we are left – thirdly – with the *consequentialist* reasons. Löw's argument in favour of the embryo's personality – 'otherwise a newborn child would have less right to protection than a fully grown Alsatian' – points to one of the key motives behind the sub-stantialist approach, and for this reason deserves to be examined a little more closely. It has to do with the fear that only 'categorical foundations', a deontological principle, an unshakeable human nature, could guarantee that everything human and of value will not be undermined during the further developmental course of gene and reproduction technology. Here the chance to relativise our view of humanity, there a piece of *humanum* made accessible to technology – and ultimately there will be nothing left of what used to be connected with the concept of the 'human being'.

> If scientific research managed to put an end to continual striving towards the ideal human being, which is always accompanied by the risks of failure however good the intentions behind gene surgery might be, then we would have before us a totally different creature, which would only be physically similar to the human being we are familiar with. This creature would no longer be the human being assumed by the German Constitution, since it would lose not only the necessity of having to take responsibility for defining its own life itself, but also the ability to do so.
>
> (Benda 1985, p. 158)

This is the *slippery slope* argument, which states the fear that, by giving way just a little, we could arrive at a stage of moral crookedness, ending in the legitimisation of total technological control.

It is not possible here to examine the scope of this argument. An estimation of the extent to which our society is susceptible to such undermining tendencies would be more empirical than ethical, and working to *prevent* the feared decline is more a political than a philosophical problem. What is important is that this argument – as well as the link to consequentialist ethics at all – once again relativises the relevance of referring to human *nature*. With the slippery slope argument in mind, it is no longer human nature which is the asset to be cherished; human nature tends rather to receive the rôle of its own – whatever this may be – protective barrier. It is no longer the holiness inherent within human nature which justifies respect, but stipulations of strategic prudence.

8

Metaphysics with ecological intent

Each century has its own fundamental problem,
to which it dedicates its entire strength . . .
The originality and interests of our Century
find their full expression in the problem of Nature.
Serge Moscovici

Just as the threat of gene and reproduction technology has sparked off philosophical reflection about *human* nature, with the danger of a world-wide, irreversible, ecological crisis Nature itself has become the subject of philosophical debate.

> Until a few years ago, Nature seemed to be no longer of interest to philosophers. Everything there was to research in a material sense about Nature had become the domain of the increasingly differing natural sciences. Everything there was to know in a formal sense, i.e. concerning the concept of Nature, seemed to be reduced to an analysis of scientific knowledge. A philosophy of Nature which promised to offer more than just a meta-scientific analysis revealed itself *eo ipso* as the echo of an antiquated, systematic way of thinking.
>
> (Schäfer 1986, p. 4)

Today the situation is totally different; a growing number of publications is concerned with the fundamental philosophical problems regarding the relationship between Nature and humanity, especially the pathology of this relationship. Based on the conviction that the ecological crisis is neither a coincidence, nor to be traced back to political and social causes alone, the necessity of philosophically *diagnosing* its spiritual causes – and of developing a therapy to heal our sick relationship to Nature – is emphasised. There are similarities, both in practical appreciation of the problem and in theoretical content, between the *ecological ethics* project conceived within this context and the GenEthics project: both projects deal with preserving Nature from technological destruction, as well as the moral norms which are to guarantee this preservation.

Against anthropocentrism

This kind of ecological ethics is based on the presupposition that with the mediation of highly advanced technology the scope of human action has attained a dimension previously unknown. Whereas the range of effect of human actions used to be restricted to individual areas of Nature, today it includes the entire terrestrial biosphere, thus boasting a totally new magnitude. According to Jonas, the consequences of this expansion of human power extend beyond the theory of action to the realm of ethics: with the irreversibility and cumulativity of the effect, not only has the structure and quantitative scope of human action changed, but also – and especially – its ethical scope. Assuming 'that the nature of human action has *de facto* changed' (Jonas 1984, p. 7), we are confronted with a responsibility so large that we can hardly measure it.

> It is at least not senseless any more to ask whether the condition of extrahuman nature, the biosphere as a whole and in its parts, now subject to our power, has become a human trust and has something of a moral claim on us not only for our ulterior sake but for its own and in its own right. If this were the case it would require quite some rethinking in basic principles of ethics. It would mean to seek not only the human good but also the good of things extrahuman, that is, to extend the recognition of 'ends in themselves' beyond the sphere of man and make the human good include the care for them.
>
> (Jonas 1984, p. 8)

The quantitative extension of our practical options leads to a – carefully formulated for now – qualitatively new philosophical

human. Both are highly problematic sources of validity: the divine, because the existence of its source is contested, while its authority is hypothetically granted; the human, because authority is lacking, while existence is the given fact.

(Jonas 1984, p. 130)

Jonas believes *metaphysics* to be the only possible foundation for the ethics both necessary and sought after. Contrary to faith, which cannot simply be summoned, metaphysics has always been

a business of reason, and reason can be set to work upon demand. To be sure, here too, a tenable metaphysics can no more be conjured by a bitter need for it than can religion, but the need for it at least can move us to search after it; and for the search to be unprejudiced, the worldly philosopher struggling for an ethics must first of all hypothetically allow the *possibility* of a rational metaphysics, despite Kant's contrary verdict, if the rational is not preemptively determined by the standards of positive science.

(ibid., p. 45)

Thus what is needed is a metaphysical foundation for ecological ethics: a metaphysic with ecological intent.

Since Jonas assumes that

all proofs of validity for moral prescriptions are ultimately reduced to obtaining evidence of an 'ontological' ought

(ibid., p. 130)

he sees it as his task to construct a metaphysic which can overcome the *scandalon* throughout the field of modern ethics: the gulf between 'is' and 'ought'. His aim is to make plausible the futility of this gulf, by proving the existence of purposes within Nature. He attempts to achieve his aim with two lines of argumentation. First of all, the fact that human individuals define their purposes *subjectively* is taken as an indication of the existence of purposes throughout Nature. Since, firstly, subjectivity has emerged from organic and inorganic Nature as a product of evolution and, secondly, evolution is a gradual, developmental process, not party to sudden leaps or the surprising emergence of new characteristics, then, thirdly, subjective definitions of purpose must have their roots in pre-subjective Nature: purposes must be prevalent throughout the *whole* of Nature.

As subjectivity is in some sense a surface phenomenon of nature – the visible tip of a much larger iceberg – it speaks for the silent interior beneath. Or: The fruit betrays something of the root and the stem out of which it grew. Because subjectivity displays efficacious purpose, indeed wholly lives in it, we must concede to the silent interior which finds language only through it, that is, to matter, that it harbours purpose or its analogue within itself in nonsubjective form.

(ibid., p. 71)

Alongside this line of argumentation, which cannot be gone into in more detail here, Jonas makes a second attempt to bridge the gap between 'is' and 'ought', based on the prerequisite that a single example able to prove the coincidence of 'is' and 'ought' would refute the dogma regarding the moral neutrality of reality. Jonas has no difficulty producing an example '*ontic* paradigm':

For when asked for a single instance (one is enough to break the onto-logical dogma) where that coincidence of 'is' and 'ought' occurs, we we can point at the most familiar sight: the newborn, whose mere breathing uncontradictably addresses an ought to the world around, namely, to take care of him.

(ibid., p. 131)

Jonas emphasises strongly that this unpronounceable 'ought' is not a psychological fact – such as *feeling* sympathy for a helpless being – or a natural drive, in the sense of genetically programmed care of the brood, but a *metaphysical* fact:

I mean strictly just this: that here the plain being of a *de facto* existent imminently and evidently contains an ought for others, and would do so even if nature would not succour this ought with powerful instincts or assume its job alone.

(ibid.)

The aim of this argumentation is obvious: bridging the gulf between 'is' and 'ought' would clear the way for an ontological anchoring of moral values and norms, as was the case in former times with the teleological world view. It is therefore a case of rehabilitating teleology.

Jonas is not alone in his efforts. There have been various approaches towards a revision of modern metaphysics, and especially towards viewing Nature as an entirety of equally ranked circumstances and processes, none of which is inherently 'superior' to the others. Any evaluation of natural phenomena aimed at more than just establishing the probability of their occurrence can thus only originate from the subject: natural phenomena do not have a moral quality *per se*. Efforts to reintroduce teleological thinking are nothing other than attempts to *remoralise* Nature. Certain circumstances and processes are to be assigned inherent moral qualities, justifiying rights and claims towards acting human beings. Behind these efforts is the conviction that the problems facing us today are a consequence of the modern view of the world, according to which the human being no longer sees itself as a member of a purposeful ordering within Nature, but as a subject, confronted with a morally neutral world.

> The ecological crisis stems from the explosive expansion in human control over Nature ideologically embedded in the anti-teleological philosophy prevalent since the early Modern Ages.
>
> (Spaemann & Löw 1981, p. 287)

A universe which is governed by 'blind' natural laws and mere chance does not offer the human being any ontologically predefined, behavioural guidelines, instead burdening it with the construction of such guidelines itself.

The ecological crisis is interpreted as practical proof that the human being cannot cope with this responsibility, that an ethics which is based solely upon a human 'fiat' (Jonas 1984, p. 130) does not possess enough authority to protect Nature from human interests. The fundamental meta-ethical decision therefore consists of choosing between ethics as an *ex nihilo* – creation of mankind for the purpose of human survival – and ethics anchored, at least in some individual points, in Nature itself:

> I suspect that we may be forced to a much older classical medieval notion that there is, indeed, a nature, man is part of that nature, and that nature is teleological in some very fundamental sense.
>
> (Callahan 1975, p. 589)

In this sense, returning to a teleological world view would mean ontological support for the field of ethics. Reality would acquire an inherent meaning, and this would have to become the orientation for human action for the latter to qualify as morally legitimate. A teleologically ordered cosmos relieves humanity of the burden of building up a morality single-handedly; in this context, Nature is no longer to be considered as a mere means, as a neutral object, at the mercy of all and sundry, but must be respected as inherently valuable.

Equilibrium versus evolution

Attempts to relive a teleological understanding of Nature are usually based on two implicit, empirical prerequisites.

1. Global ecological stability is disturbed and endangered by the tremendously increased scope of human action resulting from scientific and technological progress (cf. Jonas 1984, pp. ix, 6–7, 140). However plausible this theory may appear, highly developed technologies are in no way necessary for the disturbance of even larger ecological systems. Relatively primitive technologies and seemingly small interventions in Nature are sufficient to destroy large areas of forest, transform steppes into deserts, bring about far-reaching climatic changes, etc. (Remmert 1980, pp. 191, 253). Of course, the emergence of modern hi-tech has increased the scope of human action and caused Nature to become endangered to an extent previously unknown in human history. Yet at the same time we should not forget that the landscapes in the Middle East, on the Mediterranean and in Northern Germany were destroyed by the human race long before the emergence of modern technology and industry. This is because ecosystems are not nearly as stable or constant as is usually assumed. It *is* true that Nature, as we have been able to observe her, is full of ecosystems, fluctuatingly stable and in a position to absorb disturbances elastically, up to a certain, critical point. Many of these systems have remained stable within human history, not becoming endangered until very recently. Yet it should not be forgotten that this impressive consistency within Nature is relative only to the period of human observation, which is extraordinarily short in natural historical terms.

2. Ecological ethics makes this period of observation absolute, disregarding evolution in its view of Nature. The impression that Nature is constant disappears as soon as we observe periods of time which are large enough to include evolutionary processes. The idea of a universal homoeostasis of Nature is then relativised

by numerous examples of the destruction of such homoeostases by vegetable or animal organisms (Remmert 1980, pp. 243–4). This is true not only of local systems of stability, but also of life in general. During the history of the Earth so far, the palaeontologists are aware of five faunal ages, i.e. large-scale periods of extinction of biological species. It should be assumed, despite the impression that our global ecosystem is naturally stable,

> that, even without human intervention, Nature is in no way stable or self-regenerating. Life is always being threatened and endangered, most of all by itself. The 'consistency' of Nature is largely an illusion, arising from a perspective which is temporally too short. Natural catastrophes mark the various epochs of the history of the Earth. What geologists describe as different ages of the Earth are characterised by the fossilised leftovers of different life forms in successively deposited layers of rock. During the transition from one age to the next, a whole range of previously dominant animal and plant life disappears and is replaced by a host of new life forms.
>
> (Markl 1982, p. 64d)

The extent of this 'natural' destruction of Nature becomes clearer when we consider the fact that more than 99 per cent of all the biological species that have ever lived on the Earth are now extinct. The field of ecological ethics finds its ultimate fodder in a pre-modern view of Nature, in which the concept of Nature is still closely linked to that of unalterability and harmony, and in which there is no systematic place for the concept of evolution.

Referring to the harmony and finely-tuned balance of her different parts, Nature is identified as a global idyll which can only be described using moralising vocabulary.

> Have we the right to counteract, irreversibly, the evolutionary wisdom of millions of years, in order to satisfy the ambition and curiosity of a few scientists?
>
> (Chargaff 1976, p. 940)

This is nothing other than secularised physico-theology: what was previously the wisdom of the Creator has been replaced by evolution. Considering the fact that, periodically, life forms are destroyed *en masse*, talk of an 'evolutionary wisdom' is even less plausible than of God's wisdom before it. Evolution – if one may personify it – is not aware of a planned strategy for achieving particular purposes; all of our empirical knowledge about evolution shows that its method of procedure involves opportunist advancement, under the circumstances given at a particular time, with the chances available at that time.

> There is nothing in human behaviour which corresponds to the process of natural selection. For the sake of a comparison, however, one could say that natural selection goes about its work not like an engineer, but like a D.I.Y. enthusiast, a D.I.Y. enthusiast who does not yet know what he is going to make, nevertheless collecting everything he can find which may at some stage come in handy, such as lengths of thread, pieces of wood, old boxes, etc., in other words, like a D.I.Y. enthusiast who uses what he has around him in order to create a useful object. The engineer does not commence his work until he has all the raw materials and tools exactly suited to his concept. The D.I.Y. enthusiast, on the other hand, can get by with all sorts of rubbish. Most of the objects which he creates are not part of some overall plan. They are the result of a series of coincidences, the result of all the opportunities the D.I.Y. enthusiast has had to increase his stock of junk.
>
> (Jacob 1983, p. 51)

Accordingly, Nature has no respect for the things she creates. She does not care if an organism or an entire species dies, if an entire group of species is extinguished, or even if the complete biosphere of our planet is destroyed; a collapse of this kind would merely signify the starting-point of a new phase of evolutionary development, in which new species emerge and a new biosphere is constructed.

It is not a case of contrasting idyllic emphasis on the harmony and stability within Nature to the opposite image of Nature as cruel and inconsiderate, as was common during the last century, following the modest reception of Darwinism (Bayertz 1990). This is also the line of interpretation taken up by John Stuart Mill when he writes that Nature

> impales men, breaks them as if on the wheel, casts them to be devoured by wild beasts, burns them to death, crushes them with stones like the first Christian martyr, starves them with hunger, freezes them with cold, poisons them by the quick or slow venom of her exhalations, and has hundreds of other hideous deaths in reserve, such as the ingenious cruelty of a Nabis or a Domitian never

surpassed. All this, Nature does with the most supercilious disregard both of mercy and of justice.

(Mill 1969b, p. 385)

It is difficult to contradict this description, since Nature really does do all the things that Mill accuses her of doing. Yet at the same time she gives the human being the gift of life, feeds it with precious fruits, brings it joy with beautiful flowers and magnificent sunsets, and offers it the most charming examples of caring for one's creatures. Nature is just as cruel as she is kind – and is thus neither one nor the other.

The only conclusion which we can draw from this is that Nature can be neither teleological nor a moral example for us. She gives us just as many examples worth following as ones which we should not follow. Yet we ourselves have to decide *which* of her examples are worth following, and which not. There is no 'goal' and there are no inherent 'values' within evolution which could serve as orientation for human behaviour. If the human being really were to base its actions upon Nature, it would be just as easy to deduce a postulate for preserving the environment as one for destroying the present ecological balance. It would not be 'unnatural' behaviour if the human being were one day to destroy its environment or even (for example in a nuclear war) the entire ecosystem; that is just what happened in the early stages of life on our planet, when green plants (cf. Remmert 1980, p. 1) set free huge quantities of oxygen (which gave rise to the atmosphere we know today) with their photosynthetic metabolism, causing environmental poisoning of global proportions and killing the anaerobic organisms which, until then, had dominated.

Here we obviously have a second indication for the ambivalence of referring to Nature in moral contexts. In the last chapter, we saw that we cannot conclude moral justification for the human race from such a 'natural' destruction of Nature. This pushes the idea of teleology, in the sense of a morality inherent within Nature, *ad absurdum*. The notion that we could find within Nature the criteria by which to measure or at least orientate our moral behaviour proves to be an illusion, and the hope that 'axiology [could] become a part of ontology' (Jonas 1984, p. 79) has to be dropped. In constructing its morality, the human being is referred back to the norms and values it itself has created.

Problems with holiness

Attempts to restitute teleology aim to raise Nature above the status of a value-for-us to that of a value-as-such, in other words to ascribe to her inherent moral values. It is a small step from such a remoralisation of Nature to making Nature sacred. For if individual natural phenomena, or even Nature in her entirety, possess inherent moral qualities, only a minor change of accent towards the religious is needed in order to conclude a *sacredness*.

> It is moot whether, without restoring the category of the sacred, the category most thoroughly destroyed by the scientific enlightenment, we can have an ethics able to cope with the extreme powers which we possess today and constantly increase and are almost compelled to wield.
>
> (Jonas 1984, p. 23)

A holiness of *human* nature has been pleaded for in a similar fashion, as a necessary protective barrier against its destruction by technology. Extinction of more than 99 per cent of all biological species is cause enough to question such a plea, yet more than anything it is confronted with practical difficulties.

How strongly should we interpret the term 'holiness'? Let us first assume an extensive definition, referring to the whole of Nature, to everything which is. According to this interpretation, not only every human being and every animal would be holy, but every plant, every bacterium, even every stone and every drop of water. Albert Schweitzer has philosophised along these lines:

> Human beings are only truly ethical when they obey the compulsion to help everything alive which they are able to help, and when they shrink back from inflicting harm upon the same. They do not question the extent to which this life or that is worthy, nor the extent to which it is able to feel. They perceive life itself as holy. They do not tear leaves from trees, nor do they pick flowers, and they are careful not to tread upon any insects. At work by lamplight on a Summer's night, they prefer to keep the windows closed and to breathe stale air, than to watch the insects fall one by one onto the table with their wings singed.
>
> (Schweitzer pp. 378–9)

Whereas Albert Schweitzer limits holiness to living Nature, other authors would like to see it extended to the whole of Nature, to non-living matter.

> How come we respect fish as having their own value, as well as the water lilies under which they live, but not the river surrounding both these forms of life?... Rivers have their own personality or soul, even more than they have an 'interest'.
>
> (Meyer-Abich 1984, p. 188)

Yet it is obvious that this position – carried to its radical conclusion – would make human life impossible. As a natural being, the human being depends upon a metabolism with its natural surroundings; it has to kill animals and plants in order to feed and clothe itself. If it refrained from killing them out of respect for their 'holiness', it would kill itself – thus killing a being which is no less holy than the animals and plants it has protected. We are thus faced with a choice which can be formulated as a classical dilemma: *either* we gear our actions affecting Nature towards ensuring our own survival; *then* we are forced to dismiss the holiness of many natural objects. We have to breed and slaughter animals, fight pathogens, dyke rivers or force them to flow through power plants, etc. *Or* we respect the holiness of Nature as an absolute limit for our actions; *then*, however, we bring about the sure death of the human race, thus violating its holiness. For human beings are no less holy than any other natural objects.

This dilemma has not escaped the advocates of Nature's holiness. The practical unavoidability of control over and exploitation of Nature is too obvious to be ignored. Albert Schweitzer states:

> There are thousands of ways in which my existence comes into conflict with the existence of others. The necessity of destroying and harming the lives of others has been forced upon me. Whenever I wander along a lonely path, my feet inflict destruction and pain on all the tiny creatures living there. In order to preserve my existence, I have to fend off the existences which harm it. I become the persecutor of the little mouse which lives in my house, the murderer of the insect which chooses to nest there, the mass murderer of the bacteria which could endanger my life. I destroy plants and animals in order to feed myself.
>
> (Schweitzer p. 387)

Some Asian religions have attempted to avoid this dilemma by retreating from the world, practising quietism and asceticism. Schweitzer is not in favour of this course; for not even the strictest limitation of one's needs or the most consistent passivity are able to put a complete end to the dilemma. What he does not want, however, is to take comfort in the unavoidability of this conflict. He wants to make the point that in killing the living – however unavoidable this may be – we are morally guilty, and that we have to be aware of this guilt.

> We must never become blunted. The more intensely we experience conflict, the more we remain truthful. The good conscience is an invention of the Devil.
>
> (Schweitzer p. 388)

The problem with this viewpoint is that, although it may concede the unavoidability of destroying life, it regards this as a guilty act. This abandons the traditional concept of guilt – which presupposes an intention to act, as well as the avoidability of its consequences – and dissolves the specifically *moral* dimension of the concept. Morally attributable guilt and causal 'authorship' become identical. The consequence of such an extension to the concept of guilt is the exact opposite of that intended; the concept of 'guilt' loses its moral meaning. The difference between moral and immoral behaviour vanishes. For if the human being is constantly, unavoidably and necessarily guilty, then all actions may ultimately be attributed with the same – immoral – value, and there is no longer any reason to behave morally.

Protagonists of ecological ethics have attempted to avoid this consequence and to relativise the principle of holiness in such a way that it is compatible with the human interest in self-preservation. They concede:

> that we need plants, or at least their fruit, in order to live, and that we have to protect ourselves against diseases, whether we do so by strengthening the human body's powers of resistance, or by combatting pathogenes. Living in peace with Nature may therefore not exclude combatting the smallpox pathogene, for example. I even believe, to take a very extreme example, that not even animal experiments should be fundamentally excluded, provided that they are for medical and veterinary purposes, that there are

no other methods available, and that they are not linked with terrible suffering.

(Meyer-Abich 1984, p. 146)

The idea of Nature's holiness in the sense of an absolute limit to human actions is weakened; a plea is made that Nature be respected, maybe rejecting human interests as *principally* more important, yet at the same time taking them seriously and including them in all considerations. In a particular case, the various interests would have to be weighed up against each other carefully. Thus the original intention of justifying the prescribed moral limitations to human actions with the concept of Nature's holiness has proved to be illusory. Yet again we are referred back to the necessity of conducting a calculation of interests, in which no parameter is principally untouchable. Analysis of the criticism of anthropocentric views within the field of ethics will further confirm the fact that any search for natural and absolute limitations to human action has to remain hopeless.

Subject and object

The core of ecological ethics is criticism of ethical anthropocentrism. The human being should not see itself as beyond or even above Nature, but as part of Nature: as a being which has emerged with evolution, which is related by natural history to the other living organisms, and which remains dependent upon metabolism with Nature, even within the most highly developed societies. Yet in this context two different meanings of 'anthropocentrism', which should analytically be kept separate, are constantly being confused with each other. The term 'anthropocentrism' can mean (1) concentrating on the human being as the *subject* of morality and (2) concentrating on the human being as the *object* of morality. In the first case we are interested in the instance constituting the moral norms and values, in the second in who or what may possess moral rights, and in what these rights may consist of.

A look at the first interpretation shows that the call for a refrain from the anthropocentric perspective leads to a contradiction. This call is based, on the one hand, on expressed insistence upon human naturalness: the human being is part of Nature and should regard itself in this way. This reflection of one's own naturalness aims at a world view ensuring complete consideration for, and caring treatment of, Nature. Yet we have seen that this kind of behaviour is not necessarily natural: organisms are programmed by Nature to maximise their own individual offspring, and not to preserve their species, let alone to treat the environment with consideration. Even if one has no desire to follow a vulgar Darwinist 'struggle for existence', it is nevertheless impossible to overlook the fact that the ecological ethicists' view of Nature is extremely harmonistic. No fox pays attention to the 'rights' of the rabbit, no rabbit has respect for the desire to live off grasses and herbs, and even the grasses and herbs treat the ground in which they grow solely as a resource. Organisms treat their environment exclusively from the point of view of their own survival and reproduction interests, whereby interest in the species is followed – just as it is by the human being – short-sightedly and opportunistly, sometimes resulting in long-term self-damage, even self-destruction. Examples of natural destruction in gigantic proportion by Nature herself have already been mentioned. Thus, however much ecological ethics emphasises the naturalness of the human being on the one hand, realisation of this postulate assumes, on the other hand, that the human being is *not* what it is supposed to be regarding itself as: one natural being amongst many. If the human being really were merely a natural being, no other behaviour could be expected of it than an exponential reproduction of its species and an exploitation of its natural resources to the point of a global catastrophe. The challenge to refrain from an anthropocentric point of view and to recognise equal rights for all forms of life, making them the criterion by which to measure one's own actions, only makes sense as an appeal to human reason and/or morality, thereby assuming just that special position of the human race within Nature against which it inveighs.

Critics of anthropocentrism may respond that this objection totally misses their key intention. It is not a case of reducing the human being to just any natural creature amongst many and of casting doubt on the human capacity for reason and morality; neither should it be doubted that the challenge to refrain from anthropocentrism presumes a certain special position of the human race within Nature. Something quite different is meant: precisely because the human being has a special position within Nature, it must be able to see that such a catastrophe can only be avoided if it decides – on the strength of its reason and morality – not merely to regard Nature as a resource, but to repect her as a partner with equal rights. Consequently, it is not a case of questioning the central position of the human race as the subject of its own morality, but of changing the *content* of this morality in such a way that Nature may – and must – also be respected for possessing certain rights. The ecological ethicist subtly switches at this point to the *second* interpretation of anthropocentrism: it is no longer the fact that the human being has a special position within Nature, and that this is necessary as a moral subject which is criticised, but rather the inconsiderate exploitation by the human being of this special position for its own interests.

The question is now: is it possible to have a morality in which Nature has the same rights as human beings? Whether two parties actually do have the same rights may only be established when they come into conflict with each other. We have already seen that extending morality to the realm of Nature meets with difficulties where human interests and those of Nature collide. Human interest in survival, for example, makes it necessary to kill countless plants and animals for food; these organisms (at least some of them) are interested, however, in their own survival. How is the principle of equal rights to be made valid in this everyday case? If the advocates of non-anthropocentric ethics make provision for the various rights to be weighed up against each other in such cases, allowing human interests to be put before those of micro-organisms, plants and animals, then this is a sensible, pragmatic guideline. Accordingly, refraining from the anthropocentric point of view would mean not putting human interests, whatever they may be, automatically before the interests of natural objects in every case. If, at one end of the spectrum, it is legitimate in a case of smallpox to kill the viruses in order to save the human being, it must also be possible, at the other end of the spectrum, to do without fur coats in order to prevent a species of animal from becoming extinct. Yet both examples are extreme cases: in the first, the human right to life is so significant and the 'rights' of the smallpox viruses so insignificant that it is only possible to come down in favour of the former; in the second case, the interest in fur coats is so insignificant – at least for ethicists – and the right to life of an entire species so significant that it is only plausible to decide in favour of the latter. Yet hidden behind examples such as these are not only the pragmatic difficulties forming part of all those cases in the middle, where the situation is not as clear, but also the principal problem of how to *justify* such decisions. For if we decide to abandon the anthropocentric point of view, it is not *a priori* obvious that – and, more than anything, *why* – a human being should be 'worth' more than millions of viruses. Considering 'Nature in its entirety' (Meyer-Abich 1984, p. 93), there can hardly be a grading of life according to its value; and it is precisely a division of Nature into an inherently worthy part (the human being) and an inherently worthless part (the rest) which the critics of anthropocentrism are against, believing that the *whole* of Nature must be respected as worthy.

The conclusion to be drawn from these contemplations is that criticism of the anthropocentric point of view is aiming in the right direction, insofar as it is aimed at a *pragmatic* relativisation of human interests. This means an obligation upon the human being to consider carefully, in every situation calling for a decision, whether the interests which it follows in its treatment of Nature justify the damage to Nature which this treatment possibly or surely will inflict. However, this pragmatic relativisation cannot ultimately be a *principal* one, since this would be incompatible with the human interest in self-preservation. To put it pointedly: we can afford to respect the rights of Nature only where the interests affected are relatively insignificant – as in the case of the fur coat – but not where our vital interests are touched upon – as in the example of the smallpox viruses. We can therefore only decide according to *our own* interests where and when we are to respect the interests of Nature as having equal rights to our own.

Human interests and autonomy

There are three points to be noted from our observations on ecological ethics.

1. Referring to Nature as the source and basis of moral orientation is ambivalent in its content, as well as meta-ethically untenable. Hope of discovering norms and values within Nature is futile; we cannot harvest the rules governing human life as fruits of the earth any more than we can the rules governing interaction with Nature. But:

> We do not have to learn from Nature how to live, but we should seek to evaluate in critical discussion various ideas of how to cultivate Nature.
>
> (Schäfer 1986, p. 14)

2. We therefore have to rely on ourselves and our own interests in the formation of a moral orientation. Not even the plea for teleological metaphysics can totally escape reference to human self-interest, however subtle the reference may be.

> There is a practical imperative which, as far as life within the Natural world is concerned, commands us not to relinquish our natural, teleological way of viewing things.
>
> (Spaemann & Löw 1981, pp. 287–8)

Otherwise we will be faced with the following alternative:

> Either we manage to integrate our domination over Nature into a new, at first somewhat vague, relationship between us and Nature, or we ourselves will become the victims of our domination over Nature. Either we have to decide to interpret the living world anthropomorphologically, or we ourselves will become an anthropomorphism, worldless subjects cutting the ground from under our own feet.
>
> (ibid., p. 288)

The *pointe* of this argumentation is the attempt to demobilise the naturalistic fallacy by concluding it *backwards*: from the *'ought'* survival of the human species, the *'is'* of a teleologically structured Nature is concluded. We do not need to concern ourselves here with whether this kind of conclusion is philosophically convincing; what should be emphasised is the key rôle played by human interests for ethical justification, even in a plea for the relativisation of human interests.

3. The attempt to use human survival interests as an argument against the anthropocentric point of view has met with the objection that it merely represents a 'cleansed anthropocentrism'

(Meyer-Abich 1984, pp. 65–7), which does not escape the influence of human self-interest. For Meyer-Abich, a complete acceptance of the rights of Nature cannot be the result of such argumentation, but only the result of a *decision*:

> The extent to which we have to treat our natural environment with consideration for its own sake also depends upon existential pre-decisions.
>
> (ibid., p. 24)

This is not to be taken as sheer decisionism; instead, respect for the rights of Nature presupposes that the human being recognise that it is a part of Nature, and that it make this a central part of the way it perceives itself:

> In natural historical terms, we and our natural environment, animals and plants, earth, air, fire and water, are all related. Perceiving Nature as a whole, all of them are equal to us, and we are equal to them. At peace with Nature, we have to respect our natural environment not just for its usefulness as far as we are concerned, but for its own sake.
>
> (ibid., p. 24)

Yet such evolutionary considerations may only suggest, support or motivate the decision which is called for, and never rationally enforce it. Reference to the uneliminable moment of decision, underlying the validity of norms, finally brings our attention back to the *subject* of morality and its *autonomy*. Not only the call for a revitalisation of teleology, but also the call for a refrain from anthropocentrism focus on a being which can only become their addressee due to its extraordinary, objective position within Nature. We are not relieved by metaphysics, nor by any concept of teleological or holy Nature, of our responsibility as the subjects of our actions and our morality for the preservation and formation of Nature: both of Nature itself and of human nature.

9

Playing God

Men ought not to play God
before they learn to be men,
and after they have learned to be men
they will not play God.
Paul Ramsey

The rôle of the human being as the responsible *subject* of its relationship with both Nature and human nature brings us to the second fundamental doubt which the substantialists have regarding gene and reproduction technology. A curious dialectic characterises modern development in science and technology. On the one hand, this development has systematically naturalised the human being and undermined its elevated position within Nature. On the other hand, it has rendered the human being 'master and owner' of Nature, thus emphasising its special status. With technological control over its reproduction, the human being makes human nature a 'piece of Nature', and itself the master above it all. Copernicus and Darwin degraded the human being: now, instead of being put down, the human being is forced by science to play God. Modern biological technology has created a controlling power over life processes previously unknown and, with it, assigned to the human being a 'new rôle as creator' (Jonas 1985, p. 204). It is this temptation to 'play God' which gives rise to much of the uneasiness felt by the substantialists: it is not just the holiness of the manipulated object at stake, but also the unholiness of the manipulating subject.

Insufficient wisdom

The 'playing God' accusation is immediately plausible if we consider the ideas which emerged at the end of the 19th century regarding a control over biological evolution, and if we remember that the early eugenicists were the first to make the prospect of such extended control over human evolution their main interest. These efforts were ultimately aimed at improving the human race, and Herman Muller spoke of 'God-like beings, where we sickly creatures of today are the pathetic premonition of what is to come' (cf. Chapter 4). Finally, we should not forget Stanislaw Lem's concept of autoevolution, which goes beyond even the most ambitious eugenic plans, marking the flight path for eugenic philosophy: Lem's concept follows through to its radical end an idea which is inherent to all modern biological technological procedures, and – most importantly – which forms part of most eugenic strategies: the notion of a *new creation*.

The uneasiness experienced by some at the notion of a revised creation is not only because of the violation of the holiness of human nature, which it necessarily implies, but also because it carries human subjectivity too far. With the advent of gene and reproduction technology, human subjectivity begins to rotate on its own foundations: it begins to modify and shape its own natural basis. This self-shaping bestows upon the human being a rôle which Western mythical and religious tradition had previously reserved for the Gods. In Greek mythology, Prometheus was cruelly punished for forming the first human beings out of clay and introducing them to fire. In the subtitle of her book on Frankenstein, Mary Shelley characterises her biological engineer as a 'modern Prometheus'. In Jewish and Christian mythology, God himself creates the human beings:

> And the Lord God formed man of the dust of the ground, and breathed into his nostrils the breath of life; and man became a living soul.
>
> (Genesis 2: 7)

With the new gene and reproduction technological options available, and especially in the futuristic projects aimed at improving humanity, the human being changes from being the mere procreator of its descendants to being their *creator*: it no longer simply brings children into the world, but also determines, the more it learns to control the relevant natural processes and thus to influence the characteristics of the children, *which* children it brings into the world. In the Bible, God created the human being in his image, and in a similar way we are gaining the ability to create, i.e. design, our descendants in our image. It is therefore understandable that primarily Christian writers (e.g. Ramsey 1970, pp. 138–40) refer to the topos 'playing God', and that they do so critically.

Beyond the theological problems involved in this accusation, it may be understood in a *moral* sense for referring to the fundamental limitations of human knowledge. In his *Republic*, Plato made the following comment concerning the eugenic arrangement of 'marriages and children' by the ruling elite of the Utopian Republic:

> Dear friend, how imperative, then, is our need of the highest skill in our rulers, if the principle holds also for mankind.
>
> (V, 459b)

Interventions in human reproduction, especially those involving an alteration to the genetic constitution of the future human being, presume a knowledge both vast and reliable. Whereas our concept of God includes that of omniscience, i.e. whereas we assume that a heavenly creator possesses complete knowledge about the consequences of the act of creation, we know of ourselves that we do not possess this kind of knowledge, and that we never will. However progressive science may be, human decisions are always made with incomplete information.

> The term 'playing God', used pejoratively, implies that we are making Godlike decisions without Godlike omniscience.
>
> (Grobstein 1981, p. 67)

The critics have good reason to draw attention to the experiences we have had with 'conquering' Nature. The world-wide ecological catastrophe we face today is a clear indication that our actions can have, and actually do have, unforeseen consequences. Where is the guarantee that conquering our own nature will turn out better than conquering Nature has? The human race did not possess enough wisdom in its treatment of Nature to avoid a catastrophe, so it is logical to fear that its treatment of human nature will end the same way. 'When we lack sufficient wisdom to do, wisdom consists in not doing.' (Kass 1972, p. 62).

Risk

Of course, it did not take reproduction technology for the human being to start playing God. It has been said that human beings play God each time they spray pesticides or carry out surgery; it has even been maintained that each one of us is only here because two human beings played God, creating life. It is not playing God which is new, but the extent to which it is played. In addition, each of these actions took place in uncertain circumstances; for we are never in a position to assess anticipatively all the consequences of an action – regardless of whether technology has increased the strength and effects of this action or not. Yet uncertainty as to the result of *all* human actions has never been accepted as a reasonable objection to human activity. Far more, the human race has dealt with the risks involved in its actions in a way described by Grobstein as 'pragmatic'. A step is taken and then its effect is evaluated; progress is usually made in stages, with the expected risks involved at each individual stage being weighed up – albeit with incomplete information – against the expected benefits.

> What is now happening with external fertilization, it can be argued, is dramatized but not clarified by invoking comparison with acts of God. To seek to understand and then to apply this understanding to human problems has always been and remains the human way. Given socially acceptable purpose, responsible human beings do not avoid all fore-seeable risk, let alone succumb to fear of speculative risk. They pro-ceed sequentially by probing consequences as far into the future as possible, making the appropriate decision for the time, and assuming that a later decision will be better informed by the knowledge that greater experience will bring. This is not playing God; it is being human, often in areas that previously were subject to religious or other taboos that entered tradition during a less knowledgeable time.
>
> (Grobstein 1981, p. 68)

This riposte is nevertheless unsatisfactory. There can be no doubt that every human action is laden with risk; yet a reference to the risks involved in all actions does not free us from the responsibility of weighing up whether the risks involved in each individual action are bearable. The fact that we cannot avoid *every* risk certainly does not mean that we must or may take *all* the risks involved. Even reminding ourselves of the stepwise character of our progress cannot fully remove doubts about the sufficiency of our wisdom; for, as is obvious enough from our current ecological problems, even single steps can add to an overall effect with a new quality and unseen consequences. There is another reason why we should be *especially* cautious with gene and reproduction technology. Unlike other technologies, the possible, maybe even probable negative consequences of gene and reproduction technology directly affect human beings. It is no coincidence that the critics of this technology are forever referring to the potential mishaps involved:

> Those dazzled by the vision of a glorious specimen emerging from the try should also think of the inevitable failures – abnormal embryos to be discarded, or malformed beings to be guilty for – even if they lack the imagination to foresee the glorious specimen itself (perhaps most of all) become their accuser for abuse of power.
>
> (Jonas 1974, p. 163)

There can be no doubting the prickliness of this argument. Gene and reproduction technology involves a *specific* dimension of risk which distinguishes it from other technologies. There is a very grave difference between an unsuccessfully constructed machine and an unsuccessfully constructed human being. Nevertheless, there are two reasons why this argument does not justify a *principal* objection to technological intervention in human reproduction.

1. The *specific* dimension of risk involved in gene and reproduction technology may be attributed to the direct effect it has on the lives and health of human beings; in this respect there is no distinction to be made between it and other *medical* technologies, which we believe should be applied even when we cannot exclude all the possible risks. The risk argument simply draws attention to a condition which has to be fulfilled by all applications of gene and reproduction technology: they have to meet the bioethical criteria to be met by all therapeutic interventions.

2. Even though it is definitely morally relevant to refer to potential risks, since it can be considered immoral to take an unjustifiable risk, especially when others are affected, it is not a *moral* argument which is at stake in the narrower sense referred to here; we are far more concerned with whether it is 'prudent' to carry out a particular action or to apply a particular technology, than with whether it is 'moral' to do so. The difference becomes apparent when there is a debate on whether to permit a technology which involves no risks at all, or only very minor ones. Does this also make it *morally* justifiable? – The risk argument is merely capable of justifying a condition necessarily to be fulfilled before technological interventions in human reproduction may be permitted, but is not capable of justifying a sufficient condition.

Values

Yet the importance of the concept of 'wisdom' does not end with a thorough knowledge of the *empirical* consequences of particular interventions in human reproduction. Wisdom is more than anything a matter of deciding whether the factual consequences of such interventions, and indeed of controlling reproduction at all, are 'good' for humanity. Each intervention of this kind implies a decision about ourselves and about our descendants; it is up to us not only whether, but also *how* our descendants will live. Questioning our wisdom draws attention to the fact that our descendants' quality of life, and the chances they will have in life, depend more than anything on the *values* which we take as orientation for our manipulations. Of course, the soundness and completeness of our knowledge, as well as the scope and safety of our technology, play an important rôle. Yet, with the assumption that proceeding in stages would solve these scientific and technological problems, the values involved in our decisions immediately become central. Do we really possess a system of values which is sufficiently secure, reliable and agreed upon to enable us to reach responsible decisions of such proportion? The answer to this question is obviously no, we do not. One only has to think of the decisions we would be faced with if we opted for a strategy of positive eugenics. In this case we would have to decide at least some of the characteristics of our descendants: are they to be athletic and sporty, or highly intelligent and interested in scientific and technological problems? Maybe we should aim at a generation of sensitive beings, finding fulfilment in the formation of human relationships. A further goal could be musical skill, and ultimately various combinations of these and other variations. We should not forget how different aspirations have been in the past – in Ancient Greece, the Middle Ages or the 19th century – and still are in different countries today – in the U.S.A. or Russia, in the Vatican or Iran. In other words, there is not a universally accepted system of values which could be taken as a basis for the decisions at stake, meaning that these decisions depend upon contingent factors: upon individual arbitrariness, fashions or orders from the Government.

The scope of such decisions, and the key rôle played by the values underlying them, are especially apparent in the example of positive eugenics, but are on no account restricted to this one field. Far removed from all the futuristic possibilities involved in improving the human race, decisions are being made today about the 'whether' and the 'how' of our descendants' lives, without this being considered particularly spectacular. We already decide the 'whether' with our desire to have children or not to have children; and, from time to time, we make decisions about the life or death of children which have already been conceived. Every year, thousands of amniocenteses are carried out in Germany alone, often leading to an abortion when the test result is positive – in a case of Down's syndrome, for example, or a similarly grave disease. With the constant perfection of genetic prognostics, there will be a continual increase over the next few years in the number of predictable human characteristics. This will also mean an increase in the chances we have of determining our descendants' characteristics through selective abortion.

It seems obvious that future practice in this field will largely be determined by our values, and by the picture which we have of a fulfilled life. There are many ways in which we decide the 'how' of our descendants' lives: indirectly, through all of our actions, since they establish facts which outlive us and affect the lives of our descendants; directly, more than anything through the socialisation and upbringing of our offspring. Strength of habit often leads us to overlook the profound effect of socialisation and upbringing; they affect not only our descendants' knowledge and convictions, but also their characters and personalities. And this effect does not take place on the basis of a universally valid system of values, but according to the values which we happen to adhere to at the time in question, values which are thus contingent. If 'playing God' means making decisions about human lives, then we are already doing so, and always have done. Even though bringing up children unreflectedly and even irresponsibly may be regarded as immoral, there is no way that omniscience or wisdom is called for here to the extent with which it is assumed in the accusation that gene and reproduction technologicists are 'playing God'.

This is not meant to smooth out all the differences between socialisation and upbringing on the one hand, and technological intervention in reproduction on the other. These differences exist, and must form the basis for a moral orientation in both areas. One difference which must be named is the fact that it is very difficult to avoid socialisation and upbringing – of whatever kind – since we cannot avoid having some kind of influence on our offspring, whereas there is no such unavoidability in the case of gene and reproduction technology. Nevertheless, the comparison with bringing up children makes it clear that there is nothing new about human control over human life *per se*. We are always deciding about the lives of the next generation and their chances in life, especially those of our own children: first of all by bringing them into the world (or not); then by giving them emotional security (or not), bringing them up in a certain religious faith (or not), giving them the chance of a good education (or not), etc. – without making ourselves prone to the accusation that we have assumed the rôle of the Gods. We make all of these decisions according to our *own* values, influenced by individual experiences and historical trends or fashions; and we also expose our children to the influence of social institutions (the State, the Church, the media, etc.) with their convergingly or divergingly orientated values, without calling for universally valid and accepted values. Talk of insufficient wisdom draws attention to a problem connected with intervention in human reproduction; yet it does not constitute a decisive objection, at least not until it is plausible that the dangers looming due to insufficient wisdom are greater than the chances provided by our existing and – humanly – fallible wisdom.

Increasing responsibility

Independently of any form of reproduction technology, we are already responsible for our descendants. The fact that we make decisions about their lives and their chances in life means that we have moral responsibilities. We are not only legally, but also morally obliged to keep them, to bring them up to be independent and well-mannered, to give them a good education – in other words to give them as good a 'social constitution' in life as possible. The fact that modern biology and medicine also enable us to influence their 'natural constitution' means more responsibility. In the past, the birth of a handicapped child had to be accepted as an unfortunate stroke of Fate. The knowledge we possess today about the statistical correlation between the age of the mother and the frequency with which Down's syndrome occurs, for example, changes the situation: a woman over the age of 35 is now able to anticipate the increased risk which she takes of giving birth to a handicapped child if she becomes pregnant. This knowledge is not morally neutral; every woman (couple) is morally obliged to take note of this risk, to weigh up the pros and cons involved and to take them into consideration when deciding how to act. *How* she/they should decide, whether a severely handicapped foetus should be brought into the world or aborted, is another matter; various responsible decisions are conceivable and viable. It would be irresponsible, however, purposely to ignore the relevant statistics, to disregard the risk of having a handicapped child, and to leave everything to chance.

With our expanding empirical knowledge and opportunities to intervene with technology, we lose our innocence and acquire responsibility where previously we had none. With the progress being made in reproduction technology, we necessarily increase our obligations towards our children; optimising their 'social constitution' is no longer sufficient when we also have the opportunity to influence their 'natural constitution'. This stretching of responsibility has always accompanied technological development,

and it reaches into all fields. The explosive increase in the technological options available within the field of human reproduction is
particularly dramatic, however, since the innovations which have
emerged so far are merely the start of a technological revolution,
the conclusion of this revolution being left to our imagination.
Joseph Fletcher's prognosis (1974, p. xiv) has hinted at where this
development might lead, with our moral responsibility for human
reproduction extending from a mere control over how many
children we have

> to the trickier business of controlling the genetic or physical *quality* of
> our children. It would be quite a jump to go from the blind chances
> of sexual roulette or 'taking what you get' in baby making to the care-
> ful production of prefabricated babies.

If we ignore both the slovenly terminology of the quality control
propagated here and the problems contained within it, an important
point still remains: what is extolled here by Fletcher as a magnificent prospect can also be seen as cumbersome. Increasing the size
and range of our responsibility to cover additional technological
options will not necessarily be easy to bear. Very often the decisions
to be made are complicated ones, not made any easier by the fact
that they always directly affect human life. How serious must an
embryo's prenatally diagnosed disease be – to take a realistic example – in order to justify an abortion? In the light of such life-
and-death decisions, or potential decisions concerning the quality of
our descendants, the 'playing God' accusation does not appear out
of place, and it is also fuelled by fears that the human being cannot
cope with the moral burden of such decisions. Seen like this, modern reproduction technology represents an attempt to dispute the
fact that both the beginning and the end of life are events beyond
human control, indeed events which form the limits of this control.

> Whenever the human being ignores this 'dependence', the limitations
> of its existence as a creature, it threatens and easily perverts its own
> nature, setting itself up as its own creator.
>
> (Eibach 1983, p. 148)

It is not only a linguistic criticism when talk of 'making' children
is criticised for being a linguistic indication of the objectivisation
of the procreative process; neither is it a factual observation – disregarding for now the choice of vocabulary – that children

'emerge, they become, and all during a process where procreation is not usually the aim in mind', a process where reproduction is 'an unintentional side-effect, one which cannot even be forced or produced when it *is* intended' (ibid. p. 146). The fact that procreation is often not intentional, but happens 'during something quite different' (Löw 1983, p. 39) is often seen as being *morally* significant, which may be formulated as follows: the greater the spontaneity, the lesser the danger of 'making' and 'controlling' – and the lesser our responsibility.

Yet this overlooks the fact that a mere concentration on the 'quite different' and on a thoughtless begetting and bearing of children did not even relate to moral norms when the concept of responsibility was more traditional and there was no such thing as GenEthics. We may not have to justify to a third party whether we have children, or how many we have; but this does not mean that we have the right to reproduce *al gusto*, without wasting a thought on whether we can feed these children and bring them up in a fit manner. In this sense, it is misleading to speak of reproduction as a

'natural event' not deducible from human action alone.

(Eibach 1983, p. 146)

Since natural processes are involved in every human action, and there is no event which may be deduced 'solely' from human action, then this argument, were it to be taken seriously, would carry the concept of responsibility *ad absurdum*, eventually dissolving it altogether. Our responsibility for an action does not actually depend at all upon the extent to which natural laws are *also* involved, but rather upon the fact that our actions cause results which could be avoided. There can be no doubt that the two people involved in an act of reproduction are the causal originators of the 'natural event' which then takes place, nor doubt that they had the chance of avoiding being the originators; an act of procreation from beginning to end may only be described as a 'natural event' in the sense that a violent punch or a car journey are 'natural events': the natural processes involved in all of these actions do not change the fact that we are responsible for the consequences. Insisting upon the fact that the human being passes on life 'as a natural being' (Löw 1983, p. 39) proves to be an attempt to turn the natural act of procreation into a mere natural process, in order to contrast idyllic freedom from responsibility all the more effectively with the oppressive burden of responsibility with which artificial methods of procreation weigh us down.

> If life is controlled, the human being is fully responsible for its actions. What it is and what it will be is of its own doing, and if this turns out to be an evil then it is the human being's fault that it is an evil. The human being is then burdened with a far greater ethical responsibility than it is when overcome by an unavoidable fate.
>
> (Eibach 1983, p. 136)

However, there are several reasons why this kind of interpretation is unconvincing.

1. The assumption that paradisial irresponsibility used to prevail within the field of human reproduction is by no means tenable. The reason for this is not least the necessity, forever being emphasised by Christian sexual ethics, of releasing sexual processes from the status of mere natural processes and moralising them to give them the dignity of genuinely humane behaviour. When Löw talks of the human being passing on life 'as a natural being', we should remember Rousseau's description of the natural state, especially his description of the reproductive habits of the 'natural beings' living in this state.

> His appetite satisfied, the man has no longer any need for a particular woman, nor the woman for a particular man. The man has not the least care, nor perhaps the least idea, of the consequences of his action. One goes off in one direction, the other in another, and there is no likelihood that at the end of nine months either will remember having known the other . . .
>
> (Rousseau 1984, p. 165)

Procreation results 'during something quite different' (Löw), it is 'an unintended side-effect' (Eibach) of satisfying the sexual drive. Bearing this 'natural' attitude to the process of reproduction in mind, the following two questions are easy to answer:

> If a certain woman is indifferent to the man during these nine months, if indeed she becomes a stranger to him, why should he help her after the birth? Why would he help her to raise a child he does not know is his, and whose birth he has neither desired nor foreseen?
>
> (ibid., p. 165)

It is not a question of whether Rousseau has described the natural state appropriately, but of whether this is behaviour which we are prepared to accept as moral.

2. If this is not the case, as we may assume, then the sharp dividing line between the supposedly pure and natural reproductive process and the artificial forms of reproduction loaded with responsibility crumbles. Instead of creating new responsibility in a void, the progress of science and technology merely increases responsibility which has been around for a long time. If this is a problem which we have not yet learnt to deal with, and which in many cases confronts us with difficult decisions, then this does not necessarily mean that the problem is an insoluble one.

3. We should not forget that the growing burden of responsibility is counterbalanced by a growing number of opportunities. Gene and reproduction technology *can* contribute to a reduction in human suffering. Its moral evaluation should not only take into account the burdens involved, but must also weigh up these burdens against the possible benefits.

4. Finally, we have to face the fact that this long and drawn-out increase in responsibility is *unavoidable*; not only because everything points to the fact that this process cannot be reversed, but also because it is *logically* irreversible. If responsibility is a function of our ability to anticipate cognitively and control technologically, then we are also responsible for events which we anticipate, but then cannot control because we have not created the necessary technology. In concrete terms, this means: if today we were to decide to stop all further research and development in the fields of gene technology and reproductive medicine, then this would not free us of our responsibility for the suffering of all those people who would then come into the world with grave genetic disorders. They could accuse us of consciously prohibiting development of the means to help them, of ignoring their suffering, although we were able to anticipate it. This does not mean that we are bound to support the progress of science and technology indefinitely. We may well decide as the result of ethical reflection that we can prevent genetic diseases only at the cost of other, unacceptable consequences, in other words that we will have to accept the genetic suffering of many future human beings in order to avoid an even

greater evil. This thought does not relieve us of the obligation, however, to weigh up carefully all the relevant points of view, and to discard from the outset this option or that if we are not capable of taking on the responsibility associated with it. Even reaching no decision is a decision, the results of which we are responsible for; whether we like it or not, there is no way back to the idyll of irresponsibility.

Meta-responsibility

Yet, however difficult the decisions associated with modern gene and reproduction technology may be: are we not confronted with similar difficulties in all areas of human activity? Growth in human responsibility is not limited to the field of reproduction, but is a *universal* consequence of progress within science and technology. A steadily increasing range of action automatically leads to an increase in responsibility. A car driver has more responsibility to bear than a pedestrian, and the management of a modern chemical company more than an 18th century soap manufacturer. It has been the looming ecological catastrophe which has – more than anything else – drastically drawn attention to this moral reverse of technological progress. Whereas in former times the range of effect of our actions was limited to individual parts of Nature, today it encompasses the entire terrestrial biosphere – with the potential destruction of the entire terrestrial biosphere as a consequence. This magnitude of human action, previously inconceivable, has become a central point of interest in modern technological philosophy; it is the starting point for Hans Jonas' theory on the necessity of developing a new ethics based on the *Imperative of Responsibility*. Modern technology has

> introduced actions of such novel scale, objects, and consequences that the framework of former ethics can no longer contain them . . . To be sure, the old prescriptions of the 'neighbor' ethics – of justice, charity, honesty, and so on – still hold in their intimate immediacy for the nearest, day-by-day sphere of human interaction. But this sphere is overshadowed by a growing realm of collective action where doer, deed, and effect are no longer the same as they were in the proximate

sphere, and which by the enormity of its powers forces upon ethics a new dimension of responsibility never dreamed of before.

(Jonas 1984, p. 6)

Maybe this new dimension of responsibility becomes clearer if we consider a nuclear destruction of all the higher forms of life on this planet, including the direct extermination of humanity. In this light, reproduction technology appears as one moment in a development across *all* the fields of human activity in which the 'imperative of responsibility' is becoming more and more important, due to progress in science and technology.

And yet the problems involved are different from those connected with other technologies. If we take another look at the car driver, his/her increased responsibility results from the increased damage which he/she is in a position to inflict. The increase is only quantitative, since no *new* moral problems have arisen. The case of the chemical company is more difficult. Yet even these difficulties may be traced back to two problems: to the practical problem of *carrying through and accomplishing* valid norms, and to the problem of weighing up *competing* norms and values. Yet the problems posed by gene and reproduction technology have a qualitatively new dimension. When is a prenatally diagnosed disease grave enough to justify an abortion? Competing values are at stake: on the one hand the value 'life', on the other the value 'health'. The difference from any other problematic situation in which we have to decide between competing values is that, before we can choose one value or the other, we have to make a fundamental decision as to whether we are allowed to weigh up such values *at all*. Doing so would, after all, place the value 'life' at our disposal. A similar case is that of cloning. This is not simply a case of deciding between a 'right of the child to genetic individuality' on the one hand, and a 'right of the parents to choose how they would like to reproduce' on the other, but a case of whether such rights actually *exist*. In dealing with gene and reproduction technology, we are not only confronted with *applying* valid norms and values to a concrete case, but also with deciding about the *validity or invalidity* of these norms and values.

If we take a look at the normative problems raised by the global environmental catastrophe and by nuclear war, the specificity of gene and reproduction technology quickly becomes clear. It *is* possible to find moral arguments why the human race should extend and perfect its control over reproduction; it is *not* possible to find any to explain why the human race should destroy its environment and wage atomic war. Of course, this is by no means the final solution to all the ethical and moral problems surrounding ecology and the combat of international conflict. Totally diverging political and philosophical opinions exist as to *how* the environment can and is to be saved, and nuclear war avoided. And yet everyone agrees that these are goals at which we should be aiming. Both cases involve problems where we already possess the moral norms required to solve them; the norm 'thou shalt not kill' is as relevant to nuclear weapons as to truncheons and guns. Gene and reproduction technology is a different case altogether. Whereas there can be no discussion about whether we should leave the natural world totally desolate for the generations to come, we certainly can discuss the moral permissibility of extracorporeal fertilisation and an improved human race. Thus the difference is that in the case of ecology and nuclear arms technology we are 'only' faced with the task of putting existing and agreed upon moral norms into operation in a concrete case, together with practical instructions for use. Yet we do not have corresponding norms for the field of reproduction technology. With the help of GenEthics, we have to create them.

This brings into play a new type of responsibility which forces us to differentiate between two different levels of responsibility. (1) On the one hand, we take responsibility for our actions with regard to valid values and norms. Every car driver is responsible for all the avoidable inconveniences or dangers suffered by other road users as a result of his/her driving; every chemical company manager is responsible for potential damage caused to the environment and for risks to the health of his/her employees. (2) A different kind of responsibility is called for in all the situations where there is no valid moral orientation by which to judge a particular action, where we – as in the case of technological intervention in human reproduction – are not faced with the problem of how to evaluate certain interventions, but with the problem of deciding which norms and values should be taken as the basis for such an evaluation. This calls for something which we may term *meta-responsibility*: responsibility not only at the level of certain actions, but also at the level of a moral orientation for the evaluation of these actions (Bayertz 1987). There are many indications that meta-responsibility is central to the substantialist uneasiness at 'playing God'.

GenEthics and a new morality

When human beings are born, they are confronted with a morality which is historically determined and socially established. The acquisition and internalisation of this morality forms a significant part of their socialisation. Moral norms and values are never at our disposal: anybody is free to lie or steal, but nobody can seriously debate whether it is morally correct to lie or steal. Traditionally, part of the task of ethics is to make systematic and to justify *valid* morality. For modern Western moral philosophers this means: making systematic and justifying the morality characterising Christianity, as outlined in the Biblical Decalogue. Apart from anti-moralistic hardliners, atheist moral philosophers have never, not even programmatically, attempted to doubt or replace the fundamental norms and values underlying this morality. 'Thou shalt not kill' and 'thou shalt not lie' are the paradigmatic moral norms which are forever being discussed and *presumed* valid, even without this validity being philosophically justified. Ethics was comprehended as being the rational reconstruction of valid morality, but not as the 're-evaluation of all values' or the discovery of *new* norms and values.[1] Kant formulated this exclusively reconstructive

---

[1] It was this limitation to rational reconstruction which caused Nietzsche to poke fun at moral philosophy. For example in *Jenseits von Gut und Böse* (Beyond Good and Evil), where he writes: 'As soon as they occupied themselves with morality as a science, all the philosophers demanded higher, greater, more solemn things of themselves, with a stiffness and seriousness which made one laugh: they wanted the *justification* of morality, – and every philosopher to date believed to have justified morality; yet morality itself was considered as "given" . . . Still *missing* in all the "science of morality" to date, however surprising it may seem, was the problem of morality itself: the suspicion that something here could be problematic. What the philosophers termed "justification of morality" and what they demanded of themselves was, seen in its true light, merely an educated form of good *faith* in existing morality, a new means of *expressing* it, an actuality within a particular morality, even a kind of denial that this morality *could possibly* be seen as a problem: and in any case the opposite of an examination, dissection, doubt, vivisection of precisely this faith' (Nietzsche pp. 105–6).

claim very fittingly in a famous riposte to a critical review of his *The Moral Law*:

> A critic who wished to say something against that work really did better than he intended when he said that there was no new principle of morality in it but only a new formula. Who would want to introduce a new principle of morality and, as it were, be its inventor, as if the world had hitherto been ignorant of what duty is or had been thoroughly wrong about it? Those who know what a formula means to a mathematician, in determining what is to be done in solving a problem without letting him go astray, will not regard a formula which will do this for all duties as something insignificant and unnecessary.
>
> (Kant 1949, p. 123)

Bernard Gert defines the task of moral philosophy similarly: as a reconstruction and explication, as a reformulation and precise statement of valid moral rules (Gert 1973, p. 5). Habermas likewise comprehends

> practical discourse as a procedure which does not serve to create justified norms, but to examine the validity of exisiting norms which have become problematic and which are deliberated hypothetically.
>
> (Habermas 1984, pp. 220–1)

Finally, despite all the pathos of moral renewal, even current efforts to reconstruct 'ecological ethics' follow in this tradition. The revision of modern ethics called for in connection with the environmental crisis aims to enhance and extend the 'principle of responsibility' and to adapt traditional, moral behavioural norms to suit the new technological options available. Morality, traditionally limited to human relationships, is to be extended to include norms and values regulating the relationship between the human race and Nature. This extension to morality's range of validity does not form the philosophical core of ecological ethics, however, but rather the postulate of overcoming the anthropocentric point of view. And this is a problem of *justifying* norms.

GenEthics is, however, not only aimed at systematising, explaining and justifying existing moral norms governing technological intervention in human reproduction. For the advocates of reproduction technology at least, GenEthics calls for a revision of existing norms and values, as well as the *creation of new ones*. This moral revisionism can be found throughout the history of eugenic philosophy. As already cited in Chapter 2, Campanella was one of the first to describe the contrast between existing Western morality and his idea of Utopian State control:

> They deny what we hold – viz., that it is natural for man to recognize his offspring and to educate them, and to use his wife and horse and children as his own. For they say that children are bred for the preservation of the species and not for individual pleasure, as St. Thomas also asserts. Therefore the breeding of children has reference to the commonwealth and not to individuals, except in as far as they are constituents of the commonwealth.
>
> (Campanella 1885, p. 235)

The eugenic criticism of Western Christian morality which was to follow in the 19th and 20th centuries, combined with the call for a 'generative morality of the future' to replace it, did not have much to add to this description of a reproductive ethics. When the notion of a total revision of existing morality was taken up again at a later date, even Herman Muller considered it essential that we

> rid ourselves of preconceptions based on our traditional behaviour in matters of parentage, and open our minds to the possibilities afforded by our scientific knowledge and techniques.
>
> (Muller 1967, p. 257)

This reference to new scientific and technological options also gives voice to the driving force behind current demands for a GenEthics: scientific and technological progress. Revising 'old' morality, and replacing it with a new one, is a considerable step towards adapting moral standards to suit the current state of science and technology.

> Our traditional morality of baby making is based on heterosexual intercourse or coital conception, and on uterine gestation or fetal nurture in the human womb. This has been superseded or at least become supersedable. Since mores and values always change as conditions and situations change, our morality will and should change too.
>
> (Fletcher 1974, p. xiv)

It is no longer the progress of science and technology which is being evaluated in the light of morality; it is the validity of morality which is being debated, with regard to science and technology. Morality is declared the dependent variable of scientific and technological progress.

With this in mind, it becomes clear why the substantialists feel uneasy about GenEthics. *Theologically* speaking, GenEthics implies a usurpation of heavenly privileges. For, in all religions, moral norms are accepted as having heavenly origins. This is also true of Jewish-Christian mythology, where the Ten Commandments are not invented by human beings, but passed on by God. It is therefore presumptuous and hubristic when human beings start playing God by making themselves the creators of a new morality. If scientific and technological progress forces us to create a new moral orientation, then this means in *philsophical* terms that the human being recognises itself as the subject of morality, and thus as a being which is not only responsible for its actions, but also meta-responsible for the morality it adheres to. The gene ethicist should not forget Sartre's comment that

> there is no legislator but himself; that he himself, thus abandoned, must decide for himself.
>
> (Sartre 1973, pp. 55–6)

It is this sense of abandonment which makes the substantialists uneasy, as well as the fear that human beings cannot cope with their heavenly rôle as creator of a new morality.

Losing ground

We should remember that not only theological and philosophical *theories* are at stake here, but also the moral evaluation of the *practice* of technological intervention in human reproduction. Uneasiness regarding the attempt to play God is fuelled not least by the fear that we will lose the ground from beneath our feet if not only all the stages of human life become controllable, but also the moral norms and values which we use to evaluate this control. Morality had an indubitable certainty from its heavenly origins; yet as the mere work of human beings it will fall prey to all sorts of criticism, fundamental scepticism or even total despair. Neither a norm nor a value may claim the dignity of inviolability if human beings are not only free to act as they please, but also to decide about the morality of their actions. This is exactly the conclusion that Sartre came to:

Dostoievsky once wrote 'If God did not exist, everything would be permitted'; and that, for existentialism, is the starting point. Everything is indeed permitted if God does not exist, and man is in consequence forlorn, for he cannot find anything to depend upon either within or without himself.

(Sartre 1973, pp. 33–4)

What is here formulated as philosophical theory comes into practical effect with GenEthics. This is most obvious in the discussions about who or what may or must be regarded as a 'human being'. Joseph Fletcher, for example, states:

Human beings, in order to qualify as human, have to be something more than just biologically classifiable as organisms of the species *Homo sapiens*. They have to have individual or separate existence ('viability') and they have to be actually 'sapient' – that is, possessed of a functioning cerebral cortex – some minimal level of intelligence.

(Fletcher 1974, pp. 170–1)

On another occasion, Fletcher gives a precise and quantitative definition of this minimal level:

Any individual of the species *Homo sapiens* who falls below the I.Q. 40-mark in a standard Stanford–Binet test, amplified if you like by other tests, is questionably a person; below the 20-mark, not a person . . . Mere biological life, before minimal intelligence is achieved or after it is lost irretrievably, is without personal status.

(1972, p. 1)

This definition is top of a list of fifteen positive and five negative criteria, collectively presented as 'indicators of the status human being'. We do not need to go into detail regarding this 'tentative profile of the human being' in order to realise the problems associated with it: if we start to discuss what we are to accept as a human being, and what not, then everything may be regarded as plausible. The demand from molecular biologists that: 'no newborn infant shall be declared human until it has passed certain tests regarding its genetic endowment' (quoted from Etzioni 1973, p. 70) can no longer come as a surprise. More and more philosophers are coming to the conclusion that not only abortion, but also infanticide is morally permissible (Tooley 1983; Kuhse & Singer 1985). Engelhardt's reflections upon the moral standing of persons have led him also to

a reconsideration of our moral rules regarding the active and passive
euthanasia of infants born with significant mental and physical handicaps. It is clear that the categorical prohibition of such practices cannot be justified in terms of general moral principles.

(Engelhardt 1986, p. 236)

Are these trends not a clear indication that the meta-responsibility involved is too much for the human being to cope with? Do we
need further proof that, in making themselves the subject of
morality, human beings will, far from introducing new and better
norms, destroy that morality? It seems so. The beginning and the
end of human life are becoming particularly prone to conceptual
reformulation and normative alteration, leading in turn to fundamental changes of traditional morality. A further example is the
introduction of brain criteria to define human death. Although it is
now a recognised definition throughout almost the entire world,
brain death remains the subject of fierce controversy and deep
uneasiness. One of the reasons for this is surely the fact that (more
or less) *anything* seems to be possible and *allowed* when the difference between life and death is dependent upon an (arbitrary) definition. In the past, death used to be a natural event which was
established as fact: cardiac or respiratory arrest could be taken as a
sharp dividing line between life and death. The progress of medical technology has blurred this dividing line; the greater our medical know-how, the more dying replaces death. The clarity which
used to be part of the *concept* of death is dispelled. We find ourselves faced with the necessity of establishing a sharp dividing line
where, 'in reality', there is no such line. In this sense we may
speak of a 'denaturalisation' of morality (cf. Bayertz 1992). The
definition of death is no longer dependent upon 'ontologically' pre-
determined limits: it becomes dependent upon the state of medical
art, upon the availability of certain technologies, upon moral convictions and ethical arguments, upon social agreement, etc. In
other words: the 'natural basis' of our morality becomes narrower,
and the human being increasingly becomes its own creator and
designer. Especially unnerving is the fact that the permissibility of
certain actions is now dependent upon a definition – and that *we*
make these definitions. The removal and reuse of organs is certainly legitimate according to the brain death definition: adhering
to the cardiac arrest definition it amounts to human vivisection.

Substantialist criticism of the attempt to play God has the same goal as substantialist reference to human nature: both cases involve a search for a pre-determined, and thus *unshakeable* moral orientation. Characteristic of this yearning for an unshakeable moral orientation is a comment by the biologist, Robert Sinsheimer, quoted by Leon Kass, according to which the prospective chances of gene technology lie more than anything in the human being's consequent ability to transcend its own nature. Even in ancient mythology the human being was limited by its 'essence', it was unable to rise above its own nature and determine freely its own fate. Yet what Sinsheimer considers a 'cosmic event', is for Kass a threat to all things human:

> The idea of man as that creature who is free to create himself is purely formal, not to say empty. It provides no boundaries that would indicate when what was subhuman became truly human, or when what was at first human became less than human; moreover, the freedom to destroy (by genetic manipulation or brain modification) one's nature, including the capacity and desire for freedom. It is, literally, a freedom which can end all freedom. And it provides no standards by which to measure whether the changes made are in fact improvements.
>
> (Kass 1972, pp. 60–1)

The feeling of losing ground could hardly be made clearer, equally the conviction that only *pre-determined* – whether by God or by Nature – criteria can deliver an effective orientation for human action, and that losing such pre-determined criteria also means the loss of moral orientation altogether. Yet there can be no doubt that it is illusory to trust in such pre-determinism. In actual fact, the human being has always been the subject of its morality, just unknowingly. Values and norms came into being spontaneously. They are the expression of thousands of years of interactive human experience, passed on within the cultural tradition of each epoch from generation to generation, so that each generation was presented with a pattern of moral orientation which it was expected to adopt, but not – consciously – to alter. The necessity of adapting to new developments, and especially scientific and technological innovations, is a phenomenon which was unknown until the recent past, or maybe even the present. The fact that the human being is the subject of morality is nothing new; what is new – expressing the increasing reflexivity of modern societies – is the human being becoming *conscious* of being the subject of morality. It is correct to say that we are not only free to act, but also to establish the moral criteria for our actions: we are the masters of our morality.

Yet existentialist pathos of freedom is just as rash as substantialist fear of losing ground. The fact that we are the subjects of our morality does not necessarily mean that we are 'free' to treat that morality as we please; and the fact that the foundations of our morality are not unshakeable does not mean that morality is unfounded. In exceeding the framework of philosophical debate, and carrying out moral discourse not only within, but also with society, we quickly become aware that not 'everything is allowed'. In modern societies, a fair share of the valid moral norms and values are legally institutionalised; in this sense, morality is a *social fact* which may not have the dignity of being indubitable and inviolable, but which nevertheless exists, and which must be taken into account with every action which is put into practice. This is also true of the way in which many writers believe scientific and technological progress to be eroding morality:

> Technological possibilities seen as *social options* are always possibilities under normative conditions . . . . Thus the technological prospects within society do not simply increase at the same rate with which we are able to control Nature with scientific explanations and experiments. New methods of killing or destroying human beings are just as contemptible as past methods, and are therefore ruled out as viable options from the start. To put it pointedly: the social problems connected with technological dynamism arise from an increase in the *legitimate* options available.
>
> (van den Daele 1986, p. 161)

Whatever the GenEthicist or the reproduction technologist may think of valid and institutionalised morality, he/she may always put it to debate, but never at human disposal. Talk of human beings as the subject of morality is thus misleading whenever it abstracts from the concrete social and historical circumstances in which this subjectivity has to unfold, from the fact that it is not the single individual which is the subject of morality, but the moral community at any one time, and from the fact that an alteration to morality cannot be presented as the decision of an individual, but only as the result of a more or less intense process of rational discourse and negotiation of opinions and interests. It is, of course, conceivable that this discourse could conclude problematically; that the individuals involved in discussion and negotiation agree upon the adoption of a 'morality' which selfishly overlooks the interests of generations to come. The introduction of such a morality is just as conceivable as an ecological catastrophe which would hinder further human life upon this planet. Yet is this any worse than saying that the introduction of an 'immoral morality' would conflict with our meta-responsibility to the same extent as the destruction of our environment would our responsibility?

Part III

Subjectivity and self-alteration

10

The human being as subject

As we have seen, the anthropological concepts formulated in Western philosophical tradition are located in the area of tension between two opposed poles: human nature and human subjectivity. Dividing this area of conflict is the philosophical front line between the two competing GenEthical movements. Whereas substantialism emphasises the natural side of the human being and concentrates its ethical efforts on protecting natural 'substance' from intervention by technology, the various variations on anti-substantialism emphasise the opposite pole. Here the human being is above all *subject*: a rational, self-determining being capable of controlling Nature.

Human nature as an outside world

The newborn baby is totally wrapped up in its own nature, and its behaviour follows physical drives and needs. Yet soon a self-awareness begins to form, constituted not only in a differentiation between Self and Outside World, but also in a consciousness of its own body. The body does not coincide with the Self; far more, it confronts the Self as a kind of highly complex machine, functioning according to many different physiological and mechanical laws, a machine which we then have to learn how to 'operate'. An infant is not capable of coordinating its limbs to grasp an object or to crawl – let alone walk; neither is it able to speak, instead gradually shaping its spontaneous garbles through mimicry and practice. Later on, it is time to train precise movements, without which it would be impossible to learn the 'cultural technique' of writing. To put it briefly: we have to learn to control our own nature. Since Freud, if not before, we have also been aware that this control is not limited to our bodies. In every society, and especially industrial civilisation, individuals have to learn how to control their spontaneous needs and drives, whether these drives are brutally suppressed or sophisticatedly sublimated. These are all indications that the human being and human nature are not the same thing; the human body functions according to its own laws, these laws constituting human naturalness. We take it for granted – unconsciously – that this nature has to be *controlled*. It may seem strange that we have to control human nature, but it is plausible if we compare it with the much more common expression 'physical control' used in sport and acrobatics. Human beings – in contrast to animals, which also have to learn to control their bodies – are able to make endless demands of their nature, not restricted by their instincts and drives, but endowed with free will and consciousness. Sport and acrobatics have already been mentioned as examples of this diversity; 'spiritual' forms of training the body and its drives include autogenous training, yoga, celibacy and religious asceticism.

Our relationship to human nature is two-sided. On the one hand, there can be no doubt that human nature is the material basis of our existence and our subjectivity. Without it there would be no thinking, feeling or hoping, not even the most primitive vital expression. On the other hand, there can be just as little doubt that, as far as our subjectivity is concerned, human nature appears to be part of the outside world. However much human nature might be the natural basis of our subjectivity, it is also to be seen separately. According to its 'ontological' status, it is more a part of Nature than part of our subjectivity. A quick reference to the evolutionary theory of anthropogenesis since Darwin shows that human nature emerged from Nature. Biologically speaking, we are mammals. Independent of evolutionary origins, our continued existence as natural beings – and thus *also* our continued existence as human subjects – depends as much upon Nature as upon our own nature; if it comes to it, we can do without individual parts of our own nature (hair, finger nails, even limbs or organs) more easily than without parts of Nature (oxygen, water, food). Our own nature especially seems to be part of the outside world when it is confronted by our desires, our goals, our will or our needs. We never have absolute control over our bodies and our drives: both retain an element of independence which we are not capable of removing. However hard we try, we will never be able to fly, or to run 100 metres in two seconds; however much we would like to, we will never be able to survive for 24 hours without oxygen, or to solve complicated equations in our heads. Even when carrying out normal tasks, the body does not always obey as it should; when we are tired or unable to concentrate, when we are under the influence of alcohol or drugs, and especially when we grow old, the body often ignores our will and intentions, and reminds us that it can be a law unto itself. Even when the spirit is really willing, the flesh remains weak.

This is especially true in times of illness, probably the most obvious and painful reminder of how little coincidence there can be between our subjectivity and our nature. This also goes for genetic diseases. Pathology aside, who we are with regard to race, family, build, attractiveness, etc., is influenced not solely, yet partly by our genes; this becomes particularly apparent in a case of disease. Clinical experience confirms that diseases seem to gain a whole new dimension when prefixed by the word 'genetic' (Lappé 1979, pp. 40–1). Knowledge of 'bad genes' can sometimes be devastating. A common, somatic disease can often damage self-esteem and lead to a feeling of powerlessness, yet knowing that this disease is intrinsically connected with one's own biological constitution often leads to a feeling that one has been condemned by Fate. As early as the last century, the psychiatrist, Jean Marie Charcot, wrote about two cases of hysteria which he had examined and which he had chosen as typical of very many others:

> One might say that both have been touched by the finger of Ancient Fate, nowadays replaced by hereditary determination. Both might cry: What have we done, O Zeus, to deserve this Fate? Our fathers may have erred, but we, what have we done?
>
> (quoted from Leibbrand & Wettley, p. 533)

Today this feeling has not changed; genes seem to be a modern substitute for the furies of Greek mythology, or a secularised synonym for Original Sin (Lappé 1979, pp. 32, 45). This feeling is shared not only by those who are affected by genetic diseases themselves, but also by those who, as carriers of particular recessive genes, are themselves perfectly healthy, but whose children are potentially endangered. One's personal genetic constitution in general, and a genetic disease in particular, are experienced as *fated*. They appear not as part of one's identity, but as something foreign, threatening this identity.

Evaluating human nature

If, in a *first* definition, we characterise 'subjectivity' as the human ability to distance oneself from one's environment, to gain awareness of oneself, and to set oneself goals, human nature appears to be part of the outside world: it is 'ontologically' separate from subjectivity, and we reflect upon it as something external. It obstructs, if not bars us from practically realising our subjectivity. This implies that a study of human nature need not, and cannot, be valueless or disinterested. We can judge and evaluate our own nature according to our ideals and interests in just the same way as we can Nature herself. If we further consider the grave restrictions which human nature poses upon our subjectivity, then it can be no surprise that this kind of evaluation does not always end positively. There are many written accounts of negative evaluations of human nature. According to one famous episode, King Alfonso of Castile, whose Alfonsinian Tables went down in astronomical history, is supposed to have said that the world would have turned out better had God taken his advice whilst creating it. Considering the complexity and vagueness of Ptolemaic astronomy, such censure of creation may in retrospect seem plausible; nevertheless, it proves to be an historical myth. Whatever this 12th century anthropological censure might have been referring to in concrete terms, the topos of the incompleteness of human nature draws our attention to the fact that the self-aware human being may experience its own nature – just as Nature herself – as the basis of its existence, but that it also experiences it as the limit of its subjectivity.

It must be said, however, that the mere desire to fly, and the disappointment experienced when it proves to be impossible, are somewhat childish. As long as we simply continue to think up things of which we are not capable, the incompleteness of human nature will remain abstract and fantastic. In order to be taken seriously, it needs a criterion which is detached from mere dreamt-up desirables. The first, and maybe most significant, criterion is human nature itself. In its 'normal' form, it plastically demonstrates how and what the human being can be, and how and what it should be. The fully developed, strong and healthy human body forms the norm by which to assess the incompleteness of the underdeveloped body, the diseased body or the body which is worn out with age and use. The physiological achievements of animals are a second criterion. The eagle's sharp eyesight, the ability of owls and cats to see in the dark, the dog's fine sense of smell, the lion's strength, the gazelle's speed – how often have they all been used to measure human abilities? Here are many criteria which make corresponding human achievements pale in comparison, and yet they are not fantastic, for we know that they are biologically possible. Thirdly, and finally, technology has recently turned out to be such a criterion.

Human nature often comes off badly in comparison with the products of our own engineering skills. In a lecture on the human eye, for example, Hermann von Helmholtz, one of the founders of physiological optics, made an impressive list of this organ's insufficiencies and inadequacies:

> Now, it is not too much to say that if an optician wanted to sell me an instrument which had all these defects, I should think myself quite justified in blaming his carelessness in the strongest terms, and giving him back his instrument.
>
> (1893, p. 194)

If Helmholtz's criticism seems a little homespun, then this is not because of his chosen technological point of view, but because of the stage of development of modern technology. Nobody familiar with infra-red cameras would use the *camera obscura* to measure the efficiency of the human eye. If Helmholtz had compared the human eye with the technology available today, his censure would have been even more severe. It would also have to be generalised to cover all of human nature's inadequacies. This has been done on several occasions, for example by Stanislaw Lem in his *Summa technologiae*. Of all the inadequacies which Lem takes note of, I shall list three.

1. Owing to minimal redundancy during the transfer of genetic information from one generation to the next, a high risk factor is involved. Evolution:

> behaves like a constructor who is not concerned about all his cars reaching the finish, as long as the majority of them gets there. Our mentality is not familiar with this 'statistical principle of construction', according to which success does not depend upon all of the results, but upon the relative majority of them. This principle is particularly foreign when minimal informational redundancy has to be paid for not with defect machines, but with defect organisms, including human ones. Every year, 250 000 children are born with considerable genetic defects.
>
> (Lem 1976, p. 561)

2. Blood is kept in circulation by a rhythmically contracting mechanical pump; the muscle pushes against the vessels which supply it, narrowing their diameter and temporarily reducing its own supply of blood and oxygen – at the very moment when it requires the most. The consequence of this is that coronary artery disease is currently one of the most common causes of death. A much more elegant solution to the circulation problem would be one based on the electromagnetic pump principle, with the heart as an electric pump, and the blood corpuscles as electric dipoles. Through the buildup of electromagnetic fields, an even circulation of blood could be achieved, requiring less effort, fully independent of the elasticity of the artery walls and compensating for the variations in pressure caused by a mechanical pump (ibid., pp. 564–5).

3. Evolution's building blocks are 'tiny, sticky drops of protein'. It uses them to create an astonishing variety of substances and structures – bones, blood, glands, muscles, coats of hair, shells, brains, nectars and poisons – yet this choice of building material nevertheless limits, both quantitatively and qualitatively, the range of products available.

What would an organism have to be like in order to be more perfect than a biological organism? As a determined system – thus similar to natural organisms – it could be a system which maintains its ultrastability by absorbing energy in its most economic form, in other words as nuclear energy. Without oxidation, not only would the formation and transportation of blood become superfluous, but also the lungs, the entire pyramid of the central respiratory system, the entire chemical apparatus of tissue enzymes, muscular metabolism, and the relatively slight and severely limited strength of our muscles. Nuclear energy permits universal changes; a fluid medium is not the most appropriate (although such a homoeostasis could be built if somebody really wanted one); it opens up the most various possibilities of action at a distance, whether by lines ('cables' corresponding to nerves) and in discreet form, or in analogue form (radiation would, for example, be the equivalent of analogue, information-carrying, hormonal links); radiation and force fields are also able to influence the environment of the homoeostases, rendering the primitive mechanisms of our limbs, with their balls and sockets, superfluous.

(ibid., pp. 574–5)

We do not need to discuss here whether Lem's deliberations are convincing, nor whether the idea of a human organism driven by nuclear energy could possibly be realistic. Neither do we need to go into the fact that it has taken only two decades – by Lem's standards an extremely short space of time – for atomic energy to be considered a very dubious choice. Far more important – and here Lem agrees with Helmholtz – is that human nature is observed and evaluated 'from the point of view of the constructor' (ibid., p. 560): criticism and suggested alternatives are equally *'technocentric'*. Unlike Helmholtz's observation of the human eye, Lem does not primarily criticise the inadequacies of individual organs; his digressions to the heart or to other constituents of human nature have a merely illustrative function within an argumentation which is aimed at something far less specific: the constructive process of evolution in general. With this, Lem is referring to the second fundamental characteristic of recent expositions on the incompleteness of human nature.

Helmholtz's observations already signified an *evolutionistic* point of view. Yet – by emphasising the adaption aspect – they use Darwin's theory in order to redress the balance and hold on to the perfection of the human eye after all: 'The adaptation of the eye to its function is, therefore, most complete' (Helmholtz 1893, p. 201). This is, of course, only possible if the theory of evolution is interpreted teleologically, as was often the case in the 19th century. Nowadays, reference to the theory of evolution usually serves the opposite purpose: it is no longer perfect adaption which is emphasised, but imperfection. There are two arguments which are used to explain the inadequacies within human nature, the first referring to evolution in general, and the second specifically to human evolution. Evolution in general is no longer understood as being a process, the results of which are marked by increasing perfection, but as a procedure, always based on the contingent historical conditions of the time, and developing them both step by step and 'opportunistically', i.e. according to the options available at the time. This was what François Jacob was referring to when he characterised natural selection as 'D.I.Y.', and what Theodosius Dobzhansky meant by 'automatic, mechanical, planless and opportunistic' (Dobzhansky 1962, p. 393). Superfluous characteristics, adopted from past stages of phylogenetic development, are often passed on for tens of thousands of years; natural selection does not necessarily get rid of damaging characteristics, especially not if they exist in combination with other characteristics which we need to survive. Evolution's only 'goal' is the survival of the species, and not the perfection of the organism.

With regard to the human race and its evolution, we have to remember that we are dealing with a very new species. According to Julian Huxley, *Homo sapiens* emerged less than 500 000 years ago, and did not become a dominant species until after the Neolithic revolution, about 10 000 years ago.

> All new dominant types begin their career in a crude and imperfect form, which then needs drastic polishing and improvement before it can reveal its full potentialities and achieve full evolutionary success. Man is no exception to this rule. He is not merely exceedingly young; he is also exceedingly imperfect, an unfinished and often botched product of evolutionary improvisation.
>
> (Huxley 1964, pp. 253–4)

This becomes even clearer if we consider that the human being emerged during a period of radical evolutionary change; in several respects it represents a totally new species of animal. Yet the more fundamental and radical the phylogenetically novel construction proves to be, the greater the likelihood that it will display weaknesses and insufficiencies.

> As a product of evolution, man is only roughhewn: he lacks the biological polish that comes from a long and slow adaptive improvement through natural selection.
>
> (Dobzhansky 1962, p. 396)

It is not possible here to examine how empirically convincing this interpretation of evolution may be; far more important is the fact that, with the theory of evolution, the topos of human incompleteness became scientifically significant in a manner previously unknown. For the first time, insufficiencies within human nature, such as the birth pains peculiar to *Homo sapiens*, or the frequency with which complications arise during child delivery (ibid.), or some less well known insufficiencies such as the susceptibility of newborn babies to haemolytic diseases, or the insufficient healing of wounds to the skin (Medawar 1955, pp. 123–3), all became potentially explainable in theoretical terms. Even the ancient theory about the inferiority of the human being because of its inefficient individual organs, or because of its increased susceptibility to disease, could finally be explained in theoretical terms with the help of the theory of evolution. This is especially clear if we take the example of upright gait, which, as we are already aware, is considered one of the most important features of the human genus, both biologically and symbolically.

Critique of upright gait

The human being's upright gait may, as Medawar writes, 'be a constant source of moral satisfaction, but it has certain serious mechanical drawbacks' (1955, p. 127). We have been aware of many of these disadvantages for as long as we have known that they are not to be found in the anatomical structure of any other mammal, including our nearest relation the primate. In the 18th century, independently of any thought that the human being could be phylogenetically originated from the animal kingdom, it was possible to prove the disadvantages of upright gait with comparative anatomy. This was done in an academic speech held by the Italian anatomist, Peter Moscati, reviewed in German translation by Immanuel Kant in 1771. Kant begins his discussion with an ironic reference to a precursory philosophical theory, and then goes on to examine Moscati's speech in minute detail:

> Here again, we have 'natural Man' on all fours, brought back into this condition by an anatomist, since Rousseau as a philosopher did not succeed. Dr. Moscati proves that the upright gait of Man is enforced and against nature. Man can maintain himself and move in an upright posture only with discomfort and disease. This proves that he has been misled by Reason to deviate from his first animal organization. |
> In his interior organization Man does not differ from those animals which stand on four legs. If he raises himself up, his bowels, particularly the foetus in pregnant persons, assume a hanging and half-inverted position which, if constantly maintained, can cause deformation. When the heart is compelled to hang down, it assumes a sloping position, resting on the diaphragm, and its point slides towards the left side. This inclines Man unavoidably to suffer from palpitation, asthma, dropsy in the chest, &c.
>
> (Kant 1963a)

We shall skip the additional diseases and hardships on Kant's list, and go straight to the end of his discussion, a brief and conclusive philosophical interpretation of the problem.

> We see from this thesis that nature was first bent on preserving Man as an animal species; but the germ of Reason was also implanted in him. Then he assumed the position best fitted for this purpose, which is the upright one. By this he gains enormously over the animal, but he must resign himself to some discomfort as a retribution for having raised his head so proudly over his old comrades.
>
> (ibid.)

If we compare this list of inadequacies with the disadvantageous consequences of our upright gait reported by modern biological scientists, we notice that, although some of the details may have changed, the overall diagnosis remains the same (Dobzhansky 1962, pp. 336–7; Medawar 1955, pp. 122–33). The important difference is not in the description, but in the theoretical explanation. From the evolutionary point of view of the modern biological scientist, these inadequacies are the result of the opportunist manner in which natural selection tends to proceed. The human being's anatomical, physiological structure has emerged from a redrafting of the 'plans' otherwise used to build mammals; these 'plans' are based on four legs and a horizontal spine, so that numerous compromises and provisions were necessary in order to redesign it to include upright gait.

> As Evolution shaped our genus, she worked extraordinarily fast. Her specific tendency to preserve constructional solutions from an earlier genus has burdened our organisms with a series of defects unknown to our four-legged ancestors. In the latter, the pelvis does not have to support the weight of the inner organs. Because the human pelvis does, muscles have formed which are a considerable hinderance to the birth process. Upright gait has also had a negative effect on our blood circulation. Animals do not suffer from varicose veins, one of the plagues of the human body. The enormously increased brain capsule has led to a 90° twist in the pharynx (at the joining point with the gullet), causing a build up of air. As a result, many aerosols and microorganisms become deposited along the walls of the pharynx, rendering the pharynx a trap for a great number of infectious diseases. Evolution has attempted to combat this by surrounding the critical point with a ring of lymphatic tissue, but not only has this improvisa-tion not had any effect: it has become a cause for new complaints, since this build up of tissue is the focus for permanent infections. I do not maintain that our animal ancestors were ideally constructed. From an evolutionary point of view, every genus which is capable of surviving is 'ideal'. I merely maintain that, even with our miserable level of knowledge, it is possible to think of solutions, whether or not they can yet be put into practice, which would free human beings from count-less causes of suffering.
>
> (Lem 1976, pp. 508–9)

No further explanation of the evolutionary background of this pas-sage is necessary, nor of the 'naturalising' philosophy resulting from it, in which the human biological constitution appears to be the result of a specifically opportunistic constructional procedure, characteristic of evolution, the result of an historical process marked by chance. Human nature did not have to turn out the way it is today; it could have developed differently. And since we cannot simply assume that human evolution has come to a stand-still, we may not see human nature as it is today as a finished product. We are dealing with a certain stage in the development of our biological constitution. Thus human nature is contingent in two ways: (a) because of the fortuitousness of the historical process from which it has emerged and (b) with regard to the point in time at which we are observing it.

Subjectivity

The diagnosis of a 'naturalisation' of human nature would be commonplace if the options becoming available through gene and reproduction technology did not lend it a practical accent, one previously unknown and subtly introduced by Lem in his last sentence. Lem's philosophy is characterised by an amalgamation of evolutionistic and 'technocentric' observations of human nature. Terminologically, this is clear from his constant references to the 'constructional solutions' for human nature favoured by evolution. For 'constructional solutions' can end in more than one way, and each one contains an element of randomness. This is the deciding factor in the situation at stake here: the moment that alternatives are hinted at, the human being's present biological constitution becomes disposable.

Here the historical distance between Lem's and Kant's texts becomes clear – a distance which, due to the noticeable correlations in both diagnoses, is easily overlooked. According to Kant, the upright gait of the human being is a prerequisite for human subjectivity, and we 'must resign [ourselves] to some discomfort'. Lem would certainly support the first half of this argument, but not the second. Upright gait, he might argue, may be the biological basis of human subjectivity, but this does not mean that we have to put up with its disadvantages. Precisely because we as human beings are endowed with subjectivity, we are in a position to overcome such hardships, and the source of suffering and boundary to our subjectivity which they entail. We are rational beings, capable of self-reflection, beings in a position to articulate our needs, beings with sufficient technological imagination and skill at our disposal to dream up and put into practice – if not just yet – alternative solutions to the constructional problems of human nature: as such beings, we should not be prepared to 'put up with' any facet of nature, but should use our subjectivity to improve it. Hegel described the transition from the merely subjective to the objective as unavoidable: For him the subject is

> the total, not only the internal, but also the realisation of the internal through and in the external.
>
> (*Ästh.* I, p. 104)

Human subjectivity no longer appears as a theoretical ability, as self-reflection and self-determination, but as a practical ability: more than anything the ability to assert oneself against Nature, and actively to shape and to alter one's objective living conditions.

In a *second* definition, we could therefore comprehend 'subjectivity' as the epitome of all those capabilities which put human beings in a position not simply to adapt to their environment, but to alter it to meet their needs. This definition of subjectivity revolves around the ability to use technology to control Nature, as human beings have been bent on doing since they began making tools and building shelters in the early stages of their development. What we have learnt to take for granted in the context of Nature – our search to protect ourselves from Nature's 'blows of Fate' through technological control – seems new and unfamiliar when applied to our own nature. Bearing the 'naturalisation' of human nature in mind, it seems logical to extend subjectivity beyond the rest of Nature to cover our own. After learning how to protect ourselves from the hardships of the weather with clothing and shelter, we have now begun to learn how to protect ourselves from the hardships of our own nature. From the hand-axe used by our forefathers for various tasks to the laparoscope used by modern surgeons use to aspirate the ovaries, technological development has been a continous process. If we consider in sufficiently abstract terms the purpose served by technology through all the stages of this long process, it has not changed from the Stone Age to the present day.

> Our basic ethical choice as we consider man's new control over himself, over his body and his mind as well as over his society and environment, is still what it was when primitive men holed up in caves and made fires. Chance versus control. Should we leave the fruits of human reproduction to take shape at random, keeping our children dependent on the accidents of romance and genetic endowment, of

sexual lottery or what one physician calls 'the meiotic roulette of his parents' chromosomes'? Or should we be responsible about it, that is, exercise our rational and human choice, no longer submissively trusting to the blind worship of raw nature?

(Fletcher 1974, p. 36)

Practical subjectivity is not viewed as just one human characteristic amongst many, but as an *essential* human characteristic. In this sense, Fletcher's dictum 'Control is human and rational; submission, the opposite of control, is subhuman' (1974, p. 157) is not aimed at describing factual human behaviour, but at a much more significant and wide-ranging definition. In other words, the ability to use technology to control not only subjective but also objective living conditions is a human characteristic, and the specifically human dimension of the human being is realised in this characteristic. It is of secondary importance whether this control over living conditions refers to Nature herself or to human nature. Far more important is that in this control, subjectivity is manifested as one – if not *the* – expression of human being. In a moral theological essay on the subject of gene manipulation, Karl Rahner reinforces the view that the human being has always been a being which has manipulated itself, and that this self-manipulation will continue with the present and future technologies aimed at controlling evolution:

It is impossible to reject on principle the idea of human 'genetic manipulation' as an immoral project. Christianity perceives the human being not just as a product of 'Nature', with Nature as the *only* entity able and entitled to define and shape it. The human being is not just the being which may and should, on behalf of God and in continuation of His task of creation, 'subjugate the Earth' (in other words, the environment). Far more, it is the being which is committed and changed in its freedom to itself. In this respect, it has to 'manipulate' itself. Freedom is the unavoidable *necessity* of self-determination, through which the human being – albeit from a given starting-point and within an horizon of available possibilities – 'makes' *itself* what and whom it wants to be, and will ultimately be within the remaining validity and eternity of its free decision. The fact that this planned self-determination ('self-manipulation') used to extend only to the individual, morally transcendent realm of convictions and conscience, may at first hinder our views about the human being in this respect, but it does not alter this fact of transcendental necessity: insofar as the human being is committed to itself, it is (within the limits of its 'nature' and its 'history') a 'self-manipulating' being. Today, its basic essence has entered the dimension of historical and social experience: the human being is now able to manipulate itself with regard to its incarnate and social tangibility, and – even more of a contrast to before – to plan this manipulation rationally and guide it technologically.

(Rahner 1967b, pp. 289–90)

Self-alteration

Whereas substantialism declares the conservation of human nature to be a central ethical principle, subjectivity implies that human nature is not a value *per se*. As the natural basis of subjectivity, human nature may not be totally value-free; but it does not have a value in its own right, rather gaining one in relation to subjectivity. Insofar as the attribution of a value can be expressed in quantitative terms at all, it could be formulated thus: the more human nature enables subjectivity to unfold, the more value it has; and the less it does so, the less value it has. Human nature *can* therefore be worthy of protection, but it is not necessarily so: not when it restricts subjectivity, and obstructs its free unfolding. The crassest examples of this kind of restriction are disease and death. A dead human being is robbed of all its subjectivity, and the subjectivity of the diseased is more or less severely curtailed. The latter are restricted in their actions and movements, maybe even in their capacity to think and decide. Disease not only limits the subject in its feeling of well-being; it also prevents it from fully exploiting its self-determination. It is easy to see why such limitations to subjectivity constitute a good reason to use technology to intervene in human nature.

But our subjectivity is not only limited by a pathological deviation from the norm. There are many ways in which normal, healthy human nature also restricts the satisfaction of our needs and the free development of our goals. The human being's physical and spiritual capabilities are as limited as its days, and there are many things which we would like to do as individuals or as a genus which we are not able to do, because our inner natural conditioning prevents us. It can hardly come as a surprise that this factual limitation of human subjectivity is the impetus for projects aimed at removing these natural barriers, at first partially, and then maybe totally.

Self-alteration is a result of human subjectivity, and also of the way the human being is. The human being creates itself. In a *third* definition, subjectivity may be seen as a dynamic principle of continual self-alteration and enhancement, entering a new dimension with the advent of gene technology. In this sense, the newer concept of subjectivity, to be found in particular in the works of Kant and Hegel, extends and radicalises the concept of human self-preservation with the concept of human self-enhancement throughout history.

This definition of the human being does more than merely describe what the human being is; it has a normative dimension. If, as subject, the human being is capable only of unfolding the possibilities which it and only it possesses, thus becoming a 'human being' in the full sense of the word, then the normative conclusion to be drawn from this would be that human beings *ought to* strive to control their living conditions as comprehensively as possible. Realising the options open to them is not simply an option which can be accepted or rejected at will. It is morally expected of humanity, as well as of each human being individually, that such potentialities are not neglected, but developed, using all the powers at our disposal. This is Kant's argument in the passage quoted above, deeming it to be Nature's will that the human being develops its ablities all on its own in order to prove itself worthy of living. Also to be viewed in this respect are the 'duties towards oneself', which every human individual possesses, and which prevent him from committing suicide when life becomes too much, or from 'preferring indulgence in pleasure to troubling himself with broadening and improving his fortunate natural gifts' (Kant 1949, p. 82) through sheer idleness. According to Kant, neither of these actions would stand the test of the categorical imperative: not suicide, because as a maxim it leads to a contradiction, and not the neglect of individual abilities because this cannot be desirable as a universal law: 'For, as a rational being, he necessarily wills that all his faculties should be developed, inasmuch as they are given to him for all sorts of possible purposes' (ibid.). There is no need here to go into the difficulties which Kant's examples raise, or the extent to which the categorical imperative can be a valid universalisation test for moral rules. What we should take note of is the fact that, starting from a self-definition of the human being as a subject, subjectivity acquires a normative dimension. If the human being only becomes a human being when and insofar as it is a subject, then it has to comprehend its subjectivity as a moral obligation.

For the substantialists the idea of self-alteration is unacceptable because it presupposes the reduction of human nature to a piece of matter without inherent value. Yet substantialism is also mistrusting of emphasis upon human subjectivity, fearing – and understandably so – that the prospect of self-alteration is a corollary of accentuating human freedom and self-determination. The more we take subjectivity as the basis for our image of humanity, the less we are able to tolerate the factual limits of this subjectivity. Yet, from the substantialist point of view, such tolerance is necessary and salutary. In total contrast to the position defended by Karl Rahner, other Christian writers have, especially, strictly condemned the idea of autoevolution or self-manipulation:

> Christian *faith* desires to teach human existence within the relationships which make life possible, and which at the same time limit it. Christian *ethics* has to describe these relationships and outline these limits. This should be maintained despite the frequent assertion – including from theologians – that a decisive characteristic of the human species is its constant drive to go further, to transcend itself, in order to search for an as yet unfound identity with itself and its history. Because it is not satisfied with itself, the human being is constantly to exceed its limitations. If similar demands are made of the human mind, then there is no reason why an attempt should not be made to take the human *physis* further, to construct a better, more powerful human being. Yet will the human being not discover new dissatisfaction and problems every time another border is crossed? Instead of constantly calling for limitations to be exceeded, Christian ethics should teach recognition of life's limitations through God, and modesty within the limits which God has deemed it beneficial to set, so that within these limits the human being is capable of doing what is good and what may reduce human suffering.
>
> (Eibach 1983, pp. 190–1)

This statement puts forward the anthropological view that renunciation and moderation are more fundamental to the human being than subjectivity is. The concept of essential human limitation is used to counter that of self-determination and, especially, *self-alteration*. The concept of 'limitation' – whether set by God or Nature – acquires a key position in the criticism of gene technology.

Autonomy

Emphasis upon salutary limitations raises the matter of where they are to be found. We can only distinguish clearly between what may (legitimately) be done within the limitations, and which actions would (illegitimately) exceed these limitations, if we have exact knowledge as to the location of these limitations. The substantialists believe that only human nature may serve as orientation for establishing these limitations. Even if the 'naturalistic fallacy' is avoided, and the human freedom to decide for or against this orientation emphasised, this strategy still encounters not only the practical difficulties discussed above, but also serious problems of justification. Kant rejected any structuring of ethics according to actualities in Nature or human nature:

> Empirical principles are not at all suited to serve as the basis of moral laws. For if the basis of the universality by which they should be valid for all rational beings without distinction (the unconditional practical necessity which is thereby imposed upon them) is derived from a particular tendency of human nature or the particular circumstance in which it is found, that universality is lost.
>
> (Kant 1949, p. 98)

He defines practical reason as the ability to act exclusively according to laws one has chosen oneself, independently of all natural actualities. Put another way, this means that only those values and norms which have their origins in the free decision of the subjects may be deemed moral, whereby 'freedom' should not be understood as subjectivistic arbitrariness, nor as decisionistic randomness. It is supposed that moral self-determination is structured according to the standards of reason, which lead to the obligation inherent to practical reason, characterised by Kant as the 'categorical imperative'.

This insistence that morality is independent of all natural actualities complies with the various strains of subjectivistic GenEthics – regardless of the individual extent to which these variations are prepared to follow Kant's moral philosophy. The principle of subjectivity, once formulated and introduced, cannot remain restricted to the relationship between the human race and Nature; in order to be consequent, it must also cover morality. It is no coincidence that, in their works on the problems involved in gene and reproduction technology, as well as ecology, various authors have emphasised the unavoidability of human decision making. As long as this emphasis is not radicalised to decisionism, bent on revealing every justification to be the mere rationalisation of resolutions, it can only be interpreted as confirmation of Kant's principle of human moral *autonomy*.

> Autonomy of the will is that property of it by which it is a law to itself independently of any property of objects of volition.
>
> (Kant 1949, p. 97)

Introduced by Kant as 'the sole principle of morals' (ibid.), the concept of autonomy is directed against any external determination (heteronomy) of the practical will, whether through the dogmatic establishment of morality, or whether through empirical facts, including – for Kant – human nature. Human subjectivity is the only source of morality and the only basis for its validity.

In a *fourth* definition, human subjectivity may therefore be defined as the possibility – and necessity – of moral self-legislation. The human being is the subject of its morality; it is unable to find this morality set out anywhere, not in Nature, nor in a heavenly book of rules, and is thus forced to create it itself. The human being is not only subject to this morality: it is also its designer. It should be emphasised that the notion of autonomy does not necessarily involve that hubristic presumption included as a warning in critical references to 'playing God'. With his categorical imperative, Kant's autonomy excludes not only any arbitrariness and randomness within moral legislation, but also any egotism, whether individual or collective. The only thing which is really autonomous is the will, not allowing itself to be influenced by contingent, external impetus, preferring to follow freely the criteria of practical reason. Without such freedom, *responsibility* would be impossible, whilst any reduction in autonomy limits the freedom to decide and to act, thus removing responsibility. This is the reason why all attempts to derive moral obligations towards Nature from Nature herself prove to be counter-productive.

> Each Naturalism – regardless of its motivation – is geared against the idea of autonomy. For whatever could possibly be justified as 'a duty' is to be traced back to something resulting 'from Nature'. That is why I believe that Naturalism – even if it is intended to strengthen the basis of moral argumentation for a desired alteration of human prac- tice – ultimately flouts the imperative of responsibility. The attempt to base an ethics of responsibility on the concept of Nature seems to me to be a contradiction in itself. For, wherever it has been attempted in the past, Naturalism has proved relieving of responsibility, or even eliminating of responsibility . . . An ethics of responsibility, of responsible interaction with Nature, will – so I believe – only make sense if the idea of autonomy is strengthened.
>
> (Schäfer 1986, pp. 10/13)

The insistence upon the idea of autonomy, as well as the relevant criticism of naturalising strategies to justify morality, are not lim- ited to the reproach of 'naturalistic fallacy' as one of the invalid modes of argumentation, logically and methodologically speaking, but also have a deep moral and practical importance. This is the only way of philosophically anchoring the notion of responsibility; for if one is not recognised as subject and not assumed to be autonomous, one cannot be burdened with responsibility.

GenEthical subjectivism

Analagous to the 'substantialistic' point of view, it seems appropri- ate to characterise each approach within GenEthics which takes up this fourfold definition of human subjectivity as *subjectivistic*. GenEthical subjectivism is characterised by its strict insistence upon human subjectivity. It considers the human being not merely as factual subject, but sees subjectivity as an obligation. Its central task is the ethical legitimation and support of this subjectivity. With regard to this approach, 'subjectivism' does not imply a prin- cipal scepticism as to the possibility of justifying moral norms objectively and rationally; it implies neither that each moral judgment is merely the expression of an individual's subjective approval nor disapproval. Rather it is based upon a specific interpretation of the human being, according to which the latter is essentially subject. The moral autonomy of the human being plays a key rôle here, and its direct corollary is the delegitimation of all pre-determined sources of moral norms, whether they originate from Nature, from metaphysics or from religion.

This in turn includes a premise of considerable scope, characteristic of subjectivistic GenEthics, and separating it from its substantialistic competitor. If the human being is autonomous, the moral legitimacy of technological intervention in reproduction – including the most fantastic measures within an autoevolutive strategy – may no longer be disputed *a priori*. Reference to the 'holiness' of human nature can no longer be used as an argument against such intervention or against an autoevolutive project; all of these things are fundamentally worthy and capable of being discussed. Yet this is exactly what the substantialist contests:

> Just imagine parents who would like a child with three eyes, four arms or a tail. There is nothing to discuss or weigh up responsibly in such a case. A human discussion about the desirability of other, as yet uncreated 'human beings' is really a discussion with God. He chose to create the human being in His image.
>
> (Löw 1983, p. 47)

In contrast to this substantialistic taboo, subjectivism assumes that not even suggestions in favour of the most adventurous and radical manipulations may simply be rejected *a priori*, having instead to become the object of a process of moral discussion and evaluation. The result of this evaluative process is open, and a decision as to the moral legitimacy of such interventions is yet to be met; nevertheless, the subjectivist renders human nature disposable. As long as a contradiction exists between human nature and human subjectivity, the alteration and even total reconstruction of Nature is legitimate.

> In the future our ability to constrain and manipulate human nature to follow the goals set by persons will increase. As we develop the capacities to engage in genetic engineering not only of somatic cells but of the human germ line, we will be able to shape and fashion our human

nature in the image and likeness of goals chosen by persons. In the end, this may mean so radically changing our human nature that our descendants may be seen by subsequent taxonomists as a new species. If there is nothing sacred about human nature (and no merely secular argument could show it to be sacred), there is no reason why, with proper reasons and with proper caution, it should not be radically changed.

(Engelhardt 1986, p. 377)

11

From substance to consequence

Morality is made for man,
not man for morality.
William K. Frankena

If the subjectivistic GenEthical approach emphasises self-determination and self-alteration as the fundamental definitions of *humanum*, then this is not only an anthropological and theoretical antithesis to substantialism, but also a moral and practical one. For advocates of subjectivism, emphasising the subject side of the Western view of humanity is a matter of philosophical principle, as well as a humanistic attitude towards the purpose of morality. The entire point of morality is the benefit to be gained from it by humanity, and not to serve given authorities or 'higher' purposes. Protection of human substance is therefore replaced by evaluation of the consequences of human action, for it is here that the aforementioned benefits must ultimately find expression.

Suffering

In his programmatic writing on utilitarianism, John Stuart Mill attributed to every human being the ability to live a fulfilling and happy life, as well as the chance of doing so,

> if he escape the positive evils of life, the great sources of physical and mental suffering – such as indigence, disease, and the unkindness, worthlessness, or premature loss of objects of affection.
>
> (Mill 1969a, p. 216)

He accepts that one has to be fairly lucky to avoid 'these calamities' completely.

> Yet no one whose opinion deserves a moment's consideration can doubt that most of the great positive evils of the world are in themselves removable, and will, if human affairs continue to improve, be in the end reduced within narrow limits. Poverty, in any sense implying suffering, may be completely extinguished by the wisdom of society, combined with the good sense and providence of individuals. Even that most intractable of enemies, disease, may be indefinitely reduced in dimensions by good physical and moral education, and proper control of noxious influences; while the progress of science holds out a promise for the future of still more direct conquests over this detestable foe . . . All the grand sources, in short, of human suffering are in a great degree, many of them almost entirely, conquerable by human care and effort.
>
> (ibid., pp. 216–17)

This is a programmatic declaration of war against all kinds of human suffering. The causes of such suffering include the diseases which may be prevented, cured or at least relieved using gene and reproduction technology. Take infertility, for instance, often viewed by those affected as a severe limitation to their practical options, maybe even experienced as a traumatic catastrophe. Women suffer particularly in cases of unwanted childlessness, as reported in numerous eye-witness accounts, for example in the Old Testament:

> And when Rachel saw that she bare Jacob no children, Rachel envied her sister; and said unto Jacob, Give me children, or else I die. And Jacob's anger was kindled against Rachel: and he said, Am I in God's stead, who hath withheld from thee the fruit of the womb? And she said, Behold my maid Bilhah, go in unto her; and she shall bear upon my knees, that I may also have children by her. And she gave him Bilhah her handmaid to wife: and Jacob went in unto her. And Bilhah conceived, and bare Jacob a son. And Rachel said, God hath judged me, and hath also heard my voice, and hath given me a son: therefore called she his name Dan. And Bilhah Rachel's maid conceived again, and bare Jacob a second son. And Rachel said, With great wrestlings have I wrestled with my sister, and I have prevailed: and she called his name Naphtali.
>
> (Genesis, 30: 1–8)

Two points should be noted in this passage. Childlessness is experienced as a serious blow of Fate, as a personal catastrophe. Yet instead of simply accepting Fate, an attempt is made to circumvent it with a procedure which today we would term 'surrogate motherhood'. More modern literary accounts (Bainbridge 1982) show that the attitude of those affected nowadays is the same as it was then.

Genetic diseases are a second, perhaps more serious source of human suffering. Let us consider briefly the following examples of serious hereditary illnesses. (1) *Cystic fibrosis* is the most common congenital, autosomally recessive, metabolic disease, and the most common paediatric chronic respiratory disease (1:1000). It leads to over-production in various exocrine glands, especially the pancreatic and bronchial glands. Because of the high viscosity of these secretions, the respiratory tracts become congested, in turn leading to pathological and often fatal changes in heart frequency. From the time they are born, the patients often suffer from a painful cough similar to whooping cough. At the same time they suffer from digestive trouble, rendering them particularly susceptible to infection, regularly affecting the respiratory organs. Discovering the disease early is crucial if treatment is to have a chance of success; about 80 per cent of the patients suffering from the disease today live to see their 19th birthday. (2) *Tay–Sachs syndrome* is an autosomally recessive enzyme defect which leads to an accumulation of ganglioside GMA in renal and cardiac tissue, destroying nerve and muscle cells. Symptoms of this disease are muscular hypotonia, reflex jumpiness and cramps. The central nervous system decays rapidly, accompanied by blindness and dementia to the stage of idiocy; there is no way of treating the disease, which ends in death after two or three years. (3) *Huntington's chorea* becomes apparent in muscular hypotonia, especially in rapid, uncontrolled and arrhythmic contractions of muscles or muscle groups in all regions of the body. The patients are constantly fidgeting and grimacing. The disease advances chronically and leads to personality loss and dementure. The most pernicious thing about this disease is that it does not break out until the sufferers are between 35 and 55 years of age. By this time most of them have children, who – because Huntington's chorea is an autosomal-dominant disease with full penetrance – are all affected. (4) *Lesch–Nyhan syndrome* is

an X-chromosomal recessive enzyme defect which leads to an accumulation of uric acid in the body of the patient. The consequences
are uncontrolled movements and a strong tendency towards self-
mutilation, through scratching and biting of fingers and lips.

In the light of such diseases, and the suffering they inflict upon
the diseased and their relatives, the human race seems called upon
to combat them with all the options available. It also seems consistent to relate Mill's declaration of war against the causes of disease
to human reproduction, and to call for a comprehensive employment of all the achievements made within the field of gene and
reproduction technology. In medicine, the fundamental ethical
principle is conscious control, in order to minimise suffering:

> Producing our children by 'sexual roulette' without preconceptive and
> uterine control, simply taking 'pot luck' from random sexual combina-
> tions, is irresponsible − now that we can be genetically selective and
> know how to monitor against congenital infirmities. As we learn to
> direct mutations medically we should do so. Not to control when we
> can is immoral. This way it will be much easier to assure our children
> that they really are here because they were *wanted*, that they were
> born 'on purpose'.
>
> (Fletcher 1974, p. 158)

Fletcher is not concerned with control for its own sake, with
realising technological potential merely in order to do everything
which may be done, but with helping to prevent concrete cases of
human suffering. The subjectivity manifested in technological
control is a human obligation, because true human essence is
realised within it, and because it serves, or can be used to serve,
human needs and interests. These needs and interests are the
highest value according to which human action may be measured.

Control or renunciation?

From a substantialistic point of view, this programmatic declaration of war against human suffering is fundamentally inappropriate. It is not that the substantialist rejects any attempt to reduce
human suffering; yet the substantialist does have three objections
to a programme of the kind put forward by Mill and Fletcher.

The latter is based on a melioristic hope which is *factually* illusionary, for we will never be able to exercise total control over all of our living conditions. This goes for external natural conditions influencing our existence as much as for causes of suffering which are embedded in our own nature. Not even extremely progressive medicine or a perfect health system would be able to put an end to all the existing genetic diseases. Thus when individual writers appeal for a crusade to exterminate hereditary diseases –

> Society should vote to extinguish muscular dystrophy, Tay Sachs disease, cystic fibrosis and sickle cell anaemia, just as it has practically put an end to smallpox, polio and measles
>
> (quoted from van den Daele 1985, p. 87)

– realisation is impossible purely for technical reasons. A significant number of genetic indispositions are not transferred to the children directly by the parents, but emerge as the result of an 'error' in the union of the parents' germ cells. This kind of mutation could only be registered by extending the practice of prenatal diagnostics to include (a) every single foetus, and (b) each of the *c.* 4500 genetic indispositions presently known. This would be more or less impossible for economical reasons.

> There can hardly be any doubt that desiring to reduce the number of severely handicapped persons within the Federal Republic of Germany by 5% (approx. 50 000) via genetic prevention would be a legitimate political goal, or that the achievement of this goal would mean considerable financial relief for the health system. At the same time, we must not forget that this strategy ignores 95% of the cases at stake.
>
> (ibid., p. 89)

The substantialists have convincing arguments to counter the exaggerated hope of a human race free from genetically conditioned suffering. The question is, however, whether the limitations affecting our chances of success can be a valid argument against attempts to make the utmost of these chances.

Yet it is not primarily for empirical reasons that the substantialists reject the general declaration of war against human suffering and its consequent overrating of health and quality of life. The main reason that they issue warning against Utopian visions of absolute health is because notions of health and quality of life which focus solely upon achievement and enjoyment, and which disregard renunciation, limitation, suffering and sympathy, represent a genuine threat to humanity.

(Eibach 1983, p. 208)

Important in this argumentation is not doubt as to the factual possibility of realising the ideal of absolute health, but that absolute health *as an ideal* is questioned. This is based on a view of humanity in which 'renunciation, limitation, suffering and sympathy' play a constitutive rôle: human existence is unavoidably fated; it necessarily involves renunciation and suffering. It is, however, not merely a case of stating the facts: there can hardly be any empirical doubt that human life usually involves suffering, nor that it usually demands renunciation to some degree, even from those who are not party to the worst suffering. The central argument of the substantialists is not that the human being will never be able to circumvent this fate, but that it is not supposed to.

The third objection is that an attempt to remove suffering completely would mean an arbitrariness of the means used to achieve this end. If we take seriously the principle which states that morality should always serve humanity, and if the service of humanity, the satisfaction of human needs and interests, is taken as being the highest moral value, then there can be no technology, no means which is bad *per se* and thus principally illegitimate, providing that it only serves this purpose. Fletcher, for example, reaffirms that the end justifies the means (1974, p. 121). Even if this may not be interpreted as confirmation that every end justifies every means, for the substantialists this point of view is nevertheless unacceptable. Paul Ramsey chose the means problem as the central point of interest in his examination of Muller's apocalyptic vision of a genetic decline of humanity, a decline which Muller claimed could only be stopped with the realisation of his gigantic eugenic project. Whereas Muller deduces a moral obligation to act (eugenically) from his prognosis of catastrophe, Ramsey maintains that a Christian or a Jew is no more obliged to combat a worsening of the human gene pool than to slow down entropy, to prevent the Earth colliding with another planet, or to prevent the sun from losing its heat (Ramsey 1970, p. 29). Christians are not aware of a single absolute goal which justifies every means; and were they to attempt to solve the problem of human genetic decline, they would constantly be aware of the premise that there may be a whole series of effective means, but that they are all inherently wrong, morally speaking.

> He knows that there may be a great many actions that would be wrong to put forth in this world, no matter what good consequences are expected to follow from them – especially if these consequences are thought of simply along the line of temporal history where, according to the Christian, success is not promised mankind by either Scripture or sound reason. He will approach the question of genetic control with a category of 'cruel and unusual means' that he is prohibited to employ, just as he knows there are 'cruel and unusual punishments' that are not to be employed in the penal code. He will ask, What are the right means? no less than he asks, What are the proper objectives?
>
> (ibid., p. 30)

It is only the first of these three objections which the subjectivists attach any importance to. Yet it is in this point that they tend to agree with Sigmund Freud, who did not doubt the necessity of fighting unhappiness, although he was pessimistic as to this fight's chances of success:

> We shall never completely master nature; and our bodily organism, itself a part of that nature, will always remain a transient structure with a limited capacity for adaption and achievement. This recognition does not have a paralyzing effect. On the contrary, it points the direction for our activity. If we cannot remove all suffering, we can remove some, and we can mitigate some: the experience of many thousands of years has convinced us of that.
>
> (Freud 1969, p. 23)

Thus however severe the limitations may be, we are not relieved of the obligation to make full use of the chances which remain. Only five per cent of all genetic diseases may actually be avoidable; but this small number affects the fates of 50 000 people in West Germany alone.

From a subjectivistic point of view, the other two objections are open to vehement contradiction. The obvious consequence of the first is that Fate acquires a normative solemnity, with suffering and renunciation acquiring an inherent *moral value*. Whereas the substantialists regret

the disappearing human readiness and ability to *accept* an unplanned
or even unwanted fate, to view it positively and bear it

(Eibach 1983, p. 148)

subjectivistic ethicists reject a glorification of Fate, suffering and
renunciation. Not only does this contradict the ideal behind subjectivity; it also contradicts the 'humanistic' orientation towards
human interests and needs. Instead of attributing an independent
moral value to suffering, we should combat it – and this is directed
against the third objection – with all our might and means. In
order for this to be possible, all the factors which influence human
life have to be controlled as closely as possible; this naturally
includes all the possible ways of deliberately controlling human
reproduction which achievements in the field of gene and reproduction technology have opened up. In this sense, subjectivity is
not an abstract philosophical principle; its practical application is
not a means to its own end, but a means of realising human needs
and interests, and of preventing human suffering. By applying its
subjectivity, the human being unfolds its essence and creates the
conditions which are necessary if its own needs are to be satisfied
and the living conditions of its fellow human beings and offspring
are to be improved. With this in mind, we not only have the right
to control our internal and external living conditions, but are
morally obliged to do so.

Increasing happiness

Probably the most consistent strain of ethics based on the consequences of human actions or rules of action is *utilitarianism*. Based
on the premise that all human beings endeavour to find happiness
and to avoid unhappiness, utilitarianism sees the maximisation of
happiness and the minimisation of unhappiness as the highest
principle or criterion of consequentialist evaluation.

> The creed which accepts as the foundation of morals, Utility, or the
> Greatest Happiness Principle, holds that actions are right in propor-
> tion as they tend to promote happiness, wrong as they tend to pro-
> duce the reverse of happiness.
>
> (Mill 1969a, p. 210)

Following a well-known formula, it is the greatest happiness of the greatest number which is at stake, whereby 'happiness' is usually interpreted in the hedonistic sense as desire, joy, pleasure, and 'unhappiness' as hurt or displeasure. It is not possible here to go into detail about the various nuances of this approach or, in particular, the problems behind the utilitarian concept of happiness. However, utilitarianism does seem to be very suited to the ethics of a profession which, as it is, involves activities geared towards helping other people: it is reasonable to expect that, to the best of their ability, physicians should increase the happiness and decrease the pain and displeasure experienced by the patients in their care. Utilitarianism seems to be more or less made for the field of medical ethics, and it can come as no surprise that Joseph Fletcher describes his moral point of view as

> motivated by human well-being. In this approach what is right will be what is most humane, what is most conducive to human welfare and happiness. It is based on loving concern. The issue is between obedience to abstract principles and service to concrete human needs; one is dogmatic, the other is compassionate.
>
> (Fletcher 1974, p. 120)

Human needs must form the basis for every moral evaluation; rights may be deduced from needs, but not *vice versa*: 'The sanction for our humanistic ethics lies in need; need is the court of appeal' (pp. 124–5). The main objection of utilitarian humanism is the subordination of human needs to abstract moral principles; it is not compliance with principles which is decisive for the morality of actions or rules of action, but solely the question of whether their consequences contribute to satisfying human needs, and thus to an increase in human well-being.

In evaluating an action or a rule of action, the utilitarian will first examine its positive goals, the needs to be satisfied as a result of this action, and then – assuming the goal has been deemed beneficial – the potential side-effects, and whether they are damaging enough to destroy the expected benefit. In addition, the utilitarian will consider all the means of reaching the desired goal which are available, not ruling out any on principle. On the one hand, the utilitarians believe that the permissibility of a particular means cannot be decided upon independently of the context (Fletcher

1974, pp. 121–3). On the other, the 'costs' involved in employing a particular means become part of the total benefit calculation. Thus, even though not every end justifies every means, for the utilitarians there is no means which is inherently bad.

With regard to gene and reproduction technology, there is therefore a significant distinction to be made between the utilitarian point of view and the approaches discussed so far. The utilitarians are less interested in the moral feelings which these technologies could come into conflict with, and more interested in the benefit to be gained for the human being from their application. In actual fact, it is mostly *objections* to these technologies which have been formulated within deontological analyses; their potential benefits have been rather disregarded. If morality is not to be an abstract set of rules, but an institution which is there for us, and there to secure collective and individual human interests, it seems necessary to make the goals of these technologies, and especially the human needs which they are to satisfy, our primary concern, using this information as a basis for all further evaluation. These goals and needs are as easy to list as the objections (cf. Chapter 5):

1. Probably the oldest and most frequently practised intervention in human reproduction is the prevention of unwanted children. There is widespread consensus that contraception and birth control are legitimate practices in the face of the overpopulation threatening our planet and the individual right to self-determination. Despite religious objections, sexuality is usually viewed as the physical demonstration of love between partners, or as lust for its own sake, and seldom in terms of biological reproduction.

2. A second group of goals covers the aspects of gene technology aimed – in a broad sense – at the therapy of diseases. They include the various types of prenatal diagnosis, as well as the various attempts to cure genetic diseases, at present still few in number, and finally all the interventions aimed at curing infertility.

3. The 'improvement' of the human being can be a speculative goal behind technological interventions in human reproduction, whether through the alteration of particular characteristics of individuals or whether in the sense of 'reconstructing' the entire human race.

Rationalising the evaluation procedure

This emphasis upon the positive goals behind gene technological manipulations is in no way intended to suggest that they alone would have a systematic status within a utilitarian evaluative procedure, excluding from the start the possiblity of disastrous developments. Utilitarianism is very much concerned with both aspects. The basic idea behind it is not reduced to the theory that human action should serve human happiness, but, at the same time, includes a procedure which operationalises this idea. The utilitarian evaluative procedure consists in listing as thoroughly as possible the non-moral consequences of an action or rule of action, and in weighing up the number of positive consequences against the number of negative ones. Thus neither the positive nor the negative consequences may be suppressed. The action or rule of action at stake may not be deemed morally legitimate until the positive consequences are established as weighing more. This procedure is obviously based on a *rational* viewpoint, with a threefold definition.

1. First of all, rationality means the lack of prejudice involved in evaluation. Rationality can result only from a procedure which comes up to the standards customary within science (empirical convincingness, logical exactness, etc.) Utilitarians mistrust moral feelings; at least, they are not prepared to endow them with a higher status than psychological motives, which could give rise to a consequentialist evaluative procedure. For example, as long as the uneasiness surrounding technological intervention in human reproduction described earlier cannot be confirmed by the results of such a procedure it will maintain the status of a prejudice. As we have already seen from Fletcher's critique of 'abstract principles', the same goes for the implicit obligations postulated by deontological ethics, insofar as they may not be traced back to a spreading of human happiness. Utilitarianism strictly rejects reference to super-empirical bodies in order to justify moral norms, as philosophers have traditionally tended to do, for two reasons.

Firstly, they conflict with its fundamental presupposition that the highest moral principle is the maximisation of happiness. Secondly, all these 'higher' justificatory instances – God or Nature

– prove to be unjustifiable themselves and thus susceptible to modern suspicion of the metaphysical. Utilitarianism also requires certain values upon which to base its evaluative procedures; yet these are non-moral values which do not have to be introduced and justified with moral philosophy, but which can be ascertained empirically. Health is one such non-moral value which is doubtlessly held in equal esteem by almost all human beings. From a utilitarian point of view, every action or rule of action which serves to safekeep or reinstate health must be considered morally good (providing, of course, that the potential harm inflicted by this action does not weigh more). Utilitarianism thus continues in the anti-metaphysical tradition of modern philosophy, on the one hand rejecting as misanthropic every subordination of human interests and needs to abstract, 'higher' principles, and, on the other, showing a way in which moral evaluations may be made without any reference to metaphysical instances, solely by concentrating on empirically establishable, non-moral values. Utilitarianism thus avoids the difficulties involved in the substantialist assumption that human nature is unalterable; the non-moral values are not deduced from some substantialist assumptions about human nature, but may (at least in principle) be created anew for each evaluative procedure. If the majority of human beings should begin to favour disease instead of health as a desirable state – in the interests of a decadent increase in aesthetical sensitivity, for example – then the evaluative procedure could be adjusted to suit this change in values without a problem; the procedure is neutral with regard to the criteria upon which it is based, and therefore recipient to every historical alteration in human 'substance'.

2. Utilitarianism's claim to rationality rests upon its limiting the objects to be morally evaluated to actions and the results of actions. Whereas various other moral philosophies are concerned with the subjective side of morality, i.e. the basic convictions or intentions of the acting subjects, utilitarianism concentrates on the objective side of morality: on the actions of the subjects and their non-moral consequences. This shift in the object for moral evaluation may be traced back to the view that the morality of a character and the basic convictions of a person do not necessarily coincide with the morality of an action,

that a right action does not necessarily indicate a virtuous character, and that actions which are blameable often proceed from qualities entitled to praise.

(Mill 1969a, p. 221)

The advantage of such a shift is that any speculation about the good or bad subjective intentions behind an action is pushed aside to allow the action itself – as an objective, empirical fact – to become the object for evaluation. Such an 'objectivisation' is essential for the medical problems discussed here; for it cannot be the evaluation of the medical staff's characters and intentions which is at stake, but the evaluation of their actions. Whether a surgeon carries out an appendectomy for career or financial reasons, or whether he does so out of love and sympathy, is important for the moral evaluation of the surgeon, but not for the moral evaluation of the appendectomy. In the same way, GenEthicists are concerned with evaluating the *technologies*, and not with a moral assessment of the people developing and using them. Even the anti-utilitarian, Leon Kass, voices the fear that the greatest danger to humanity may be the 'well-wishers',

> for folly is much harder to detect than wickedness... The road to Brave New World is paved with sentimentality – yes, with love and charity.
>
> (1972, pp. 39/63)

This does not mean that ethics is not at all concerned with the subjective motives behind actions; insofar as the latter form empirical side-conditions, realistic ethicists will have to take them into consideration. But they do not constitute their actual object of evaluation.

3. Finally, utilitarianism may stake a claim to rationality in that it considerably extends the scope and significance of empirically decidable questions. By elevating the non-moral consequences of an action or rule of action to the highest evaluative criterion, utilitarian evaluative procedures are mainly concerned with observable facts: the sum of positive and negative consequences. The rest of the procedure is reduced to a calculation which then reveals whether the sum of positive consequences outweighs the sum of negative consequences, or not. Muller's criticism of negative eugenics by sterilisation outlined in Chapter 3 is an instructive example of the efficiency of this manner of observation.

Similar doubts may be expressed concerning Muller's concept of positive eugenics by germinal choice. Using a relatively simple mathematical model, it is possible to calculate the effect which a practical realisation of this concept would have upon the reproduction of single genetic characteristics. Since for the eugenicists the most favoured human characteristic – apart from health – is intelligence, we will take a look at the following example: a strict selection process, in which only the sperm from men with an I.Q. of 130 is used, would lead to a 1.5 increase in the average I.Q. of the next generation, assuming participation in the programme of 20 per cent of the female population. If 50 per cent of the female population were to participate, the increase would be 3.8. Yet in the generations to come, this growth would gradually dwindle until finally more or less disappearing altogether. This effect is obviously fairly minimal, suggesting that a similarly strict selection process should take place within the female population; the increase in intelligence would then double (Cavalli-Sforza & Bodmer 1971, pp. 768–70). This calculation provides us with conclusive results: since only 6 per cent of men have an I.Q. of 130, such a strict selection process would mean excluding 94 per cent of the male population – with the modest effect of increasing the I.Q. of the following generation by 1.5. For an increase of 3 it would be necessary to exclude 94 per cent of the *entire* population. It goes without saying that such a massive intervention in the reproductive behaviour of our society – apart from the fact that it would not be feasible – would mean a spectacular imbalance between the trenchant behavioural restrictions upon individuals and the non-moral benefits gained, so that from a consequentialist point of view it would have to be condemned. The great advantage of the utilitarian approach is that it is largely able to replace abstract, controversial ethical considerations with empirical analyses.

Utilitarian difficulties

Utilitarianism, with its emphasis upon rationality, lack of prejudice, science, etc., may have a significant strategic advantage over its deontological competitors with regard to *Weltanschauung*. Yet it is not without its own – and, as we shall see, unsoluble – share of problems, problems which are closely connected with this advantageous position. One of these advantages is the presupposition that ethical and moral differences of opinion may be settled empirically and quantitatively. If, in a particular situation, different points of view exist, then, according to utilitarian theory, they can (and must) be settled by carefully examining the consequences. This theory permits not only rational decisions between single actions and maxims governing actions, but also rational decisions between complex moral attitudes and *Weltanschauungen*. According to Fletcher (1974, pp. 138–9), the heavily controversial matter of abortion, for example, including the inextricably interwoven problems concerning the moral status of the embryo, may be decided by examining the consequences which each moral attitude towards abortion would lead to if carried through. And when Fletcher postulates that ultimately the position should be chosen which would contribute the most to human well-being, he presupposes something needy of proof: namely the possibility of comparing quantitatively positive and negative consequences.

The utilitarian calculus of interests assumes the existence of a universally accepted hierarchy of values, enabling the satisfaction of differing needs, the experience of happiness, pain or listlessness to be added up against each other to produce a definite – positive or negative – result. Yet precisely this is not the case. A quick look back at negative eugenics proves the point: would it not be just as possible to view an increase of 3 per cent in the average I.Q. as far more useful than an exclusion from reproduction of 94 per cent of the population would be harmful? – We just have to visualise two things. Firstly, such an increase in the average intelligence would not result in an even spread across all individuals; instead, the increase would be accumulated individually by a growing number of geniuses. In view of the growing complexity of modern societies and the progressively acute situation caused by industrial civilisation, an increase in intelligence, and especially in highly intelligent problem solvers, seems to have become necessary if the human race is to survive. This is, at any rate, Julian Huxley's main line of argumentation:

> The improvement of human genetic quality by eugenic methods would take a great load of suffering and frustration off the shoulders of evolving humanity, and would much increase both enjoyment and efficiency. Let me give one example. The general level of genetic intelligence could theoretically be raised by eugenic selection; and even a slight rise in its average level would give a marked increase in the number of the outstandingly intelligent and capable people needed to run our increasingly complex societies. Thus a 1.5% increase in mean genetic intelligence quotient (I.Q.), from 100 to 101.5, would increase the production of those with an I.Q. of 160 and over by about 50%.
>
> (1967a, p. 17)

The utilitarian might argue that, although restricting the rights of more than 90 per cent of the population is a high price, it is one which is worth paying in order for the human race to survive, for the sum of happiness produced by such a eugenic strategy is greater than the sum of listlessness.

This calculation in favour of eugenics is, of course, just as incomplete as the earlier one against it. A comprehensive utilitarian evaluative procedure would certainly have to take into account a whole series of additional factors. Yet regardless of how precise we choose to become, we will always come up against the question of whether it is possible to weigh up quantitatively such different values as the survival of the human race and the individual right to reproduce. And even if it were possible to render them comparable through the construction of a universal set of values, this would not remove the difficulties involved in utilitarianism. A simple mental experiment from the field of biomedicine may help to clarify the point.

> You have five patients in the hospital who are dying, each in need of a separate organ. One needs a kidney, another a lung, a third a heart, and so forth. You can save all five if you take a single healthy person and remove his heart, lungs, kidneys, and so forth, to distribute to these five patients. Just such a healthy person is in Room 306. He is in the hospital for routine tests. Having seen his test results, you know that he is perfectly healthy and of the right tissue compatibility. If you do nothing, he will survive without incident; the other patients will die, however. The other five patients can be saved only if the person in Room 306 is cut up and his organs distributed. In that case, there would be one dead but five saved.
>
> (Harman 1977, pp. 3–4)

It should be noted that this martial example concerns a decision between values which are materially exactly the same (human life) and different only in quantitative terms. If we take the utilitarian principle of maximising happiness seriously, then the only possible option in this case is to sacrifice the patient in Room 306: five human lives happen to be more than just one human life.

Avoiding evil

It is obvious that this conclusion would be contra-intuitive: it is immoral to kill a human being willingly even if this sacrifice could lead to many others being saved. The basic utilitarian theory of being able to balance out evil consequences with good ones, and *vice versa*, contradicts the asymmetry between good and evil which is characteristic of our morality. Consciously committed evil deeds cannot be justified through the good which they simultaneously produce. An alternative moral philosophy may be developed from this asymmetry, adhering to two fundamental achievements of utilitarianism: concentration on actions or rules of action and their consequences, and orientation towards human interests, avoiding the problems mentioned.

Bernard Gert put forward a most elaborate version of such a moral philosophy, based on the assumption that the *moral rules* forever being discussed in the various ethical systems, yet never without missing the point, actually form the centre of morality. Without going into the various characteristics of these rules, I would like to mention their fundamental substantive definition. Just their usual formulation – 'Thou shalt not kill!' – draws attention to the fact that they prohibit particular actions.

> Moral rules do not tell one to promote good, but to avoid causing evil. Thus it is not an accident that all moral rules are, or can be, stated as prohibitions.
>
> (Gert 1973, p. 69)

It is impossible to conclude from such a negative variant of consequentialist ethics that inflicting harm is justified in order to promote a larger quantity of good. One of this variant's cornerstones is the insight that 'the causing of evil cannot be balanced by the promotion of good' (ibid., p. 72). A grave restriction of the purpose and scope of morality is the price paid for the precision of its essence offered by this approach. According to Gert, the essence of morality cannot be defined – as in utilitarianism – as a general guideline for human action, as a kind of comprehensive and rational 'philosophy of life'. Gert believes that the definition should be far more precise. Morality is defined by a set of rules which postulates particular behavioural limitations, but which does not prescribe any positive behavioural goals. 'Morality has as its task the lessening of evil' (ibid., p. 149), and not the formulation of general acting instructions or goals in life.

In recognising moral rules as the highest principles, constituting inviolable duties, Gert includes a deontological element within his theory. Yet the reason why these rules are accepted is that everybody (with the possible exception of masochists) would like to avoid the consequences of overstepping the boundaries within them: death, pain, unfitness, loss of freedom or opportunity, unfulfilled desire, etc. Moral rules may thus be defined as 'rules that prohibit causing the kinds of consequences that rational men want to avoid' (ibid., p. 87). Free from all the other criticism of utilitarianism, this moral philosophy nevertheless remains obliged to the notion that the purpose of morality is the maintenance of human interests.

An operationalisation of this orientation of interests, which is not only ambitious but also illusory, is represented by utilitarianism, with its appeal for 'the greatest happiness of the greatest number'. Here a more modest, but much more realistic interpretation is suggested, emphasising avoidance and restriction of the harm which we are capable of inflicting upon our fellow human beings. Morality is not comprehended as being an institution for the promotion of social happiness, but 'as a protective device' (Habermas 1986, p. 20), protecting the rights of individuals from harm inflicted by other individuals. Such a negative variant of consequentialist ethics may serve as very convincing justification for one of the fundamental principles of medical ethics: the *primum non nocere* derived from the Hippocratic oath (cf. Beauchamp & Childress 1989). Morality's protective function must acquire particular significance within the field of biomedicine, for here the individuals expose themselves to potential harm from others.

More important than all the good which physicians or bio-engineers are capable of spreading is the worry that they could inflict harm upon the individuals at their mercy, or increase the suffering these individuals are already experiencing.

Discourse ethics

The premise that the purpose of morality is not to provide instructions for universal happiness, but 'to combat the *extreme vulnerability* of persons through care and consideration' (Habermas 1986, p. 20) is, anthropologically speaking, the basis of discourse ethics, a branch of ethics developed by Jürgen Habermas. Otherwise, Habermas rather tends to follow in the footsteps of Kant's moral philosophy, taking up the latter's basic notion that morality can be philosophically justified only on the basis of a universalistic moral principle, independent of empirical circumstances, and ensuring that norms of action are capable of being generalised. Habermas replaces the judgmental criterion for moral norms formulated within the categorical imperative with a 'discourse ethical principle', according to which a norm is only valid

> if, as *participants within a practical discourse*, all those potentially affected by this norm reach (or would reach) agreement concerning its validity.
>
> (Habermas 1983, p. 76)

With his discourse ethics, Habermas therefore goes further than Kant, localising the subject of morality not in an individually perceivable sensible being, but in subjects communicating with one another, attempting within this communication to settle their conflicts consensually. It is no longer a case of each individual adopting his/her own moral point of view: a moral viewpoint is adopted *collectively* in an exchange of practical arguments.

> A viewpoint is only impartial if it may serve as the basis for a generalisation of those norms which, since they obviously represent an interest common to all those affected, may expect to find common consensus – and which thus merit intersubjective acceptance. Impartial judgment is partly expressed in the principle which forces *each*

individual within the circle of those affected to take up the point of
view of *all the others* during the process of weighing interests.

(Habermas 1983, p. 75)

Habermas' moral philosophy is therefore a programme with two
levels. Firstly, it represents a *deontological* theory of the validity of
norms: only those norms able to pass the discursive test may stake
a legitimate claim to validity. Yet, unlike Kant, Habermas bases his
theory not on an individual, but on a collective subject of morality:
autonomy has become socialised.

On the second level, within the discourse, passing of judgment
is orientated towards the *consequences* of the norms of action. This
is because discourse ethics does not consider the subjects as mere
incarnations of 'pure, practical reason' (Kant 1949, p. 97) and
because it has no desire to extend the universalistic validity of the
norms beyond human beings to 'all rational beings without distinction' (p. 98), instead assuming real, empirical human beings
with needs and interests, who attempt to come to an agreement
regarding these needs and interests in practical discourse. The
concept of interest has a central position in Habermas' formulation
of the principle of universalisation. In order for a norm to be
valid, it is postulated

that the consequences and side-effects which could (foreseeably) affect
the satisfaction of the interests of each *individual* from a *common*
adherence to that norm must be acceptable to *all* those affected (and
preferred to the consequences of familiar alternatives).

(Habermas 1983, pp. 75–6)

There are therefore two reasons why discourse ethics – beyond its
deontological criterion of validity – represents a consequentialist
concept of evaluation. Firstly, it cannot permit any obligations
which have not been accepted as valid within the discourse. If the
discourse were presented with a predetermined validity, this
would impose severe limitations on the autonomy of the discourse
community, thus destroying the central premise of discourse
ethics, which states that the rational validity of moral norms can
be perceived only as the result of practical consensus, which
means that discourse can be its only foundation. Discourse ethics
could therefore only adopt pre-determined metaphysical, religious
or natural obligations at the cost of their very essence.

Secondly, discourse ethics directly follows the 'humanistic' definition of the function of morality, according to which we have no moral obligations

> to do anything that does not, directly or indirectly, have some connection with what makes somebody's life good or bad, better or worse. If not our particular actions, then at least our rules must have some bearing on the increase of good or decrease of evil or on their distribution. Morality was made for man, not man for morality.
>
> (Frankena 1973, p. 44)

As soon as, on the one hand, a realistic view of the human being and its actions is taken as a foundation, a picture which does not only take human orientation towards needs and towards human conveyance by interests into account as empirical fact, but which considers them to be principally legitimate, and, on the other hand, the function of morality is seen as the satisfaction of the needs of as many people as possible, as well as the ensurance of their legitimate interests, then weighing up the potential consequences becomes the central task of practical discourse.

> As shown by the formulation of the principle of universalisation, which takes into account the results and consequences of norms being commonly followed when considering the well-being of each individual, discourse ethics has included an orientation towards consequence within its procedure from the outset.
>
> (Habermas 1986, p. 27)

As an institution which exists to serve not abstract principles or supernatural bodies, but human beings, their interests and needs, moral discourse must refer to the consequences of norms of action. What is necessary to serve these – imparticular – interests, and to satisfy these needs, cannot be decided abstractly, but only by establishing before or afterwards the empirical consequences resulting from actions or rules of action.

Procedures and values

With its distinction between two very strictly separate levels, discourse ethics makes a general tendency within modern ethics explicit: the separation of rational evaluative *procedures* from the constitution of – not totally rational – *values*, stemming from historically changing needs. Utilitarianism always presented itself as a uniform moral philosophy, comprising a generally accepted theory of values, and providing an evaluative procedure. However, the history of utilitarianism sheds light on the fundamental independence of the consequentialist procedure from the frequently changing theories of happiness: the procedure can be carried out with any values. Discourse ethics therefore no longer claims to have a universally valid concept of happiness or the good life, from which a hierarchy of values may be deduced, instead programmatically denying this claim by leaving the constitution of values to concrete human beings and their historically changeable and individually different needs, and by concentrating on the rationally decidable, universally valid and deontologically binding *processes* upon which the validity of moral norms is based. According to Habermas, origin of the 'moral point of view' must thus be seen in connection with a differentiation within the practical sphere:

> the *moral questions*, which, with regard to the generalisability of interests or to *justice*, may always be decided rationally, may now be distinguished from the *evaluative questions*, which, taken very generally, represent questions concerning the *good life* (or self-realisation), and which may only be explored rationally within the unproblematic horizon of an historically concrete or a strictly individual form of life.
>
> (Habermas 1984, p. 225)

Behind the strict separation of the constitution of values from matters of morality in the narrower sense, there is an interest in securing the objectivity of morality. The definition of happiness and the good life can now be left to the discretion of historical change and individual preference within a pluralism of values, without having to doubt the deontological character of procedures involving moral decision making.

This kind of obligation, separated from all the problems involving values, is also called for within medical ethics. Without following Habermas' model of discourse, Tristram Engelhardt (1986) put forward a concept of a bioethics based on a similar distinction between two different tiers of morality.

The moral life is lived within two tiers or dimensions: (1) that of a content-poor secular ethics, which has the ability to span numerous divergent moral communities, and (2) the particular moral communities within which one can achieve a contentful understanding of the good life. The first is defensible in terms of general moral arguments regarding the nature of ethics. This tier offers some absolute and universal moral conclusions, even if they are content-poor. The second tier offers competing versions of the good life, including concrete accounts of virtues and vices. Here arguments are not conclusive and often, if not usually, require accepting certain basic premises that cannot be secured by argument.

(Engelhardt 1986, p. 54)

In pluralistic societies, this separation of a hard procedural core of morality from the soft dimension of competing convictions is the only way of retaining to the compulsion of norms without resorting to power and force.

Even with the failure to establish generally the authority of a particular moral sense, one can still have authority for common actions in pursuit of particular moral goods. One can secure a justification for moral judgments for certain biomedical policies. The authority is that of common assent. There is general meaning in the assertions, 'We may do this for all involved have agreed'; 'No one may use force with authority against the unconsenting innocent, for they have not consented either directly or indirectly through refusing to forbear from the use of unconsented-to force against other innocents'; 'If other individuals act against moral agents without their consent, their action is without authority and rational beings anywhere in the cosmos can see that such actions place those individuals outside of a community with moral authority. Such persons are then blameworthy in that one is justified in using force in defense against them. That is, they are worthy of having their wishes thwarted in such a circumstance.' In short, a form of moral discourse is secured for secular ethics, even though a general justification of traditional concrete ethical viewpoints fails. One is able to establish a procedural ethic, based on respect of the freedom of the moral agents involved, even without establishing the correctness of any particular moral sense.

(ibid., p. 45)

12

The problems of subjectivism

*It is better to be a human being dissatisfied
than a pig satisfied*
John Stuart Mill

The term 'subjectivity' signifies the philosophical foundation of an alternative to substantialism within the field of GenEthics. The concept of consequentialist ethics, geared towards the satisfaction of human interests and needs, sketchily defines the function of morality, and an appropriate moral evaluative procedure. The effects of gene and reproduction technology still have to be examined from the various points of view represented within subjectivistic ethics.

Discourse with the unborn

Whereas the substantialists tend to view new technological options as a burden, the subjectivists tend to evaluate them positively. The achievements of reproduction technology enable

> free individuals to achieve the biological destinies they choose, as, for example, within the area of reproduction. Thus, far from simply tolerating the free choices of individuals concerning themselves and consenting associates, biomedicine enables those choices, and secular bioethics supports that contribution as a proper one.
>
> (Engelhardt 1982, p. 72)

In connection with technological interventions in human reproduction, the somewhat casual reference to 'consenting relatives' is

something of a surprise, however. For how are the children created or manipulated by such interventions supposed to give their
consent? Gene and reproduction technology does create the
chance to make new, free, human decisions; yet one of the fundamental ethical problems of this extended decisional scope is that a
significant group of the persons affected by these decisions is
unable *per definitionem* to give its consent. A child which does not
yet exist is neither able to give, nor to withold its consent regarding its creation by *in vitro* fertilisation; and this exclusion from the
'informed consent' so important within medical ethics becomes
even more dramatic if we consider the prospective possibilities of
cloning or creating human/animal hybrids – not to mention a
transition to other states, as envisaged by Lem.

This situation is primarily a challenge for discourse ethics.
According to its basic idea, all the rules of action underlying interventions in human reproduction should be made the object of a
discourse, and be accepted by all those affected. Yet how can a discourse take place with the unborn? The extent of the problem
becomes clear if we consider that in many cases it is not even possible for those affected to give their consent belatedly. Take the
genetic diseases which lead either to a premature death or to a
premature mental disability, for example. The possibility of prenatally diagnosing such a disease presents us with the following
alternatives: either we decree that the foetuses affected by the disease should be aborted, or not. In either case, those actually
affected are unable to give their consent; neither an aborted foetus
nor a mentally retarded child can be accepted as a competent discourse partner. The discourse orientated GenEthicist is therefore
confronted with the problem of whether interventions which are
fundamentally incapable of finding consent should be permitted at
all. This sheds doubt on the concept of consensus itself.
Particularly when applied within the realm of GenEthics, this concept comes up against several serious problems (cf. Bayertz 1994).

Yet a fundamental disqualification of gene and reproduction
technology would be very difficult to bring into line with
Habermas' definition of the anthropological function of morality.
The latter stems from the vulnerability of human beings towards
other human beings and is designed to provide 'a guarantee of
mutual mercy' (Habermas 1986, p. 20). Yet we may assume that

this 'fundamental motive behind an ethics of sympathy' (p. 21) is difficult to restrict to human relationships: the human being is vulnerable not only to its fellow human beings, but also to Nature. Morality should also cover the actions and norms of action which are motivated by sympathy for the human beings who suffer within, and because of Nature, and it should aim to help these human beings. Yet the therapy of genetic diseases regularly leads to a situation of conflict. On the one hand, we would like to adhere to the sympathy principle and protect an unborn human being from a severe disease; on the other hand, this would violate the principle of consent, for the unborn human being is unable to give its consent, either to a special therapeutic intervention or to the norm of action regulating it. If we take seriously Habermas's reference to a traditional ethics of sympathy, then there is no easy way of solving this conflict in favour of the principle behind discourse ethics. Doing so would also infringe upon a long established and long accepted practice; in the field of paediatrics, many interventions are carried out where only the parents are able to give their consent, and not the children themselves. There are also many psychiatric patients who are not capable of giving their own consent, where other persons are required to make decisions *for them*.

Advocatory ethics

This practice of making decisions for other people seems to point the way to a solution. The principle of consensus is not abandoned, but merely loosened. Instead of the persons affected having to give their own consent to a particular treatment, it is their next of kin who have to do so. This assumes that (a) the next of kin reach a decision in the interests of the person affected, and (b) the person affected would reach the same decision if he/she were able to. This could be the model for a procedure of GenEthical justification. Habermas (1983, p. 104) agreed with this kind of 'advocatory' deputisation: where those directly affected are unable to be included in the discourse, the discourse community must try and put itself in that person's position, anticipating and validating the latter's interests within the debate and during the process of reaching consensus.

However plausible this solution may appear, the fact that it touches the central nerve of discourse ethics should not be overlooked. After all, this advocatory practice does abandon the principle that *only* norms consented to by *all* those concerned may be considered valid. The price to be paid for agreeing to advocatory solutions – pragmatically perfectly understandable – is admitting that at least some of the very important norms – after all, life and death are at stake – are not justifiable in strictly discourse ethical terms. By, on the one hand, connecting the concept of justification with the concept of consensus and, on the other, having to concede legitimate validity even when in some cases persons directly affected are excluded from this consensus, discourse ethicists tangle themselves in a dilemma. Either they maintain that the concept of justification and the concept of consensus are connected, rendering GenEthical maxims unjustifiable; or they agree to an advocatory practice, destroying the foundations of the discourse ethical concept of justification.

This may concern only a limited number of cases, compared with others where the persons directly affected are at least able to make their opinions known belatedly; yet it still raises a fundamental discourse ethical problem. The root of the dilemma is the discourse ethical link between the universalistic claim, characteristic of all modern ethics, and the democratic principle of being affected.

> If discourse ethics takes seriously its claim to include all the potential participants of a discourse, and if at the same time it is clear that the temporal and spatial existence of discourse participants at a particular time is contingent, in other words, that life at a particular time, in the form of a mature person, may not represent an (ontological) privilege (temporal distance is just as inessential for moral judgment as spatial distance), then discourse ethics is forced first to become advocatory, ultimately to become paradox, in addition gradually to lose its amoral, purely procedural character.
>
> (Brumlik 1986, pp. 295–6)

This relativisation of the purely procedural character of discourse ethics becomes clear if we accept the advocatory limitation to the discourse ethical principle, and enquire as to the criteria by which such a deputy decision – assuming one is unavoidable – is to be justified. This can be only through reference to particular values. In a relatively unproblematic case, a particular therapeutic procedure may be justified by referring to the value 'health'; it is fairly plausible that the person affected will consent belatedly. The situation becomes more difficult when therapeutic means are not available and the only option open is, say, an abortion. In this type of case we are forced to decide whether a certain kind of life is worth living or not: a decision which is not only morally difficult, but which also exceeds the scope of procedural ethics, since the problem is obviously an *evaluative* one. In cases of handicapped children suing doctors and genetic advisors, U.S. courts have ruled on occasions that it would have been better not to have been born at all than to have been born handicapped. These rulings are based on a legal right to begin life with a healthy mind and a healthy body, as well as a child's fundamental right to be born 'as a whole, functional human being'. This right is obviously based on a particular ideal in life: it is not only the universally accepted value of health which is assumed here, but also the view that only a healthy life is worth living. The idea behind the term 'wrongful life', formed during these trials, is that there are at least some serious diseases which make life not worth living.

The reverse position implies a particular view regarding the meaning and value of life, too – namely, that no form of suffering is terrible enough to render life meaningless and to justify ending it. Regardless of which maxims we decide to adopt, each decision implies an imposition of our ideals in life upon our descendants. In one case we impose a life full of suffering because *we* are of the opinion that every human life is holy. In the other case we impose death because *we* are of the opinion that it is not worth living that kind of life. Thus trying to draw a strict dividing line between the procedurally hard core of morality and the individually random and historically alterable matter of evaluation proves to be problematic. At least some of the important norms to be developed and justified within the scope of a GenEthics include pre-decisions of an evaluative nature, as well as outlining a fundamental ideal of life.

What is an 'evil'?

Bernard Gert's ethics demonstrates how difficult it is to prepare a hard core of morality which is independent of historically or indi-

vidually chosen values. According to Gert, morality is always concerned with avoiding evil, i.e. it forbids actions considered to have
bad consequences (Gert 1973, p. 74). This assumes that everybody
knows what is subsumed in terms such as 'evil' or 'harm'. One of
the characteristics which a person has to have in order to be considered morally competent, and which every normal, adult member of society has, is general knowledge:

> Men are mortal, they can be killed by other men, and they do not
> generally wish to be killed. One man can inflict pain on another or
> disable him; men do not generally wish to have pain inflicted on them
> or to be disabled. Men generally wish to have the freedom and oppor-
> tunity to satisfy their desires, and it is possible for some men to
> deprive others of their freedom or opportunity.
>
> (ibid., pp. 24–5)

This knowledge is morally significant, however trivial it may seem
at first glance. The human race has gained this knowledge step by
step, in a long historical process, and even today each individual
has to acquire it anew within a complicated socialisation process.
In everyday life, there will seldom be any doubt as to whether my
actions are harming a fellow human being. Even in this context
differences of opinion may occur, since there will not always be
agreement as to which of several evils is the worst, or which of
several goods the best (ibid., p. 50). Yet such differences of opinion nearly always refer to a particular point. They do not infringe
upon fundamental agreement as to what constitutes an evil and
what a good.

The problems to be solved by GenEthics are obviously of a different kind. There is no clear hierarchy of evils and goods, and
there is no consensus as to what is evil and what good. Is it a good
or an evil, for example, to be born with three eyes instead of just
two? Or with a genetically manipulated I.Q. of 150? Or from a
single genome due to cloning? If we forget the substantialists' general objection to all interventions in reproduction for the moment,
and concentrate on the 'harm or benefit' question, the answer
seems to be clear. An I.Q. of 150 can hardly be an 'evil' for the
person concerned. And, with a view to its benefits, a third eye can
hardly be considered 'harmful'. It could be a problem from an aesthetical point of view; yet this is more a problem of getting used to

the unfamiliar, a problem which would disappear all the more quickly, the more three-eyed children were to be born. The clone is the last one to suffer; his/her genetically conditioned characteristics render him/her not in the least disadvantaged with respect to his/her 'parent'. Before we can conclude that none of these manipulations is immoral, the substantialist will point out that the above argumentation is based on a very crude concept of 'harm'. It is not only 'material' harm which has to be taken into consideration, but also 'ideal' harm, for example through a violation of moral rights. There are actually two kinds of 'evil', neither reducible to the other, which have to be taken into consideration when evaluating technological interventions in human reproduction.

1. The first kind consists of all the harm which, in normal circumstances, is unequivocal: it is harmful to be killed, injured, robbed or restricted in one's personality. With regard to gene and reproduction technology, we have to examine whether the manipulations involved inflict this kind of harm upon the affected individuals. This may include physical damage as a result of technical error. The manipulations are carried out on highly complex and sensitive 'matter', with every false move involving potentially disastrous consequences. Paul Ramsey (1970, pp. 75–7) and Leon Kass (1972, pp. 27–9) have a principal objection to all reproduction technologies precisely because of the unavoidable risks involved. Besides physical handicaps and injuries, the term 'damage' may also refer to psychological damage, as is feared, for example, in *in vitro* children when they find out about their origins. It is conceivable that they will experience the unusual manner in which they were created as an extreme burden, under which they will suffer for the rest of their lives. A similar case is that of ectogenesis, a technology which at present is still Utopian: would an embryo growing in artificial surroundings outside the mother's body – even if there were no technical problems in imitating all the physiological processes such as nutrition, oxgen supply, etc. – not be deprived of all the psychological and emotional communication which, under normal circumstances, would have been built up prenatally between it and its mother? And would it not then become psychologically stunted? All these examples of physical and psychological harm may be included within Gert's formulation of an ethical framework. The moral rules he reconstructed as fun-

damental to all of morality may be applied to them without any difficulty at all. All of the consequences of gene and reproduction technological interventions which fall under the prohibitions stated by these rules have to be rejected as immoral.

However, it is not always possible to determine this kind of evil anticipatively. This becomes clear if we take the example of ectogenesis a bit further. The artificial uterus could be developed to supply not only food and oxygen, but also psychological stimuli. Assuming the necessary technological know-how, the mother's natural movements, her changes in mood and her emotions could all be simulated and even optimised through hormonal releases and computer controlled electrical impulses, so that the embryo is perfectly cared for, not only physically, but also 'psychologically'. It would then be wrong to talk of inflicting 'harm' on the embryo; and if an analogous procedure were also applied to the mother, then this form of ectogenesis would have to be accepted as morally permissible. This line of argumentation raises a fundamental problem regarding the consequentialist evaluation of technologies. Whenever harm is predicted as the consequence of applying a particular technology, it is always possible – with a bit of imagination – to conceive of an improvement to that technology which would prevent the predicted harm from being inflicted. The masters of this argumentational strategy, including Stanislaw Lem, are able to find a technological solution to get around any moral objection, thus forcing the consequentialist into the ungrateful rôle of the hare, which – wherever he goes – always finds a hedgehog.[1]

2. The substantialist gets around the hare and hedgehog dilemma, in which the ethicist is always forced into the rôle of the loser, by asking whether we can really accept as morally indisputable all the interventions which do not inflict manifest physical or psychological harm. If, for example, the consequentialist were to concede that the cultivation of a human embryo in a uterus machine is morally permissible, as long as the machine provides

---

[1] *Translator's note*: This refers to a German fable in which a hedgehog challenges a cocky hare to a race. The hare finds the suggestion hilarious and naturally accepts. Unbeknown to him, however, the hedgehog has a wife . . . When the hare reaches the end of the track, 'the' hedgehog is already there. Amazed and disbelieving, the hare repeats the race. Yet, regardless of the speed with which he tears past the hedgehog at the beginning of the track, it always beats him to the end.

perfect physical and psychological care, the substantialist would counter that this amounts to ethical (and moral) capitulation. The concept of evil cannot be reduced to manifest harm of the kind debated in (1). A second, different type of evil, which may be characterised as *moral* harm, must be taken into account. We consider the buying and selling of children to be immoral. Such a procedure would meet with our moral disapproval even if it meant an advantage for the children, simply because it involves an 'ideal', i.e. moral harm: selling human beings is inhumane. *Homo sapiens* is not only a physical organism with a set of psychological characteristics, but a human being with a specific *dignity* and specific *rights*. This dignity and these rights are not simply philosophical attributions, and are in no way dependent upon the viewpoint of the substantialists. The concepts of human dignity and human rights are also accepted by the subjectivists, and, as part of the German Constitution (Articles 1 and 2), may be viewed as statute law. In the same way as the buying and selling of children constitutes a violation of moral rights, particular interventions in human reproduction may be seen as a violation of human dignity. The reason given for a ban on human cloning and the creation of human–animal hybrids, recommended as part of criminal law by a German Government committee ('Benda Commission'), was that such procedures involved 'a particularly serious violation of human dignity' (Report 1985, p. 60). It is not possible here to go into the difficulties involved in interpreting this concept of human dignity; but it is important in this context to mention that consequentialist evaluation cannot be reduced to an anticipation of obvious or scientifically determinable harm. Moral harm, such as a violation of human dignity or certain human rights, has to be included in the evaluation too.

Another realistic problem posed by defining the function of morality as the avoidance of evil is the splitting of embryos. Human embryos may be split during their early stages of development; because the cells have not yet started to specialise, each of the two halves may still develop into a full individual. A four-celled embryo could be split into two two-celled embryos in order to create identical twins; this kind of splitting could also be carried out as a genetic 'consumer' test on one embryo: if the result is negative, the other embryo can still grow up normally. The ques-

tion is: can or must this kind of splitting be viewed as 'harmful'?
In the first case this is not at all clear, for the creation of identical
twins does not involve killing the embryo, and the twins do not
suffer any damage to their health. Yet if one assumes that human
embryos are not organic matter of neutral value, but that they
have a moral status – however this may be defined – then, in
theory, this kind of splitting *is* problematic. 'It does not treat
embryos as the beginning of individual, human life, but merely as
the material needed in order to create other embryos' (van den
Daele 1985, p. 35), which would mean a morally refutable instrumentalisation of human life. Whatever one's opinion: the answer
cannot be a standard reference to inflicted 'harm'. Gert's definition
of morality as protection from evil has its limits wherever the
terms 'harm' and 'evil' are ambiguous.

Rights

The debate on the moral problems connected with gene technology is largely a debate about human dignity and the rights of personality which may be derived from it. In many fields, new rights
are formulated in order to prevent people from acting in ways
made possible by scientific and technological innovation. The
development of modern information technology, for example, has
in Germany led to a 'right to informational self-determination'
becoming statute law. It will come as no surprise that new rights –
and obligations – are frequently being called for within the field of
gene and reproduction technology. One example of this is the
debates held on the subject of genetic responsibility. If, due to
modern prenatal diagnostics, we are no longer forced to accept the
birth of a handicapped child as an unavoidable fate, then we could
plausibly deduce from this that parents and physicians have an
increased responsibility for the health of their children. The question is, would such an increase in responsibility would be in accordance with a 'right to freedom from injury' for children? Various
ethicists have called for this right to be introduced, and, as has
already been mentioned, it has found its way into U.S. legislation.

German legislation has to date dismissed such *wrongful life* law-suits. One of the difficulties involved is that, whereas hardly any-body would deny that it is 'harmful' to be born handicapped, many people *do* consider death by abortion to be even more 'harmful'. Another difficulty is that a handicap is passively accepted, whereas an abortion is actively carried out: a difference which, in moral terms, is relevant, considering the asymmetry between acting and refraining maintained by Gert. Both of these objections assume not only that each embryo has a 'right to life', but also that this right counts for more than all the possible con-siderations regarding *quality* of life. Even when there can be no doubt regarding manifest physical defects, highly complex prob-lems may still arise involving the decisions which have to be made, problems which are not to be solved simply by stating that we are morally obliged to prevent harm.

These problems tend to become even more difficult when they involve rights intended to protect the individual from moral harm. With a long-term view to deliberate genetic manipulations, for example, would it be sensible – or even necessary – to demand a 'right to being unplanned', in order to prevent children from being born as, and having to exist as the total design of their par-ents, or maybe even the State? This is the context in which Hans Jonas' deliberations on a 'right to ignorance' should be viewed. On the problem of cloning, Jonas questions whether the human prod-uct of such a procedure would not know (or think it knows) far too much about itself, together with what others know (or think they know). As a genotypical copy of an already existing person, the clone would automatically be pressurised with expectations, predictions, goals, comparisons, etc., concerning the known donor archetype.

> . . . and this putative knowledge must stifle in the pre-charted subject all immediacy of the groping quest and eventual finding 'himself' with which a toiling life surprises itself for good and for ill. It is all a mat-ter much more of supposed than real knowledge, of opinion than truth. Note that it does not matter one jot whether the genotype is really, by its own force, a person's fate: it is *made* his fate by the very assumptions in cloning him, which by their imposition on all con-cerned become a force themselves.
>
> (Jonas 1974, p. 161)

On the basis of these deliberations, Jonas formulates a right not to know:

> The ethical command here entering the enlarged stage of our powers is: never to violate the right to that ignorance which is a condition for the possibility of authentic action; or: *to respect the right of each human life to find its own way and be a surprise to itself.*
>
> (ibid., p. 163)

Regardless of how discussions about these and other rights will develop, the fact that they take place at all draws attention to an important circumstance. All of these rights are the direct or indirect expression of certain values and ideals in life. A 'right to freedom from injury' will only be called for by someone who thinks more of good health than of life itself, and only somebody who, like Jonas, believes the 'enticing (also frightening) *openness*' (ibid., p. 162) of individual life to be valuable, and who would not like to see the adventure of self-discovery being taken away in advance by others, will be able to accept a 'right not to know'. But if the formulation of such rights also involves staking out guidelines for a certain way of living, then a culturally independent reconstruction of morality proves to be a somewhat questionable project. This is Gert's claim when he states at the beginning of his book that he will 'present an analysis of morality; not of this morality or that morality, but of morality' (Gert 1973, p. 4). He claims that moral rules, which for him form the key to morality, have a super-historical validity: 'A moral rule is unchanging or unchangeable; discovered rather than invented' (ibid., p. 67). In some ways this claim is unavoidable if one does not wish to lapse into a relativism simply connecting moral validity with factual validity. It is necessary to demonstrate, as Habermas has formulated, 'that our principle of morality is not simply a reflection of current, adult, white, male, middle-class, Central European prejudices' (Habermas 1986, p. 18). Neither can there be any argument that the obligation not to inflict harm upon other human beings is expression of a fundamental principle of any morality.

At the same time, the fact that such a universalistic concept of morality – and this goes for discourse ethics analogously – leads to a highly abstract and formal construct should not be overlooked. The principle 'inflict no harm on your fellow human beings!'

contains two undefined, key concepts. Firstly, it is not always and in all circumstances clear what constitutes 'harm'. Gene technology especially offers a wide variety of practical options where it is not clear-cut whether or not their consequences are 'harmful' to those affected. Or to put it more precisely: it depends upon the ideal in life favoured at the time as to whether individual consequences are to be classified as harmful or not. The second key concept is 'human being'; it defines upon *whom* we may not inflict harm – presuming we know what counts as 'harm'. However minor the problem of defining this second concept may be in everyday practice, it is a very grave one within the context of technological intervention in human reproduction. Those affected by such interventions always include the unborn, whether future generations or already existent embryos. Gert pointed out that one's opinion on abortion depends upon the level of respect which one has towards unborn human life.

> If one is as concerned with unborn children as with their prospective mothers, he will publicly advocate that no abortion be allowed, not even to save the life of the mother, just as we do not allow one innocent person to be killed in order to save another. If one is seriously concerned, but not equally concerned, he will publicly advocate that abortion be allowed only to prevent the death of the mother or where there is serious risk of her suffering other evils. As one's concern decreases he will allow abortion for less and less important reasons, till, if one has no concern at all, he will allow abortion on demand, or simply because the mother wants it. Much of the discussion on abortion involves the attempt to get people to increase or decrease their concern for the unborn child, I have nothing to add to this discussion here.
>
> (1973, pp. xxi–xxii)

Gert's moral philosophy cannot actually contribute anything towards solving this problem; it must be clear from the very beginning who is the 'object' of the moral obligation to avoid harm, or even who is the legitimate owner of rights.

The conclusion seems obvious. Even if we assume that the obligation 'inflict no harm on your fellow human beings!' successfully reconstructs the core of morality, the universality of this principle is only guaranteed because the terms 'harm' and 'human being' constitute two empty gaps which can be filled with a variety of contents. Moral rules cannot therefore be said to hold the same status as the laws of logic or mathematics (Gert 1973, p. 68). A better comparison would be with the laws of physics, which are usually just mathematical formulae until they are empirically applied and gain physical content. Similarly, one could maintain that universalistic moral principles require a definite content before they may be considered as justification for rules of action and orientation for individual actions. This is especially true of fields which are expanding at an enormous rate with the progress of science and technology. Insisting on the unlimited universality of moral rules, even in the sense 'that men in every society, at any time, might have acted upon it or broken it' (ibid., p. 66), implies a systematic underestimation of the effects of science and technology on the moral *problems* of our society. Even if we take into consideration the fact that new moral problems do not always require a 'new morality', and that these new problems may often be solved with old rules and principles, we should still remember that the latter seldom remain unaffected. The old rules and principles are frequently only viable when they are – often insignificantly – modified, made more precise or extended upon.

Satisfied pigs

For the utilitarians, protection from harm is too limited a perception of morality. According to Mill, it is in the interest of each human being that no other human being inflict harm upon it:

> The moralities which protect every individual from being harmed by others, either directly or by being hindered in his freedom of pursuing his own good, are at once those which he himself has most at heart, and those which he has the strongest interest in publishing and enforcing by word and deed.
>
> (Mill 1969a, p. 256)

Yet, for the utilitarians, protecting the individual from harm is only one – if important – facet of the general principle of utility, according to which an action or rule of action may be considered moral if it contributes to common happiness. Yet what exactly is to be understood by 'happiness'? Utilitarianism necessitates a definition of happiness as the vanishing point at which all human actions are aimed, and as the highest criterion for their evaluation. It is not possible within the framework of this book to go into the difficulties surrounding this definition of happiness. One solution is hedonism, firmly anchored in moral philosophical tradition since Ancient Greek times and interpreting happiness as a maximisation of pleasure and a minimisation of displeasure. With his assertion

> that pleasure, and freedom from pain, are the only things desirable as ends; and that all desirable things (which are as numerous in the utilitarian as in any other scheme) are desirable either for the pleasure inherent in themselves, or as means to the promotion of pleasure and the prevention of pain
>
> (ibid., p. 210)

Mill seems to follow on in the same tradition. Interpreting the utilitarian principle of utility hedonistically is also fruitful for the evaluation of gene and reproduction technology. If, for example, infertility is often a cause of displeasure, and if it is possible to help infertile couples to have children with the aid of artificial insemination, *in vitro* fertilisation or other technologies, then these technologies must be deemed morally legitimate.

The reason why hedonism is problematic will become clearer with the following example. Modern neuroendocrinology has been able to demonstrate that animal and human organisms produce *endorphine (endogenous morphin)*, or corporeal opiates, which arouse feelings of satisfaction or happiness when released into the central nervous system. The biological function of endorphin is to reward or punish certain types of behaviour. If a chick strays from its mother, for example, it loses opiates as a punishment; if it comes back, it is rewarded with a release of opiates (Hoebel 1983, p. 88). It is also known that various types of endorphin have various effects:

> Research suggests that learning is 'rewarded' in the short-term by katecholomine, whereas dopamine is responsible for the motivation to learn, and norepinephrine helps us to remember successful behaviour. Long-term satisfaction is probably a state due to the effect of opiates, stimulated by the body's own opiates within the brain.
>
> (ibid., p. 101)

However they might behave in detail, the fact that these neuro-chemical substances 'are produced via an innate, genetic system' (ibid., p. 108) means that it must be possible to increase their production with the aid of gene technological manipulations. A continual release of the right sort of endorphin would place the individual in question in a permanent state of happiness. As there can be no doubt that this kind of intervention maximises pleasure, it must, from a strictly hedonistic point of view, be deemed morally legitimate, and the technological idea behind it a highly beneficial invention. Julian Huxley hinted at a similar, if less elegant solution to the happiness problem appropriate to the state of technology at the time:

> For instance, it has now been shown that in man as well as in animals, electric stimulation of a particular area in the brain can produce an overwhelming sense of happiness or well-being in the whole organism. It has even been found possible to make one half of the body feel happy, while the other half remains in its normal state. To some people this seems somehow too materialistic; but after all, electric happiness is still happiness, and happiness is very much more important than the physical happenings with which it has correlated.
>
> (Huxley 1967a, p. 12).

We do not need to go into the reason why this conclusion is contra-intuitive. Electrical happiness may not be aligned with our moral feelings. John Stuart Mill is one of the people who considers the whole thing to be 'too materialistic'. In order to rule out precisely the conclusion which Huxley so calmly came to, Mill rejects an exclusively quantitative increase in pleasure, introducing a distinction between different *kinds* of pleasure, whereby some kinds are more valuable than others.

> Few human creatures would consent to be changed into any of the lower animals, for a promise of the fullest allowance of a beast's pleasures; no intelligent human being would consent to be a fool, no instructed person would be an ignoramus, no person of feeling and conscience would be selfish and base, even though they should be persuaded that the fool, the dunce, or the rascal is better satisfied with his lot than they are with theirs. They would not resign what they possess more than he, for the most complete satisfaction of all the desires which they have in common with him.
>
> (Mill 1969a, p. 211)

We may conclude that Mill would have rejected the electrical happiness propagated by Huxley, just as he would have rejected gene technologically programmed, neurochemical happiness. And there can be no doubt that this rejection of extreme hedonism complies with our moral intuition. Nobody, except for hardliners like Huxley, would contradict him for writing: 'It is better to be a human being dissatisfied than a pig satisfied' (ibid., p. 212). Yet how are these different levels and types of happiness to be accommodated within the utilitarians' basic ideas? According to the principle of utility, happiness – defined as pleasure – is the criterion by which to evaluate actions and rules of action. If various types of pleasure are distinguished and hierarchised, there is obviously a meta-criterion needed in order to decide which types of pleasure are to be placed higher or lower within the hierarchy. Yet utilitarianism cannot permit such a meta-criterion because this would topple the principle of utility from its position as the highest of all moral principles. The hedonistic explication of the principle of utility is in any case unacceptable.

Individual goals

This unsatisfactory hedonistic interpretation of happiness does have an alternative, referring to the satisfaction of human interests and needs. The difficult philosophical task of defining 'happiness' in general terms is disregarded in favour of a pragmatic reference to empirical interests, desires and needs. This is the utilitarian line of argumentation behind Joseph Fletcher's repeated confirmation of the fundamental *principle of beneficence*, for example, according to which the highest criterion for moral evaluation can only be the satisfaction of concrete human needs. If this criterion is fulfilled, then there can be no intervention, however dramatic, worthy of rejection: 'Morally, genetic engineering is good when it serves human needs, both health and happiness' (Fletcher 1974, p. 169). This is primarily appropriate to the fight against human suffering, such as that caused by infertility or genetic diseases; the individual may be spared pain, handicap and premature death, and society spared the costs which would otherwise have been involved. Yet it is also true of positive eugenics, in the sense of deliberately planning genotypes with desired characteristics. Our imagination does not seem to know where to stop, as shown by the example of parents ordering a child with a third eye, four arms or a tail. A further fear is that cloning could lead to 'copies' of famous football stars, adored actresses or successful politicians being 'churned out' on demand.

These horror visions, and others, are usually based on false empirical assumptions. Such assumptions include naïvety concerning the extent to which the human organism may be altered in certain points. An organism is not a conglomerate of separate organs, but an ordered structure, and an intervention in a particular area leads to a great many connected problems. The 'fitting' of two extra arms – to take this example seriously for a moment – would not mean simply adding two arms, but reconstructing the entire skeleton, including all the muscles needed to move it, plus trenchant alterations to the nervous system and the brain, since the two new arms have to be controlled. It is easy to imagine similar problems for psychological characteristics, providing they are genetically determined. Most of these ideas are based on a reduced comprehension of the manner in which genes function and take effect, a phenomenon which may be termed *genetic determinism*. Accordingly, the phenotype is merely the visible expression of the genotype; the genes are in command of ontogenetic development and clearly determine the structure of the organism to be. It is no coincidence that some of the literature, and much of the popular literature on genetics and genetic manipulations has a strong tendency to use military terminology:

> In the molecular world of the gene, it is anathema to refuse, disregard or disobey. In this sense, the genetic language adopted by the scientist is more akin to a military code than to a dialectic. Genes are said to 'direct' protein synthesis, for instance, when in fact they provide merely the first template from which a whole host of highly coordinated, and other gene-mediated activities ensue to produce the specified protein product.
>
> (Lappé 1979, pp. 115–16)

In contrast to the basic assumption behind genetic determinism, the relationships between genetic information and the organisms ultimately resulting from this information are extraordinarily complex. Not only are most phenotypical characteristics polygenic, i.e. the product of several interacting genes, but they also form under the influence of many different external conditions, so that the resulting object is conditioned by a multitude of factors. This is true of every part of the human organism, and in particular the brain. It has been proved beyond doubt that the mental content of this organ, as well as its anatomical structure, cannot be reduced to the effect of genes, but must be comprehended as a complex interchange between genetic information, epigenetic factors and environmental influences. The idea of taking the genome of Wolfgang Amadeus Mozart and reproducing it as often as one desired in order to form copies of the brilliant composer is, in view of the biological relationships described, naïve.

> To produce another Mozart, we would need not only Wolfgang's genome but mother Mozart's uterus, father Mozart's music lessons, their friends and his, the state of music in eighteenth century Austria, Haydn's patronage, and on and on, in ever-widening circles. Without his set of genes, the rest would not suffice; there has been, after all, only one Wolfgang Amadeus Mozart. But we have no right to the converse assumption: that his genome, cultivated in another world at another time, would result in an equally creative musical genius. If a particular strain of wheat yields different harvests under different conditions of climate, soil, and cultivation, how can we assume that so much more complex a genome as that of a human being would yield its desired crop of operas, symphonies and chamber music under different circumstances of nurture?
>
> (Eisenberg 1976, p. 326)

Genetic determinism is based on a model of linear causation which may be justified in terms of mechanics, but which oversimplifies the real complexity of organismic – including genetic – processes. Many of the adventurous projects referred to prove to be non-viable for purely biological reasons, let alone ethical ones.

Empirical objections do not, however, remove the moral problems involved. For a moral evaluation, not even the utilitarians believe listing the positive goals behind individual interventions to be sufficient: the expected benefit is only *one* factor involved in the utilitarian calculus of benefits, and this factor may be relativised, offset or surpassed by the expected damage. A complete evaluative procedure would thus not only take into account the positive aspects of an intervention, but also its costs, starting with its negative social consequences. One realistic example could be sex determination. There can be no doubt as to the utilitarian benefits of such a technique, since there are many parents who would gladly make use of it. At first glance, this manipulation seems fairly modest: only one genetic characteristic is selected, and that is a natural characteristic generally considered to be unproblematic. It may be disadvantageous to have a third eye or four arms, but not to be a woman or a man. Yet the probable distribution of the two characteristics involved in this manipulation could well lead to problems: it has to be assumed that the introduction of this technology would lead to the birth of more boys than girls. Even if utilitarians reject the objection of prenatal sexism, they cannot ignore the social consequences of a surplus of men.

> There would be a growing proportion of the population unable to find marriageable partners; homosexuality and prostitution would probably increase. Furthermore, since there would be fewer women, there would be fewer persons interested in culture (books, theater, art) or charged with the moral upbringing of children (which is still a woman's specialization); and there would be more people engaged in competitive, materialistic pursuits (still, more of the man's world). For the same reason, violent crimes would rise (90.4 percent of all violent crimes and 81.3 percent of all crimes against property committed in the United States in 1970 were committed by men).
>
> (Etzioni 1973, p. 16)

However convincing this prognosis may or may not be, it indicates the direction in which a utilitarian calculation of benefits would have to research. And if the prognosis should be confirmed – an empirical matter – then this would prove that the social disadvantages outweigh the individual benefits, meaning that sex determination techniques would have to be rejected as immoral.

Besides the social costs, a utilitarian evaluative procedure would also have to take into account the disadvantages which could arise for the individual being manipulated. This should include not only the physical and psychological damage mentioned above, but also the inevitable side-effects of any alteration. It is so easy to think of situations in which it would be a great advantage to have two more arms, yet this attribute can be just as much of a disadvantage in other situations – buying clothes, for example. However, if the total benefit of a manipulation outweighs the total harm, then, from a utilitarian point of view, it must be deemed justified, and accepted as morally good. This is also the case when the benefits and harm are unevenly distributed: if the parents desire a child with a third eye and a tail, then its production would be legitimate even if the child itself would suffer as a consequence; for only *one* child would suffer, compared to the joy of *two* parents. The fact that this conclusion is unacceptable draws attention to two of the frequently criticised weaknesses within the utilitarian approach. Firstly, it is hard to accept that positive and negative consequences may cancel each other out:

> It is a universally accepted criticism of utilitarianism that it would allow the infliction of evil – e.g. pain, on one person – in order to promote a great amount of good – e.g. pleasure, for many others. This criticism makes clear that the causing of evil cannot be balanced by the promotion of good . . . The promotion of good does not justify the infliction of evil; only the prevention of greater evil does that.
>
> (Gert 1973, pp. 72–3)

The asymmetry of good and evil is highly relevant to the problems behind gene technological interventions in human reproduction. It prohibits us from accepting any number of disadvantages merely because the benefits are great enough, and especially – this brings us to the second criticised weakness of the utilitarian approach – when, as in this case, the benefits and the disadvantages are to be had by different people. Utilitarianism is helpless with regard to the problem of *justice*, and is thus not capable of solving the problem of unevenly distributed benefits and/or harm. Utilitarians are thus faced with a dilemma. Either they have to introduce a criterion which is independent of the calculus of utility; this would avoid contra-intuitive conclusions being drawn, but only at the price of the central principle of utilitarianism. Or they maintain their principle and permit an uneven distribution only when the total difference between benefits and harm is positive; this would mean accepting conclusions which massively contradict our perception of justice. Even the creation of slave workers, as in Aldous Huxley's *Brave New World*, would be permitted, provided the benefits outweighed the harm. Fletcher's suggestion (1974, pp. 172–3) that human/animal hybrids could be created to do the dangerous and humiliating work is proof that these deliberations are no mere fabrication.

Intelligence and instrumentalisation

The highlight amongst the utilitarian plans for improvement seems to have remained unaffected by all of these fears. A superficial glance at the appropriate literature is enough to reveal the favourite and most promising candidate for positive eugenics in the future: intelligence. It is no coincidence that even Joseph Fletcher's favourite term 'quality control' is primarily aimed at the intelligence of the descendants to be produced: 'Quality control in birth technology will have to aim at selecting for intelligence and, where possible, lifting it' (1974, p. 75). Even if intelligence is not the only characteristic which parents would like their children to have, the majority of parents would no doubt be glad of the chance to increase their children's intelligence levels, providing no serious side-effects are involved. Which couple would refuse to raise its child's I.Q. if this could be done with the aid of a small and safe, prenatal intervention? This technique – were it ever to be realised, which does not seem very likely – would satisfy a need and, in utilitarian terms, be 'beneficial'. Intelligence grants its owner the ability to solve difficult problems, as well as social recognition from his/her fellow human beings, and is thus a desirable characteristic. One may dispute whether a more intelligent person is necessarily happier, but one can hardly maintain that it would be harmful or disadvantageous to be more intelligent. For the utilitarians, there can be no doubt that the total benefits of intelligence far outweigh the potential harm – should there be any at all.

The benefits that the utilitarian has good cause to expect from an increase in intelligence are not, however, benefits in themselves, but benefits only when viewed in the light of particular social circumstances. It is only in a civilisation characterised by science and technology that intelligence can acquire enough material and cultural significance to become *the* beneficial characteristic in the eyes of so many. Of course, mental ability is useful whatever the social circumstances are. Nevertheless, in a hunting community the relative benefits of a sharp mind would be secondary to those of sharp senses; and in Middle Europe several hundred years ago, intelligence was considered culturally less significant than piety. This not only goes to show that all the goals behind genetic manipulation are socially determined and historically relative, but also that each individual decision made by well-meaning parents for the good of their child has a social dimension, and is therefore not totally 'individual'. An increase in intelligence through genetic manipulation joins parents' desires and the anticipated interests of children with the collective interests of modern societies. This convergence of individual and collective interests makes the furthering of intelligence a perfect example of the potential benefits to be gained from genetic manipulation.

This is nevertheless problematic. Firstly, a mere calculus of the benefits cannot distinguish qualitatively between individual and collective benefits – or harm. Utilitarian argumentation has a tendency to go beyond the interests and needs of individuals and take into consideration the needs of society. Even if we may assume, in the case of intelligence, that harmony exists between the interests of individuals and those of society – whoever that may actually be – there are a great many examples of cases where the interests in question conflict. In these cases, technological interventions in human reproduction are no longer proposed in the interests of individuals, but in the interests of the 'general good', the quality of the gene pool or other entities beyond the individual. The tendency to relativise the human individual, which is commonly the result, comes in two different shapes. In a *biologistic* variation, the individual is analysed purely as the carrier of ('good' or 'bad') genes. It is then logical to assess the value of each individual primarily or exclusively according to the contribution it can make to the quality of the gene pool. Traditional eugenicists lamented 'the individualistic orientation of our humanism' (Schallmayer 1903, pp. 152–3) and called for a revision of Western morality in a more communal direction. Concern for the individual must be relativised with concern for the 'people', 'race' or 'future generations'.

> Our humanism is totally one-sided in its sole consideration for the unlucky individuals within the present generation, and is unbelievably careless or blind with regard to the suffering inflicted by such

self-righteousness upon individuals within the next and subsequent generations.

(ibid.)

In response to the demand that those 'born unlucky' be excluded from the process of reproduction, Schallmayer calculates the harm involved in a genuinely utilitarian manner:

> The sacrifice or suffering of one individual of the present generation is next to nothing compared with the total amount of misery which the next and future generations could be spared as a consequence.

(ibid., p. 153)

It is worth noting once again that emphasis upon non-individual units, such as race or gene pool, tends to reduce human individuals to gene carriers, and to qualify them according to the contribution their genes can make to the 'quality' of the next generation.

The more current and more influential relativisation of the individual avoids the crude biologism found in traditional eugenics by concentrating primarily on *social* ends. Terms such as 'species', 'race' or 'gene pool' retreat to make way for concepts such as 'technological progress', 'industrial civilisation' and 'modern society'. One example of this type of argumentation is Joseph Fletcher's suggestion that individuals possessing rare, genetically determined characteristics, which could be useful for particular purposes and jobs, should be cloned.

> Individuals might need to be selectively reproduced by cloning because of their special resistance to radiation, their small body size and weight, because they are impervious to high decibel sound waves; these things could be invaluable for professional flights at high altitudes and space travel, for example. In a stretch of imagination, a biologist could solve the weight problem by going alone to a distant planet with a supply of different somatic cells, and colonize it from a cloning start. Even without any need to specialize people we might some day have to turn to either cloning or genetic engineering to correct for the loss of quality we suffer as our recessive defects get spread around in our common gene pool. Dangerous roles within society or on its frontiers might justify cloning, to safeguard those who take risks in the social interest.

(Fletcher 1974, pp. 154–5).

This kind of suggestion raises a fundamental ethical problem.

As soon as not only individual, but also social ends become part of the calculation of benefits, and the latter is based on a quantifiable concept of benefit which makes the same technology twice as beneficial because it helps two people at once, then the utilitarian evaluative procedure must lead to a systematic subordination of individual interests to social ones. This not only permits, but also pre-programmes an *instrumentalisation* of the human being for a whole range of social purposes.

Which values?

Obviously there is one problem which is raised by every strategy bent on genetically improving the human race: what actually are the *criteria* needed to determine which characteristic would be more of an improvement than another one, and where do these criteria come from? Do we have a system of values which finds everybody's consensus, both today and in the future? Is the result not going to be that each improving generation forces its system of values on those already improved: a biological tyranny of the living by the dead? Each eugenical attempt runs the risk of cementing biologically an historically certain system of values. In *Out of the Night*, alluding to artificial semination with sperm donated by 'excellent' men, Herman Muller asks rhetorically how many woman living in an open society, free from superstitious prejudice and sexual slavery, would be proud to give birth to a child from Lenin or Darwin (Muller 1936, pp. 152–3). Anti-eugenics writers have taken pleasure in pointing out that in later publications, after he turned away from Marxism, Muller never again mentioned the name Lenin. What was beyond all doubt in 1936, was seen a decade later – the Cold War had begun – in a totally different light. Muller did not draw any conclusions from this, leading Peter Medawar to say in 1962 at the Ciba Symposium:

> What frightens me about Muller and to some extent Huxley is their extreme self-confidence, their complete conviction not only that they know what ends are desirable but also that they know how to achieve them.

> (Medawar 1967, p. 296)

The historical narrow-mindedness of the various breeding programmes becomes all the more obvious, the more temporal distance we gain to them. It is hardly necessary to go into detail
about the influence of the *Zeitgeist* at the turn of the century upon
classic eugenics; moreover, scientistic ignorance of Anglo-Saxon
eugenics between the Wars and later is becoming clearer today
than ever before. What Alex Comfort pointed out then is now, in
retrospect, very obvious: namely, that most eugenic concepts do
not only project into the future the central social significance of
scientific and technological progress, but also, in so doing – should
they be realised – *prejudice* such a development.

> We have all been assuming that the exponential progress of science
> can go on indefinitely. I would have thought from what we said earlier
> about the rates of change in society that our descendants might well
> benefit from a period of relaxation. They might have a period in
> which they have a rather less intense social drive, and perhaps become
> more shallow and superficial in some of their attitudes, by our stan-
> dards; at the same time they may have less incentive to go on adding
> to discovery at quite our rate. I wonder if the preoccupations we have
> shown here may not seem as grotesque to our descendants as some of
> Oliver Cromwell's theological discussions do to us. We may be going
> to produce a generation, not so much of scientific puritans or of scien-
> tific activists, but of beatniks who are going to enjoy, for a while at
> any rate, the proceeds of what we are now laying down . . . The
> ancient Indians cultivated the art of love for both religious and practi-
> cal reasons, and I think we may find ourselves cultivating similar
> aesthetic elaborations of pleasure. At least I hope our descendants will
> do so.
>
> (Comfort 1967, p. 363)

It has already proved difficult to define objectively the potential
harm inflicted by interventions in human nature. Here it becomes
clear that it is even more difficult to define the benefits of genetic
manipulations. The 'objectivity' of the utilitarian evaluative procedure proves to be fiction. This procedure could be objective only
within a system of values which is generally accepted, and which
lays down what is harmful and what beneficial, as well as the
quantitative weight of a particular benefit or instance of harm.

13

Process without a goal

Man, with the dead God as his copilot,
is to fly off into the wild blue yonder
of limitless self-modification
Leon R. Kass

The philosophical problem posed by gene and reproduction technology is that it enables human nature to be controlled with technology, in a dimension previously unknown. The closer we get to
autoevolution, and the more we free ourselves of substantialist
doubts, the larger the question looms as to what our *goals* are in
reconstructing the human species.

> Suppose, for example, that 'we' (biologists? or politicians?) decided
> (and had the power) to make the next human generation of type 'X'.
> So far, perhaps, so good. But when we die, our place must presumably
> be taken by a new committee – which would presumably be of type
> 'X'. The question we must ponder is what kind of changes these men
> of type 'X' would think desirable in their successors – and so on, into
> the future. If we cannot answer it, then to initiate such a process might
> show the reverse of responsibility, on any explication of the term. In
> short, to navigate by a landmark tied to your own ship's head is ulti-
> mately impossible. If we are ever to make proper use of our growing
> eugenic powers, we shall need a wisdom greater than our own.
>
> (MacKay 1967, p. 286)

As soon as the autoevolutive process is under way, and its first goal
is reached, a new goal will then be proposed and ultimately realised,
making way for a third goal, etc. The prospect of a never-ending
sequence of goals and realising goals emerges, itself goal-less in its

endlessness. This is not an argument against autoevolution, however. MacKay's assertion that it is 'ultimately impossible' to navigate by a landmark tied to one's own ship's head ignores the fact that evolution has always done just that. It has advanced without a fixed goal, and has managed to create a creature as complex as the human being on the way. The autoevolutive process could therefore also start without a fixed goal in mind. This is, after all, precisely what the term 'auto*evolution*' implies.

The great void

A look at the goals which the improvements to humanity suggested in various works of eugenic literature are aimed at reveals that many others are named besides physical health.

> When the choices are not imposed but voluntary and democratic, the sound values common to humanity nearly everywhere are bound to exert the predominant influence in guiding the directions of choice. Practically all peoples venerate creativity, wisdom, brotherliness, loving-kindness, perceptivity, expressivity, joy of life, fortitude, vigour, longevity. If presented with the opportunity to have their children approach nearer to such goals than they could do themselves, they will not turn down this golden chance, and the next generation, thus benefitted, will be able to choose better than they did.
>
> (Muller 1967, pp. 260–1)

There can hardly be anybody who would not desire the things on this list – some may even wish to extend it, to include characteristics such as a sense of beauty, a love of order, potency or piety. Nevertheless, these goals remain unsatisfactory. Naïvely and transparently they adhere to values which are both *indefinite* and *traditional*. If the most advanced and futuristic technologies are called upon to realise the most familiar and traditional values, then this may be indication of just how difficult it is to anticipate future values. Just as the future of science fiction usually turns out to be a mere extrapolation of the present, the 'future human being' is presented as the current human being, with all its positive characteristics increased.

In the light of these difficulties, it seems logical to ignore the goals and emphasise instead the openness of the autoevolutive process. In his *Summa technologiae*, Stanislaw Lem made no attempt to define any goals, instead emphasising the endlessness of the reconstruction process:

> I do not believe in an ultimate solution. After a certain period of time, even a 'superman' will probably consider himself inadequate in the face of new technologies enabling him to do something which for us is pure fantasy.
>
> (1976, p. 510)

We will return later to the implicit subject of autoevolution: not the human being and its values, but technological options determine the advance of this process. What is important for now is that, later on in his deliberations, Lem makes it clear what it is he prefers to view as a normative criterion.

> Our criterion is progress – or rather the possibility of progress. This refers to the emergence of homoeostatic solutions which are not only capable of existing despite inner and outer disturbances, but which also develop, in other words extending the field of this homoeostasis. They are systems which are perfect, not only for their ability to adapt to the state of the environment, but also their ability to change. These changes have both to satisfy the requirements of the environment and to permit further changes, since otherwise the path to successive existential solutions would be barred, and development would be at a dead-end.
>
> (ibid., pp. 524–5)

The criterion by which the success of a reconstruction of humanity is to be evaluated is its chance of leading to another reconstruction, which is then capable of leading to yet another reconstruction, etc. Doubts about autoevolution are not concerned with its chances, but with its desirability. Even if it should prove possible, this process is worryingly *empty*: its various stages are aimed solely at continuation. Without substantial values, autoevolution is merely the expression of human subjectivity for its own sake. The substantialists draw particular attention to the emptiness of the concept of freedom behind this project, for example in the passage by Leon Kass already quoted in Chapter 9:

> The idea of man as that creature who is free to create himself is purely formal, not to say empty. It provides no boundaries that would

indicate when what was subhuman became truly human, or when what was at first human became less than human. Moreover, the freedom to destroy (by genetic manipulation or brain modification) one's nature, including the capacity and desire for freedom. It is, literally, a freedom which can end all freedom. And it provides no standards by which to measure whether the changes made are in fact improvements.

(Kass 1972, pp. 60–1)

In the past, eugenicists have tried to avoid this problem by trying to create a religion. Francis Galton was a follower of this idea, and, more recently, Julian Huxley wrote:

Once the full implications of evolutionary biology are grasped, eugenics will inevitably become part of the religion of the future, or of whatever complex of sentiments may in the future take the place of organised religion. It is not merely a sane outlet for human altruism, but is of all outlets for altruism that which is most comprehensive and of longest range.

(Huxley 1947, p. 22)

Apart from the fact that this kind of religious transfiguration today seems old-fashioned and naïve, it does nothing to solve the problem. It does not provide us with the criterion called for by Kass, with which we could decide whether a concrete reconstruction of humanity should be deemed successful or not. And it is certainly not capable of telling us which overall goal a eugenic strategy should be aiming at. This is the reason why, in a later appraisal of the supermen and women to be found within the literary genre of science fiction, even Lem began to concentrate on the goals at stake.

An author who is unsure about that presents the superman as a curio, in the same way as parents present their wonderchild; if such a hero is subjected to creative or expansive pressure ('Do something!' – 'Show us what you can do!'), without this pressure being part of a meta-programme of a duly considered selection of goals, the whole thing becomes a collection of circus acts and tricks, and no amount of skill is able to conceal the void of motivation.

(Lem 1980, pp. 323–4)

The further on in the autoevolutive process we attempt to anticipate, and the more perfect we imagine the human genus to be, the harder it becomes to envisage tasks which these superhuman capabilities should be carrying out. Nearly all the activities which form part of our daily lives – education, work, leisure, keeping fit – seem inappropriate for the technically perfect human being of the future. Even if this future human being is still expected to indulge in these activities, at the very most they will be significant secondary activities in a life dedicated to very different goals. Yet which goals?

> The more generously the writer has endowed his superman with unusual talents and abilities, the more acute the problem becomes of what the hero is supposed to do with this 'embarras de richesse'.
>
> (ibid., p. 325)

Not a good life

For Lem, the fact that neither writers nor philosophers explore the goals of autoevolution in enough detail, let alone attempt to solve the connected problems, is not due to insufficient intellectual courage, but to the historical development of philosophy, which has always interpreted the human being as an invariable subject of knowledge and object of research.

> Deliberations about how the human being *should* reshape itself physically and mentally if it should manage to gain the instrumental abilities necessary to do so has never been part of philosophical or anthropological research. Such thoughts have always been, and still are regarded as fantastic, probably with the maxim *contra spem spero* in mind.
>
> (Lem p. 231)

This diagnosis is certainly not wrong, but it does not go far enough. A goal which all manipulations are geared to realise would be more or less the same thing as the *ultimate good* to be found in ancient ethics, since, as Aristotle put it, we would be striving for that goal for its own sake:

> . . . and therefore we call final without qualification that which is always desirable in itself and never for the sake of something else. Now such a thing happiness, above all else, is held to be; | for this we choose always for itself and never for the sake of something else . . .
>
> (*Eth. Nic.*, 1097a 30–b1)

It should not be forgotten that Aristotle's conception of the ultimate good is to be seen in the context of a *teleological metaphysic*, in which every thing has its natural location, every process its goal, and thus every human being its objective destination. During the course of the modern philosophical revolution, however, this metaphysic has been undermined. After the deteleologisation of our world view, it is no longer possible to attribute human actions to a pre-determined goal within the structure of the universe or within human nature. The modern human being can no longer fall back on the notion of an objective ultimate good, nor, consequently, on that of a 'good life' orientated towards this good. The modern human being has to define its own goals and, in so doing, to define not *the* but *its* 'good life'. However, this means losing any objective sense which the notion of the ultimate good may have had; replacing it with human subjectivity.

> If all the ends which human actions can aim at are based on free, human self-determination, and if even the human's own being becomes one of the things which it is able to control, then the objective context within which human actions can be an end in themselves is exceeded: the *poiesis* practically becomes absolute. This is why, after that philosophical revolution, it is so hard to pinpoint the *successfulness* in practice, i.e. the *good* life, if it is not to be the achievement of self-made goals. In modern terms, the *good life* is no longer separable from what the population voluntarily *believes to be the good life*.
>
> (Schnädelbach 1986, pp. 48–9)

Within the scope of modern metaphysics, there is no way that we will be able to anticipate the goals of action or the meaning of life for supermen and women. The ultimate good cannot be determined by anticipative knowledge, but only *decided* by an act of self-determination.

Nevertheless, striving for the ultimate good has drastically declined with modern ethics, which many consider to be a deficit in comparison to ancient ethics; in recent years it was noted that 'as beings equipped with deliberative skills, we cannot avoid raising the question of our real welfare' (Tugendhat 1984a, p. 47). In the light of a project as revolutionary as autoevolution, our 'real welfare' is a matter which needs to be settled all the more urgently. The attempt to reformulate ancient striving towards the highest goal, the truly desirable or the good life, on the basis of the modern – i.e. with a radicalised claim to justification – concept of morality therefore merits considerable interest. Yet how can the concept of an ultimate good be justified if it cannot be traced back to an objective natural tendency or to an objective human destination? If there can be no such objectivisation, and if goals are merely what human beings set themselves, then – as Kant criticised – any notion of ontological perfection necessarily becomes circular: it is always presupposed that such-and-such a life is the 'good life', and that such-and-such a person is perfect, without any justification for this presupposition. With this in mind, Ernst Tugendhat suggested a reformulation of the 'good life' concept. Based on the theory that we do have an objective criterion for whether a person is well off or not in at least *one* area of human life, namely physical health and disease, he proposed a corresponding concept of spiritual health, from which to deduce a criterion for true happiness. He is convinced that Kant's criticism would no longer apply if we stopped worrying about its content, and instead developed a formal concept of mental health. Picking up on psychoanalytical literature, Tugendhat proposes that compulsive and reflex behaviour be regarded as spiritually unhealthy, with spiritual health consisting in an uninfringed, i.e. free will.

> With regard to true happiness, it follows (as we have already learnt from existentialist philosophy) that only what I really will, in the sense that I choose it freely, is truly willed . . . the truly willed is a matter referring not to the goals of our will, but to the manner in which we will . . . I am therefore not of the opinion that the ancient question regarding true happiness is nowadays obsolete, but that it can only be answered formally, formally in a sense similar to that in which Kant's questioning of morality was answered.
>
> (Tugendhat 1984a, pp. 55–6)

If we ignore the problems behind the terms 'health' and 'disease', which Tugendhat presumed to be unproblematic, and also the problems which would no doubt arise in any attempt to find criteria by which to measure freedom of the will, then there are still two objections to be made regarding this concept of the good life. Firstly, its formal nature is a problem: if the content of the happiness concept is programmatically ignored, then this concept will no longer be able to provide material orientation of the sort needed in order to improve the human race. If freedom of the will is the only criterion, then even Lem's proposed transition to other aggregate states ('reasonable cloud'), or the bringing of happiness to individuals through a genetically programmed increase in endorphine production, would have to be accepted as morally legitimate. True, this kind of formal definition does not permit absolutely everything: freedom of the will draws attention to empirical circumstances which do not permit such freedom. This includes not only political compulsion, but also indirect social pressure, such as that emerging due to the 'restrictions' of scientific and technological progress. Yet within the limitations of free will, a formal definition of happiness is not able to provide any goals; far more, against the background of modern subjectivity, it is assumed that happiness can only be found in the self-determination of the individual and the autonomous setting of goals by the individual.

This brings us to the second problem: the individualistic limitations of Tugendhat's concept of happiness. It is ultimately nothing more than a reformulation of Kant's notion of autonomy in medical and psychiatric terms. Kant's interpretation of autonomy is that the will itself determines one's desires, remaining untouched by outside influences. In this respect, Tugendhat's 'true will' refers to the *individual* as the incorporation of autonomy or the subject of happiness. Whereas discourse ethicists attempt to overcome this individualism by socialising autonomy, this approach is an extension of 'Kant's purely personal, monologue approach' (Habermas 1986, p. 24). For freedom of the will can only be the private act of an individual. This concept of the greatest good thus proves to be an inadequate basis for GenEthics. Autoevolution would only be viable if undertaken collectively: 'collectively' not only in the obvious sense of various individuals working together, but especially in the sense of including future generations. Yet it is impossible to ascertain what will constitute the latter's formal happiness. Even if it would be *our* free will humanly giving up its organic body in order to change into the aggregate state of gases or crystals, this would by no means guarantee that those future 'reasonable clouds' affected and moulded by our will would be of the same opinion. The individuals which would primarily be affected have no chance of freely desiring their gaseous or crystalline existence.

We seem to be faced with the following alternatives. We can demand *substantial* goals as orientation for an autoevolutive strategy. Yet the formulation of such goals may be criticised for two reasons: philosophically they are exposed to the blame of circularity, and sociologically they are under suspicion of extrapolating and dogmatising an existing system of values, which – for whatever reasons – is particularly treasured. If we accept this, and are satisfied with a *formal* concept of the ultimate good, then this approach may be acceptable from a meta-ethical point of view, but the orientational marker it provides necessarily remains too vague. Norms may be formulated, yet all they do is to exclude certain types of action, not giving any clue as to positive goals. We could regard this vagueness as the price we have had to pay for the autonomy of the individual. *Politically* speaking, it would be expression of the individual's emancipation, with its right to decide freely how to shape its life; *philosophically* speaking, it would be expression of the essential freedom of the human being, which – even if it does begin to control its own evolution – is not subjected to the dominion of a given system of values. Thus nobody seems more justified in referring to Sartre's definition of human freedom than the autoevolutionist:

> I am condemned to exist forever beyond my essence, beyond the causes and motives of my act. I am condemned to be free. This means that no limits to my freedom can be found except freedom itself or, if you prefer, that we are not free to cease being free.
>
> (Sartre 1958, p. 439)

New quality

Expressed in Sartre's philosophical terminology, the human being 'designs' and 'projects' itself, and this vocabulary can be taken very literally when applied to human genetic self-alteration plans. The following passage by Sartre comes over as an infinite autoevolution devoid of goals, translated into the language of 'phenomenological ontology':

> Since freedom is a being-without-support and without-a-springboard, the project in order to be must be constantly renewed. I choose myself perpetually and can never be merely by virtue of having-been-chosen; otherwise I should fall into the pure and simple existence of the in-itself... Our particular projects, aimed at the realization in the world

of a particular end, are united in the global project which we are. But precisely because we are wholly choice and act, these partial projects are not determined by the global project. They must themselves be choices; and a certain margin of contingency, of unpredictability, and of the absurd is allowed to each of them, although each project as it is projected is the specification of the global project on the occasion of particular elements in the situation and so is always understood in relation to the totality of my being-in-the-world.

(Sartre 1958, pp. 480–1)

Apart from its parodistic flavour, Sartre's concept of human self-design may be objected to for not being linked to a particular technology, understood instead as a fundamental definition of the way in which human beings exist at all. Human 'free self-design' is not dependent upon genetic self-alteration. The human being has always, and in all circumstances, designed itself. Autoevolution would simply mean a new type of self-design, namely one affecting the biological constitution of the subject.

This interpretation has many things going for it. Human beings have manipulated human nature and controlled human reproduction whenever the means for doing so have been available. And they have also been capable, with meditation and drugs, of finding ways to influence deliberately not only the individual human spirit, but also – with social institutions such as education, religion, ideology, etc. – the collective human spirit. As the theologian, Karl Rahner, writes, active self-manipulation is as old as the human race itself:

> [the human being] has 'deliberately' drunk wine in order to combat feelings of melancholy, has consciously used coffee as a stimulant, has undertaken primitive attempts at breeding human beings, has attempted to alter its habitual appearance with various techniques – shaving being the first – has employed pedagogical methods stricter than dressage and beyond the point of acceptance, has attempted – albeit amateurishly – institutional indoctrination, etc.

(Rahner 1967a, pp. 262–3)

As parts of this world, neither the human being's biological constitution not its subjectivity have ever been beyond the scope of human action. Yet a general reference to the universality and historical continuity of human self-manipulation does not suffice to dismiss the *new quality* of gene and reproduction technology. The fact that human beings had already begun to intervene in the process of reproduction back in primitive societies, whether for contraceptive or for 'proceptive' purposes is an indication of a continuity of wishes and goals reaching into the present day. Yet if we take a look at the limited and incomplete means available then, and compare them with the technological options available today, together with those possibly available in the future, then it becomes clear how little continuity there is as far as technological means are concerned. The new quality which gene and reproduction technology has lent to human self-determination primarily consists in its technological character. Seen like this, even talk of a 'technological revolution' within the field of human reproduction loses its air of dramatic metaphor and acquires a precise meaning.

In the next section, the new quality of gene and reproduction technology is traced back to a new stage of development with regard to its technological character. I shall justify the conclusion that the advancement of technological means incurs a dynamism which increasingly detaches from, and ultimately replaces, the rational formulation and realisation of autoevolutionary goals. This conclusion is not intended to breathe new life into the *topos* 'technology as Fate'. I do not maintain that the development of technology follows an autonomous determinism, but that it involves a tendency for technologically possible options to overlap freely chosen goals involving ideas and projects of human self-alteration. An inversion of Utopia occurs: it is no longer a case of anticipating means to satisfy given needs, but of extrapolating into the future given lines of scientific and technological development, without being able to give them concrete goals. Sartre's ontology of freedom and his anthology of self-design prove to be just as abstract as Lem's announcement regarding excessive freedom of action (1980). They both abstract from the social circumstances of autoevolution, and from the consequences resulting from the technological character of this process for the structure and content of its goals. These goals will not be the result of autonomous will, but will follow the maelstrom of the 'feasible'. In absence of ontologically established values and an objectively justifiable vision of the good life, human control over human evolution will necessarily be subject to the technological imperative: orientational markers are not provided by socially constituted and rationally justified values, but by the chances provided by scientific and technological progress, together with the 'requirements' of scientific and technological civilisation.

Means as ends

1. Each technological artefact and each technological procedure is conceived and introduced in order to manipulate natural phenomena consciously and purposefully. This is also true of the earliest and most primitive interventions in human reproduction. The reforms due to current technological achievements are primarily drastic increases in the degree of consciousness and purposefulness behind the interventions, especially if we consider the scope of the manipulations and their prospects of being developed further. The past may be summarised using the following formula: either such manipulations were conscious and purposeful, and then they were limited in scope because they applied to the individual reproductive process; or – if they did have a far-reaching influence on the evolution of the human species – they were neither conscious nor purposeful since they only took effect indirectly, by influencing the conditions governing selection. To a large extent, this formula is still true today. Insofar as human beings influence human evolution at all, this influence is mainly indirect. The repercussions of civilisation and industry on the human biological constitution spring to mind, mutagenesis induced by chemicals and radiation, for example. And even the latest achievements in the field of gene technology involve individually orientated interventions with consequently negligible effects for human evolution. Yet there can hardly be any doubt that further developments in this field of technology will lead to the point where even direct influencing of human evolution will become possible. This prospect underlies each concept of eugenics and autoevolution.

2. As soon as technological artefacts and procedures have reached a certain stage of development, their application usually acquires a constructive character. They are then aimed not only at getting natural processes going or at interrupting them, but at reforming or completely redesigning whole natural systems. Modern biological technology and science confirms this by

increasingly tending not only to use existing organisms for human purposes, but to commence from purposes to be achieved, and then to construct the organisms necessary for their realisation. At the moment, there are still not many ways of applying such constructive procedures to human beings, but development is moving in this direction. Whereas manipulation of human reproduction used to be solely quantitative – offspring was prevented or created – we are now faced with the prospect of what Joseph Fletcher has termed 'quality control'. This is a direct consequence of the character of the new technologies: they are far more precise and can therefore be used more precisely; they also go 'deeper' – as far as the molecular level of human nature – and are thus capable of achieving greater, 'qualitative' effects. Just as Lem's autoevolutive strategy aims far beyond the medical prevention of harm, Lederberg's concept of 'orthobiosis' postulates the transition from the mere repair of human nature to its construction (1970, p. 40). Despite Lederberg's assurance that the distinction between repair and construction is merely an 'arbitrary definition', the consequences of such a transition are not only ethically, but also technologically extremely far-reaching. It signifies a fundamental change in the status of human nature as the object of technology. In the first case, human nature remains the focus of each manipulation; in the second, it is the mere starting point, from which the interventions extend. The trend towards a practical, or, to put it more precisely, the *technological naturalisation* of humanity outlined above will change human constitution into a plastic mass, the 'material' for technological action.

3. Technology is neutral in the sense that it provides means for arbitrary purposes. Which purposes are realisable and which are not certainly depends on technology as such; but which purposes are good and which are bad can only be decided 'aside' from technology. Technological progress is constantly increasing our means, and with them our capacity for achieving ends, but not our capacity for setting ends. The arbitrariness of purposes will also mould the constructive procedures within the field of human nature. J. B. S. Haldane presented an impressive example of this at the noteworthy Ciba Symposium, speculating about the optimisation of human beings for space travel.

The most obvious abnormalities in extra-terrestrial environments are differences in gravitation, temperature, air pressure, air composition, and radiation (including high-speed material particles). Clearly a gibbon is better preadapted than a man for a life in a low gravitational field, such as that of a space ship, an asteroid, or perhaps even the moon. A platyrrhine with a prehensile tail is even more so. Gene grafting may make it possible to incorporate such features into the human stocks. The human legs and much of the pelvis are not wanted. Men who had lost their legs by accident or mutation would be specially qualified as astronauts. If a drug is discovered with an action like that of thalidomide, but on the leg rudiments only, not the arms, it may be useful to prepare the crew of the first spaceship to the *Alpha Centauri* system, thus reducing not only their weight, but their food and oxygen requirements. A regressive mutation to the condition of our ancestors in the mid-Pliocene, with prehensile feet, no appreciable heels, and an ape-like pelvis, would be still better. There is no immediate prospect of men encountering high gravitational fields, as they will when they reach the solid or liquid surface of Jupiter. Presumably they should be short-legged or quadrupedal.

(Haldane 1967, p. 354)

These deliberations are not so much remarkable for the fact that they exceed beyond the point of parody, nor because of their technological naïvety (as if the main problem involved in human space travel were food and oxygen supplies); they are remarkable for the thoughtlessness with which human legs are removed (for the flight), then – in double quantity – put back again (for Jupiter). Haldane is prepared to carry out any sort of manipulation that could aid the success of technological projects such as space travel. Joshua Lederberg objects to this: since the time dimensions involved in genetic improvements are enormous, it would be sensible to precede genetic improvement with a phase of somatic – physiological, embryological, etc. – improvement.

If we want a man without legs, we don't have to breed him, we can chop them off; if we want a man with a tail, we will find a way of grafting it on to him.

(Lederberg 1967b, p. 362)

Technological development seems to be leading to a gulf between the precision, scope, 'maturity' of the means and the arbitrariness, randomness, 'immaturity' of the ends. Technology is not adapted to meet human interests: the human being is adapted to meet the requirements of technology.

4. It should be noted, however, that such ends can only be 'immature' according to a (moral) criterion. From a technological point of view, they are neither arbitrary nor random. The theory that technology is neutral can hardly be rejected as far as individual ends–means relationships are concerned, yet it misses the point when applied to more comprehensive techno-systems and their cultural integration.

> Logically speaking, it is correct that means are neutral ('is never implies ought'), but in sociological terms this is incorrect ('ability usually implies desire'). The non-neutrality of the means immediately becomes apparent if we remind ourselves that societies throughout history have been moulded more by the means of power and production available to them than by their changing goals. This moulding does not only include social structures, but also systems of value . . . It does not follow from the neutrality of technologies in their application that they do not have a normative influence on society. What follows is exactly the opposite: their influence is universal and comprehensive.
>
> (van den Daele & Krohn 1982, pp. 421–2)

Haldane's plans and Lederberg's comments do not really display an arbitrariness, but rather a specific 'rationality'. The interventions mentioned serve *technical* purposes which may be precisely defined; they are not arbitrary, but adhere to the criterion of technological projects. The 'heroic' character of space travel may seem to justify the manipulating away or the sawing off of legs; other writers have even considered altering human nature for the purposes of everyday technology. Once again it is Stanislaw Lem who expresses the prevailing technocratic, scientistic trend most clearly. Like Lederberg, at the early stages of 'reconstructing the genus' he demands the stepwise replacement of natural human organs with transplants ('biological prosthetics') or more efficient, mechanical aggregates ('non-biological prosthetics').

> The most important thing, however, is that not only the requirements of the human organism, but also those of the new technologies will determine the further development of biological and non-biological prosthetics.
>
> (Lem 1976, p. 504)

Technological evolution takes on the double function of forming objectives and realising objectives. The development of values and goals becomes a variable dependent upon technological progress.

Intelligence

A closer look at the relevant plans and projects shows that the values which are supposed to act as orientation for the improvement of humanity are only partly connected with the fight against suffering. These values are overlapped by suggested improvements which amount to the human race being adapted to technological civilisation. If we ignore for the moment plans to alter individual human beings for particular purposes (occupations) and take a look at more comprehensive goals, we come up against the same pattern of argumentation time and again: the human being, its biological constitution rooted in the dim and distant past, and unaltered since then, is not up to coping with modern civilisation. This is firstly true of its *body*, which may be more or less suited to life on Earth, but which is totally unsuited to space travel. As early as the 1960s, appropriate reconstructions of the human body were being suggested. With regard to the danger of nuclear war and the benefits of space travel, for example, it 'may be worth selecting resistant types when we know how to do so' (Haldane 1967, p. 355) – a suggestion which is still as relevant today with the slackening of expensive safety devices in nuclear power plants. If such a recommendation were to be realised, the autoevolutionist would still have a great deal to do. Firstly, the process of autoevolution has no natural end. Once the resistant type has been bred, it will be time to construct a new, even more perfect, human being, which is not only resistant to radiation, but which maybe – since it will be in abundant supply after a nuclear war or nuclear power plant disaster anyway – can live on radiation. Secondly, adapting the human body is only half the task. What use is the most perfect organism if the human *spirit* is still one of the 'constructional solutions' which evolution randomly came up with tens of thousands of years ago?

It is commonplace that the formation and control of a highly complex technological civilisation requires far more intellectual resources than the maintenance of a small tribal community with little technological know-how. In the future, we will require considerably more technological know-how, scientific knowledge, ability to make prognoses, ability to assess risks, etc. Yet, whereas intellectual demands seem to increase with the progress of civilisation, intellectual ability seems to be subject to biological limitations. With the emergence of *Homo sapiens*, the evolution of the brain came to a stop; the human race has managed to progress from the hand-axe to the space rocket with an unaltered brain. Since human beings are obviously no longer in a position to regulate the further development of their societies or their treatment of Nature in a planned and sensible manner, the time seems to be approaching when the requirements of an even more progressive civilisation will exceed intellectual ability once and for all. With this threatening prospect in mind, the conclusion seems obvious: if we have acquired the ability to manipulate ourselves genetically, then this ability must not stop at the human body, but must instead be deliberately used to increase human intelligence. We have already seen that an increase in the average I.Q. ranks highly in the list of individual visions regarding human genetic improvement. Intelligence is held in such high esteem within our society that most parents would view the possibility of positively influencing their children in this way as significant progress. This shows that individual evaluations of intelligence converge with a social need.

The notion of increasing intelligence with biological means has a long tradition, going back to the classical eugenics of Francis Galton, who centred his entire concept of positive eugenics around it. Besides a particular couple's individual interest in having highly intelligent children, a collective interest of society or the human species also played a decisive rôle. 'Differential fertility', diagnosed on the basis of extensive statistical research, lent great social urgency to the problem of how to increase intelligence. According to this theory, there is a negative correlation between intelligence and fertility: the higher the social rank of a couple, the fewer the children it usually has. If we assume that (a) there is a positive relationship between social status and intelligence, and (b) intelligence is hereditary, then we have to conclude that, over a considerable number of generations, the intelligence of the total population will gradually decrease. In the 1960s, prominent biologists such as Herman Muller, Julian Huxley and Jacques Monod (1972, p. 150) voiced their agreement with this theory. According to Muller (1967, pp. 253–4),

> it is not the having of children but the prevention of them which today requires the more active, responsible effort, an effort which makes demands on the participants' prudence, initiative, skill and conscience. It seems evident that persons possessed of greater foresight, and those with keener regard for their family, usually aim to have a lower than average number of children, in order that they may obtain higher benefits for those children that they do have, as well as for themselves and others near to them. Moreover, persons who experience failure in their work, their home life, or their health, are especially likely to seek compensatory gratification in having children. At the same time, as regards success in limiting conception to the extent aimed at, it is evident that ability enters in here in a negative way, in that those who are clumsier, slacker, less provident, and less thoughtful are the very ones most likely to fail in keeping the number of their children down to whatever quota they may have set.

Since the variation in size of families living in civilised countries is no longer primarily due to the biological ability to reproduce, but to the success of contraceptive devices – and thus the caution, foresight, intelligence, etc. of their users –, it is feared that a selection is taking place which will end in the population's average I.Q. being reduced. This obviously conjures up a second variation of the degeneration problem: the vision of a not only physical, but also intellectual decline of the civilised world. The empirical validity of this diagnosis is as problematic as the degeneration theory in general; yet it acquires a dramatic dimension if we consider the advancement of our scientific and technological civilisation.

> This is an ironical situation. Cultural evolution has at long last given rise to science and its technologies. It has thereby endowed itself with powers that – according to the manner in which they are used – could either wreck the human enterprise or carry it upward to unprecedented heights of being and of doing. To steer his course under these circumstances man will need his greatest collective wisdom, humanity, will to co-operate, and self-control. Moreover, he cannot muster these faculties in sufficient measure collectively unless he also possesses them in considerable measure individually. Yet in this very epoch cultural evolution has undermined the process of genetic selection in man, a process

whose active continuance is necessary for the mere maintenance of man's faculties at their present none-too-adequate level. What we need instead, at this juncture, is a means of *enhancing* genetic selection.

(Muller 1967, p. 254)

We can only solve the problems of our civilisation if the gap between these increasing requirements and the actual decline of intelligence is closed. Of course, it would be better if we could take eugenic measures in order to gain an intellectual head start. According to Julian Huxley, Francis Galton complained of a shortage of:

brains capable of dealing with the complexities of modern administration, technology and planning, and that, with the inevitable increase of our social and technical complexity, the greater that shortage will become. It is thus clear that for any major advance in national and international efficiency we cannot depend on haphazard tinkering with social or political symptoms or ad hoc patching up of the world's political machinery, or even on improving general education, but must rely increasingly on raising the genetic level of man's intellectual and practicable abiities.

(Huxley 1964, p. 255)

Within the short time of its existence, the human being has managed to create a civilisation which is developing at a far greater rate than genetic evolution. Consequently, there is a discrepancy emerging between the manifold demands made of the human being regarding control over this civilisatory development and the genetic basis of its capability to do so, formed tens of thousands of years ago. It then seems necessary to require of the human being that it attain *biologically* – as far as its physical and mental abilities are concerned – the same level of development as it has culturally. If human nature and human culture are not on a par, then both are seemingly condemned to go under.

Controlling subjectivity

Yet the difficulties do not stop here. Besides the gulf between intelligence and civilisation, there is another problem just as threatening:

. . . the disparity between the evolution of technology and the evolution of society's moral capabilities: over thousands of years, the human race has acquired technological means which could grant it individual, well-balanced access to its material environment, and yet the majority of these means is still applied in a disordered manner to satisfying predatory tendencies which can be traced back to the times when the human being's enemy was the rhinocerous.

(Leroi-Gourhan 1980, p. 287)

Once the disparity between technological ability and moral maturity has been acknowledged as fact, a search for the cause of this disparity begins. It will come as no surprise that this cause has now been located: in human genes.

Perhaps the instability, incoherences, and convulsions of our sociopolitical systems are an expression of our biological and cultural immaturity for life in large communities; evolution may have adapted us only to life in small groups. Given the rates of biological evolution, it would be somewhat hopeless to wait for biological adaptation to our new living conditions. Millions of years of hunting may have slanted us toward a behavior that is not necessarily adapted to the life we presently live. But we clearly must cope with the genotypes we have. It is, of course, encouraging to think that part at least of this adaptation may have been toward cooperation. But probably the demands for cooperative tendencies in the modern world are much greater than those that were sufficient for the smaller world of our most ancient ancestors. We can only hope that our genotypes provide us with sufficient plasticity to meet these new and challenging environments we have created for ourselves.

(Bodmer & Cavalli-Sforza 1976, pp. 554–5)

Four decades earlier, Hermann Muller had already come to a similar conclusion. He emphasised in *Out of the Night* that social evolution is dependent not only upon human intelligence, but also upon all those genetically determined dispositions and abilities which Muller sums up as 'morality'. It was not until the predecessors of the human race had evolved far enough to possess a genetic basis sufficient for social behaviour to take place that communal life began to develop, and social evolution to advance (Muller 1936, p. 120). Since this basis for cooperative behaviour has been in our genes since prehistoric times, the advance of civilisation, and especially the exponential growth of science and technology over the last few centuries, threatens to divide human nature and human culture in terms of morality in the same way as has been feared with respect to intelligence. Technologically a contemporary of the Industrial Age, the human being is morally still in the Stone Age. Yet, whereas Bodmer and Cavalli-Sforza assume that we will have to make to do with the genotypes we have, Muller is not as resigned. Human understanding of practical science and technology calls for a eugenic improvement of human morality.

> The whole course of human prehistory and history makes the necessary ideals obvious and unmistakeable; they are (aside from physical well-being) primarily two: highly developed social feeling – call it fraternal love, or sympathy, or comradeliness, as you prefer; and the highest possible intelligence – call it analytical ability or depth of understanding, or 'reason'.
>
> (ibid., p. 148)

More recently, Tristram Engelhardt has put forward similar arguments in favour of an enhancement of human morality by genetic engineering. In answer to those who fear that such procedures may contain unknown risks, he argues that a failure to re-engineer may involve similar unknown risks.

> There is evidence, for example, that human predispositions to belligerence have a genetic basis. About one-fourth of males in a state of nature (i.e. the controls of an organized state absent) die in fighting. At one point this inclination to kill competing males may have contributed to the inclusive fitness of such belligerent individuals. However, at present it may offer one of the most substantial risks for the total annihilation of mankind. In the end, the continued survival of humans may require engineering around such inclinations and such particular expressions of competitiveness.
>
> (Engelhardt 1986, pp. 380–1)

These plans to use gene technology in order to increase intelligence and morality raise a number of questions. Can we be absolutely sure that intelligence and morality are genetically determined characteristics? At the present time it seems impossible to find a clear answer to this question. Nobody is capable of giving a clear, empirical definition of 'intelligence' or 'morality'. What is clear is that both are highly complex, polygenetic characteristics, largely independent of the environment. There can be no hope of

using gene technology to modify and improve them in the foreseeable future. This book abstracts from empirical and technological
problems, however, and we shall focus now on the type of characteristics which are the focus of genetic manipulation. Intelligence
and morality are both regarded to be moments of human *subjectiv-*
ity. It is not only human nature which is being manipulated here.
A strict separation of human subjectivity and human nature is
actually only possible for analytical purposes; the real human
being is not half 'subject' and half 'a part of Nature'.

Modern scientists have repeatedly substantiated this connection.
Darwin and his supporters were amongst the first to deny that the
theory of evolution be applicable solely to the human *physis*. In
1873, the Darwinist, Oscar Schmidt, wrote:

> All of the uneasiness surrounding the theory of evolution, all the
> doubts, the anger, focus on the theory's applicability and complete
> application to the human race. And if we are forced to surrender our
> *physis*, then at least the human spiritual sphere shall remain closed to
> the researchers, a *noli tangere*.
>
> (Schmidt 1873, p. 263)

But it was already too late for a *noli tangere*. In his *Descent of Man*
and Selection in Relation to Sex, Darwin attempted to stretch his
scientific theory to include human powers of abstraction, self-
confidence, mental and spiritual individuality, language, sense of
beauty, religiousness and conviviality, and to interpret all these
instances of human subjectivity as a product of natural selection
(1974). Twentieth century scientists have successfully pushed this
research programme further, and are currently busy attacking the
bastions of the human spirit. Scientific disciplines as varied as
neurobiology, behavioural research and the computer sciences are
all bent on finding a causal explanation for the way human beings
think and make decisions.

> Under the microscope of the behavioural researcher, the intentional
> action is reduced to 'mere reflexes'; every spontaneous, voluntary step
> originates from a stimulus. Just as a ballet – an expression of the
> greatest athletic control and deep emotion – may be reduced to a
> musical score and choreography, every instance of skilled behaviour
> may be viewed as a series of reflexes.
>
> (Hoebel 1983, p. 102)

In the light of neurophysiological and neurochemical investigations, even happiness and love seem to be attributable to mere chemical reactions: even they are part of Nature.

This naturalisation of subjectivity by the empirical sciences is a challenge to human self-consciousness. As for the naturalisation of human beings in general, with the technological dimension of modern science this challenge acquires a new moral quality. The scientific explanation of a phenomenon is not just a step forward theoretically: it renders the phenomenon technologically controllable. Modern forms of biotechnology control human nature and – with this control – human subjectivity. A good example of this is electrical stimulation of the brain. Developed as a method of scientifically researching the cerebral mechanisms in humans and animals, it can be deliberately used to influence human behaviour.[1] Even if this technique in itself is fairly limited, together with other techniques such as psycho-surgery and psycho-pharmacology it

[1] 'This methodology has proved that movements, sensations, emotions, desires, ideas, and a variety of psychological phenomena may be induced, inhibited, or modified by electrical stimulation of specific areas of the brain' (Delgado 1969, p. 257). This technique makes it possible to cause people to move in a certain way or to change their feelings, the people themselves not viewing these movements and changes as the artificial results of an experiment, but as manifestations of their own, free decisions. This procedure has been perceived as more than just a means of researching the brain: 'It is reasonable to assume that just as more knowledge of natural mechanisms allows us to use and control natural forces, a clearer understanding of the central nervous system should enable us to educate and direct mental activity more intelligently' (pp. 15–16). According to Delgado, up until now the human being has concentrated on controlling its natural environment, leading to a gain in physical power, but not in happiness. Civilisation has come to a crossroads: either it continues along the familiar path of material progress, without paying any particular attention to uncovering the secrets of the brain; or it changes direction, investing some of the economical and intellectual resources available in an explanation of the mechanisms governing mental activity. 'The thesis of this book is that we now possess the necessary technology for the experimental investigation of mental activities, and that we have reached a critical turning point in the evolution of man at which the mind can be used to influence its own structure, functions and purpose, thereby ensuring both the preservation and advance of civilization. The following pages contain a discussion of what the mind is, the technical problems involved in its possible control by physical means, and the outlook for development of a future psychocivilized society' (pp. 19–20). Even if we ignore the propagandistic nature of such projects, as well as the exaggerated technological optimism behind them, we cannot ignore the significant message they contain: techniques such as electrical cerebral stimulation, psycho-surgery or psycho-pharmacology enable the brain – and thus human subjectivity – to be more or less directly influenced.

forms part of a growing ensemble of ways to control the human
brain – and ultimately human subjectivity – with the aid of
technology.

There is no direct connection between these techniques of controlling behaviour and gene and reproduction technology; nevertheless, it is obvious that if at some stage we are able to manipulate human genetic constitutions, we will also have the technology
to control the structures of the human central nervous system. It
can hardly be expected that autoevolutionists will be content to
stop at the physical alteration of human beings, and will exclude
from their improvement strategies control over all kinds of conscious processes. As early as 1936, Muller deplored how little we
know about the human brain, pointing out, however, that acquisition of the relevant facts in the future would create options for
technological intervention.

> It would be strange if advances in the study of its structure and work-
> ings (call it psychology or brain physiology, as you will) did not cause
> a succession of revolutions in our methods of controlling men's con-
> scious states and behaviour, revolutions incomparably more important
> than the relatively crude effects obtained by regulating the composi-
> tion of the blood through gland extracts or otherwise.
>
> (Muller 1936, p. 89)

A quarter of a century later, Julian Huxley made higher
demands along the same lines.

> We must explore qualitative inner space as well as quantitative outer
> space. This, of course, includes the exploration of our own individual
> minds and their operations, and also exploration of the nöosphere, the
> realm of thought and feeling which our minds create in interaction
> with the fact of experience, the psychological habitat in which we live
> and on whose resources we must draw. As regards our individual
> minds, the main aim must be to canalize their development so as to
> reconcile or transcend conflicting drives and impulses, and to develop
> effective psychological bonds with other individuals and with nature
> around us. Much of this will be psychotechnology.
>
> (Huxley 1967a, p. 11)

According to Huxley, the beneficial effects of such 'psycho-
technology' would include an abolition of the tendency – which
many people have – of transferring their responsibility to others,

of dispelling aggressive impulses in a dangerous manner, or of viewing abstractions such as 'truth' or 'virtue' as realities. It is of little significance in this context whether these effects are to be brought about through somatic manipulation or genetic alteration. What is important is the transition from human nature to human subjectivity inherent to biotechnological progress. The projects aimed at increasing the happiness of humanity using gene technology or other procedures, and especially the manifold plans deliberately to increase intelligence and morality – what is really meant is cooperativeness – are all reflections of this tendency. Once technological development reaches a certain level, the distinction between human nature and human subjectivity becomes fiction. Control over the nature and evolution of human beings then amounts to the same thing as technological control over human subjectivity.

Genetic fix and scientism

A further point worth noting is the socio-theoretical background behind plans to improve intelligence and morality. Can we really be certain that the political conflicts, economical crises and social problems of our time are due to human intelligence and morality not being able to cope with the demands of modern civilisation? The Stone Age human genome was, after all, capable of *creating* this civilisation. What makes us assume that it is not capable of controlling it sensibly and shaping it morally? The suspicion arises that that old and respected, ideological historical strategy – i.e. tracing social crises and problems back to natural causes – is rearing its head again, this time in a new disguise. A naturalistic diagnosis of this kind automatically suggests an appropriate form of therapy: political conflicts are not to be resolved politically, economical crises not to be overcome economically and social problems not to be solved socially – but with technology. In this sense,

> scientific and technological progress within Capitalist societies is gradually forming the complex of standards suitable to replace a radical reorganisation of social structures . . . Let us leave the expansion of science and technology to make up for the unavoidable imperfections

which occur in the course of socio-economic processes. Consensus exists in the following point: We have to favour control over Nature above control over society.

(Moscovici 1982, pp. 18–19)

In the case at stake, it is obviously human nature which is to be altered and controlled in place of society.

Analogous to the term 'technological fix', commonly accepted for the strategy of using technological means to solve political and social problems, the term 'genetic fix'[2] may be used to describe the proposed genetic adaption of human beings to modern civilisation. Lederberg's serious deliberations (1967a) as to whether mass cloning would make human communication easier and would overcome the generation gap – since all clones are in possession of the same 'genetically determined neurological hardware' it is reasonable to assume that they would get on with and understand each other much better – are both politically naïve and dangerous. They remove neither the difficulties connected with human communication, nor the social causes behind generation conflicts. The approach is said to be 'deeper', but the truth is that social and political conflicts are circumvented. It does not take the example of breeding radiation-resistant human beings, quoted earlier, to shed light on the doubtful social and ethical aspects of such a strategy. The possibility of subjecting applicants for particularly burdensome jobs to a genetic examination, in order to be able to select for employment only those who prove to be resistant to the danger(s) in question, is already in sight. Compared to the plans to increase the intelligence and morality of future generations, this kind of practice is fairly modest; it is not constructive, but selective, and only with regard to individual instances of susceptibility or resistance. The same logic underlies both examples, however: social conditions are not adapted to human beings, but human beings to social conditions.

If these plans to overcome the genetic limitations of intelligence and morality are taken as being in the interests of the process of civilisation, that it may continue as free from disturbance as possible, then it is easy to recognise these plans as variations of subjectivism. Based on a definition, as radical as it is one-sided, of the

---

[2] Etzioni coined this term in his book of the same name (1973).

human being as an *animal rationale*, this variation declares science and technology as belonging to those important manifestations of humanity which form the criteria according to which all areas of human action have to be governed. Since in the suspicious eye of the advocate of scientism the only things which hold water are those which meet the rational criteria of science and technology, morality is automatically suspected of being a relict from the days of superstition, and an obstruction to progress. A new morality is called for, one free of all prejudice, and promoting rather than hindering scientific and technological innovation. Intellectualistically, this new morality could be conceived of as an 'ethic of knowledge', rendering the acquisition of scientific knowledge 'by free choice the supreme value – the measure and guarantee for all other values' (Monod 1972, p. 167). Or it could have a technocratic impetus, aimed at adapting public and private morality to suit current technological options and the 'requirements' of modern civilisation. Several prominent members of this second group have been appealing to us for nearly a century to bury our prejudices about reproduction and 'making babies' (Fletcher) and to bring our attitude into line with current scientific and technological developments. Even a 'complete genetic overhaul' of Stone Age morality is being taken into consideration.

It is not possible here to make a prognosis regarding the chances a scientistic reform of morality would have of succeeding. Suffice it to say that these chances are likely to be smaller than the advocates' hope and the opponents' fear. In philosophical terms, scientism is primarily unacceptable for its attempts to declare a shortsighted concept of rationality as being the only guideline for action and the highest moral criterion. The unavoidable consequence of this position, regardless of what its advocates may maintain to the contrary, is the significant amputation of human subjectivity. Protagonists of scientism view the human being as the subject of Nature and of human nature, *but not as the subject of scientific and technological progress.* The latter becomes an independent, autonomous process, and its results are just as unquestionable a 'fate' as natural chance is for the substantialist. Scientistic subjectivism is thus, at least in one respect, closely related to substantialism: it attempts to construct the relationship between scientific and technological progress and normatively interpreted human nature according to the mathematical model of one dependent and one independent variable. Where substantialism dogmatises human nature, scientism dogmatises technology – both at the price of human subjectivity.

Epilogue

Epilogue

14

GenEthics and reproductive morality

Not even animals live without morality.
But human beings no longer know which sort . . .
Robert Musil

Modern gene and reproduction technology has provided us with practical options which we are unable to evaluate using traditional moral norms and values. The need for a GenEthics is therefore not something which has been philosophically generated, but the reflection of a problematic situation which has emerged with increasing scientific knowledge and technological ability. It was not the aim of this book to put together a detailed catalogue of norms for technological intervention in human reproduction. Instead, two fundamental positions potentially able to provide the philosophical basis for a GenEthics were discussed, and the diverging standards for action which they suggest were presented. There are seven points with which I would like to conclude.

Substantialism

In Part II of this book we became familiar with substantialism as the philosophical reformulation of a widespread, spontaneous uneasiness regarding gene and reproduction technology, its current possibilities and future prospects. Yet every attempt to make the notion of a normatively obliging human 'substance' plausible has failed. Apart from the fact that a precise definition of this substance has yet to be given, this kind of undertaking is inherently bound to end in a dilemma. Either this substance is interpreted as naturalistic, as a part of Nature which we have to accept; or it is normatively characterised from the start as the statement of an evaluating will. Since moral guidelines can only be ascertained from the first interpretation via the naturalistic fallacy, most writers tend to interpret human nature normatively, in order to avoid having to deduce an 'ought' from an 'is'. What they achieve is a shifting of the justification problem to a higher level: the reason why certain aspects of human nature are to be viewed as a normatively obliging substance is then in need of moral justification. This justification usually refers to the consequences which would ensue from another viewpoint. With this, the substantialist is deep in the wake of subjectivism, even adopting two of the fundamental subjectivistic principles: by maintaining that the human being is free to respect (human) nature as normative or not, the substantialist confirms the principle of autonomy; and with the transition to a consequentialist mode of argumentation in justifying the normativity of (human) nature, the substantialist confirms the basic rôle of human interests. In a GenEthics, the substantialist approach thus comes across as a moral philosophical diversion, ending its justification strategy at the point where subjectivism begins.

A simple mental experiment illustrates that the natural course of human reproduction cannot be merited with the dignity of inviolability. Let us assume that the eugenicists, ranging from Schallmayer and Ploetz to Muller and Huxley, were right with their degeneration theory. With changing selective conditions, civilised humanity lands up in the maelstrom of a steadily worsening gene pool. All types of genetically determined or co–determined diseases increase, whilst the average level of intelligence decreases. Under these circumstances, ambitious negative eugenics projects could obviously not be prevented; and morally viable arguments can be found to prove it. Just as ecological ethicists talk of the living having a responsibility towards the coming generations, we could also talk of our having a genetic responsibility towards our descendants. In actual fact, eugenicists have repeatedly emphasised

the existence of this kind of responsibility. It is not only the subjectivists who attack Paul Ramsey's view that the apocalyptic vision of
a slow, human genetic death does not justify eugenic counter-
measures, since Christians and Jews have no absolute obligation to
save the human race (1970, pp. 22–32). It is also countered, for
example, by Hans Jonas' 'first imperative' namely '*that* there be a
mankind' (1984, p. 43); this imperative would not only permit such
a eugenic strategy, but would demand it outright.

Criticism of the conclusiveness of substantialism is not motivated by an argumentative cavil, but by the belief that the rational
validity and binding force of moral norms depend on their being
intersubjectively and comprehensively justifiable. For a norm to be
morally valid, its foundation may not be merely in private preference. Only the norms and values which not only I personally
approve of, but which may also be recognised as obligatory for
others, and which may be legitimately sanctioned if violated, can
be deemed moral. If this validity is not to be based solely on per-
suasion or brute force, it has to be justified objectively. This leads
to my first conclusion: *Proof of meta-ethical inconsistencies leaves
substantialism merely with the status of a private morality. I personally believe that 'awe of all things holy' does not require rational justification; instead, it earns the respect and esteem which should be shown
towards each personal ideal in life. Nevertheless, substantialism cannot
be recognised as a philosophical basis for a publicly acceptable
GenEthics.*

Subjectivism

The subjectivists also have their difficulties with the problems
raised by gene and reproduction technology. We have already
looked at the impossibility of justifying long-term, material goals
for an autoevolutive strategy, the uncertain definitions of 'harm'
and 'evil', and the difficulties involved in separating a binding
hard core of morality from its soft, evaluative dimension.
Substantialism and subjectivism are alternative and incompatible
'life designs', and anyone caught between the two ultimately has
no choice but to make a *decision*.

The situation changes, however, when a public GenEthics is at stake. Subjectivism is at an advantage for three reasons. Firstly, it avoids the justification problems in which substantialism tangles itself by believing in the inviolability of human substance. Secondly, it complies with our modern comprehension of the human being as an autonomous subject, which stopped being a mere philosophical idea a long time ago, and is now politically and socially anchored, as well as legally institutionalised, in the concepts of democracy and human rights. The German Constitutional Court has, for example, confirmed the subjective quality of human beings on several occasions, as well as declaring it an essential part of human dignity, as protected in Article 1 of the German Constitution. Regardless of all the difficulties involved in establishing a precise definition of the term, there seems to be general consensus that self-determination has to be regarded as an essential element of human dignity. The modern tendency to naturalise humanity is only one side of a complex, historical process in which, conversely, the individual's personality, individuality and dignity, as well as the autonomy and subjectivity of all human beings, have been increasingly brought to the fore. This is also true of the field of medicine, in which the patient's self-determination is threatened by paternalistic tendencies; for this reason, the principle of autonomy has a key position in modern medical ethics.

Finally, subjectivism has an advantage as the basis for a public GenEthics because it has absolutely no call to doubt the individual legitimacy of substantialism, on the contrary supporting it. In this point, the two main positions are asymmetrical. Whereas a publicly binding substantialistic GenEthics would oblige individuals to refrain from intervening with technology in their reproductive processes, a publicly binding subjectivistic GenEthics would on no account oblige the individual to undertake or undergo such interventions. Subjectivism leaves room for individual, substantialistic reproductive strategies; but not *vice versa*. My second conclusion therefore reads: *Due to the fundamental significance of human autonomy, the social institutionalisation of the human being's subjectivity and the asymmetry of the two main positions, only subjectivism can be accepted as the philosophical basis for a publicly binding GenEthics.*

Self-determination

The principle of autonomy demands that individual self-determination be given as much scope as possible. Applied to the field of gene and reproduction technology, this means: each individual or each couple must be allowed to lead a sex life of its own choosing, must be allowed to determine how many children it has, and when it has them. This right of self-determination is not only to be defended against all interference from the State or a heteronomous morality, but also against potential claims from the children resulting from this self-determined sexual existence. Parents are free in all of their decisions concerning the begetting of one or more children. Just as none of the biologically conceivable children has a right to be brought into the world, none of the children actually brought into the world may claim that its right to self-determination has been violated by the birth itself. Nobody has a right to be born or not to be born. It is the sole decision of the parents, whether and how many children they bring into the world. Parents must also be granted the same freedom with regard to their chosen method of reproduction. Just as nobody has a right to be created and born, or not to be created and born, nobody has a right to be created and born in a particular manner. This applies to the use of all forms of contraceptives, as well as artificial insemination and *in vitro* fertilisation.

Thus at a fundamental level *reproduction* technology proves to be unproblematic. It aims – just like every other medical treatment – at the therapy of a physical defect, which may be accompanied by greater or lesser mental disturbances. The fact that infertility is not a disease in the same sense as tuberculosis, cancer or arteriosclerosis is just as little reason to leave those affected to their fates as the fact that most reproduction technologies do not permit a causal therapy of whatever is behind the infertility. Neither glasses nor pacemakers remove the causes of disease, and yet both are considered legitimate forms of therapy. The 'fundamental level' mentioned above refers to the fact that reproduction technology does not raise any particular medical ethical problems as a therapeutic procedure, but this does not mean that problems with moral components may not arise during the application of reproductive techniques.

One good example of this is the problem of allocating medical resources: with a mind to distributive justice, is it correct to employ such lavish and costly technology in order to fulfil the desire to have children of relatively few people, when far more children already alive in other countries around the world are dying of hunger and infectious diseases? This objection does not only apply to reproduction technology, however. Similar questions could be posed regarding numerous other forms of therapy. Further aspects connected with the use of such techniques are also cause for doubt. It has been pointed out, for example, that a strong desire to have children is often a sign of narcissism. It is therefore feasible to view 'a woman's sterility as the psychosomatic organism's useful, subconscious way of protecting her' (Petersen 1985, p. 58). Successful *in vitro* fertilisation would not dispel these psychological problems; moreover, medical intervention could expose the said child to neurotic surroundings. This draws attention to the problems involved in *applying* these techniques, problems which are not usually easy to solve. However, we must make a clear distinction here between matters of principle and problems of application. It should be a matter of principle that the patient's autonomy and self-determination have more clout than the doctors' opinions and possible doubts; reference to 'the doctor's universal responsibility' (ibid., p. 109) can on no account justify a doctor making up the patient's mind for him or her. Of course, this still means that an individual's desire to be treated may be turned down; this refusal must be justified, however, and it must be viewed as an exception to a moral rule. There is no general criterion for deciding such exceptions: in each case, there is a concrete problem involved in applying the rules. My third conclusion: *The right to individual self-determination includes the freedom to decide the number of children one has; technological interventions in reproduction aimed at regulating this number – whether through contraception or through artificial 'proception' – are therefore principally legitimate.*

Instrumentalisation

Just like every other right, the right to self-determination sometimes comes into conflict with other moral norms or legally protected rights. Parents' rights to self-determination may collide with those of their future children, for example. Even though children do not have a right to be born or not to be born, once born they have as much right to self-determination as their parents claimed to have. This kind of self-determination is never absolutely free, for it is always dependent upon all sorts of pre-given conditions. Nevertheless, it is immoral to limit the boundaries of self-control more than is really necessary. This is the case whenever parents – or others involved – take measures during the creation or prenatal development of their child which in some way or other influence the genetic constitution of that planned child, and thus indirectly its subsequent private and public life. It is not the creation of life itself which represents an intervention in human subjectivity – for the latter only comes into being with the former – but the determination of that life's 'content', as would be the case if the human genome were manipulated. Each manipulation of this kind prejudices the life of the person manipulated, channels to a certain extent his/her path through life, and restricts his/her self-determination. With and through this kind of manipulation, the emerging human being is not treated as a subject, instead being subjected to a foreign will, and made into an object. The right to self-determination can therefore also be formulated negatively: as a ban on human beings being instrumentalised by other human beings. Self-determination is violated wherever individuals are 'used' and put at the disposal of others. This principle is formulated paradigmatically in Kant's third version of the categorical imperative:

> Now, I say, man and, in general, every rational being exists as an end in himself and not merely as a means to be arbitrarily used by this or that will. In all his actions, whether they are directed to himself or to other rational beings, he must always be regarded at the same time as an end . . . The practical imperative, therefore, is the following: Act so that you treat humanity, whether in your own person or in that of another, always as an end and never as a means only.
>
> (Kant 1949, pp. 86–7)

The breeding of a caste of subhuman workers, such as the 'epsilons' in Aldous Huxley's *Brave New World*, would obviously be just such an extreme case, as would the creation of human/animal hybrids for the carrying out of primitive tasks. These projects are morally reprehensible anyway: for envisaging a total subordination of individuals to collective ends, with all the advantages coming down on one side, and all the disadvantages on the other, namely on that of the manipulated beings. The ban on instrumentalisation prohibits various projects aimed at creating human beings with particular biological characteristics. Cloning would be one example of human beings being instrumentalised for individual purposes, for example if parents wished to use this technique in order to have children who would be exact copies of themselves or of famous public figures. Independently of the fact that these wishes are unlikely to be fulfilled, for the reasons mentioned earlier, they have to be evaluated as immoral for reducing a planned human being to a copy of an already existing human being. Analogous to Jonas' 'right not to know', and taking its basic idea further, some authors are now of the opinion that each human being has a 'right to be unplanned', in the sense of not being reduced to a design chosen by its parents or other creators. Each human being must have an unrestricted right to self-determination, as well as the right to plan its own life as it chooses. He/she may not come into the world as the incarnation of a life-plan or ideal in life which somebody else has prejudiced. This is the reason why in 1982 the European Parliament declared that the rights to life and human dignity protected in Articles 2 and 3 of the European Convention for Human Rights include the right to a genome which has not been artificially manipulated.

There is therefore no need to refer to human substance or human nature in order to eliminate the topic of cloning from all the discussions in which it comes up. If a human being should attempt to create an exact copy of itself, or to 'churn out' copies of an attractive actress or an excellent soccer player, then this would not be immoral for the way it leads human reproduction down an 'unnatural' path, but for the way it plans and uses human beings for a foreign purpose or a foreign idea. It is not the intervention in human nature which is reprehensible, but the instrumentalisation of the person concerned. In desiring to prevent human individuals from being reduced by other human individuals to mere ends, the ban on instrumentalisation primarily protects not human nature, but human subjectivity. My fourth conclusion states: *The right of parents to determine freely the number of children they have and the way in which these children are created does not include a license to carry out genetic manipulation at will. A line has to be drawn at the point where technological intervention restricts the child in its right to self-determination and prejudices its course through life.*

Good reasons

Emphasising subjectivity and self-determination does not mean that the human biological constitution has to be considered as a piece of Nature, able to be manipulated in any way desired. A certain 'holiness' may be justified, even within the framework of consequentialist ethics. This is especially the case when factual conditions give rise to fears that gene and reproduction technology could be abused. In this case, even though there may be no fundamental cause for moral doubt, it would be prudent to decline certain practical options.[1] Subjectivism on no account implies that human nature is morally neutral. 'Either human nature is holy, or it is just matter': these alternatives are unnecessarily radical. As the basis of all subjectivity, human nature must have a moral status, even within the framework of subjectivism. A moral status

[1] This makes it easier to comprehend the widespread convergence between substantialists and subjectivists regarding the evaluation of individual technologies. A passage within the report by the German Parliamentary *Enquête-Kommission* for 'Gene Technology' states, for example: 'Due to the aspects at stake today, the Enquête-Kommission has come to the conclusion that therapeutic experiments involving the human germ-line are to be rejected. This rejection has been justified in different ways, partly categorically as an absolute ban, partly pragmatically as a renunciation of the option of germ-line therapy which is called for in the given circumstances. Even the members of the Kommission who do not regard every intervention in the human germ-line as fundamentally impermissible control over human nature believe that there are enough reasons why this kind of intervention should be prevented at the present time. Particular emphasis is placed upon the necessity of combatting in advance the threat of genetic technologies being abused for the breeding of human beings' (Report 1987, p. 189). In actual fact, the significant differences between the various positions usually only exist at a theoretical, philosophical level; different justifications are given for the same rules (Beauchamp & Childress 1989, pp. 40–1). This convergence should not lead to false assumptions regarding the divergences which continue to exist in other points; nevertheless, it demonstrates that differing philosophical positions do not necessarily have to hinder consensus regarding the evaluation of individual options.

does not imply inviolability, however. It implies the obligation to find good reasons to justify each intervention. This also goes for technological interventions in human reproduction. The indubitable right of each individual or couple to lead a sexual existence of its own choosing comes up against moral barriers whenever the interests of potential children are affected. This is the case with all the interventions which would affect a child's biological constitution, and such interventions therefore have to be justified. Neither the parents' desires, their rights to self-realisation and self-determination, nor State or social interests are justification enough. The *only* possible justification for technological interventions in the genetic constitution of human beings is the unequivocal interests of these human being themselves.

But is this not the gateway to manipulative arbitrariness? Can the soccer enthusiast father not point out that it would be brilliant for his son to be a famous centre-forward? And could tails and resistance to radiation not be justified with the advantages which their owners would gain from having such characteristics? All of these questions miss the main point of the argumentation set out above. There can be no doubt that a soccer-player clone could be just as successful in a career on the pitch as a tailed and radiation-resistant clone could be in a career in space travel. Yet the unequivocal interests cited as the only possible justification for genetic manipulations refer not to just any 'advantages', but to the right to choose one's own ideals and course in life as freely as possible. The centre-forward or the space traveller might 'have it made'; but they will go through life like wagons on rails. The inability to choose, the exclusion of alternatives, cannot be balanced out by other 'advantages'. These unequivocal interests are therefore not to be interpreted in a utilitarian or hedonist manner, but as referring solely to the maintenance and development of individual self-determination.

The spectrum of goals at which gene manipulative interventions may be aimed is therefore limited to the characteristics which benefit the individual concerned, and which do not pre-shape its life. These characteristics would have to increase this individual's freedom to act and to decide, and not restrict it. They could conceivably include neutral characteristics such as resistance to disease or stamina, at a physical level, and memory or communication skills at a mental level. My fifth conclusion: *The moral status held by human nature, even within the framework of a subjectivistic GenEthics, deems that good reasons must be given for any intervention in the genetic constitution of human beings; 'good reasons' can only be the unequivocal interests of the individual concerned.*

Therapeutic orientation

Since mental characteristics, such as a good memory, communication skills and, of course, 'intelligence' have a complex genetic basis and are formed in close interaction with the environment, we cannot assume that they will be controllable with the aid of technology in the foreseeable future. To be realistic, improving them phenotypically is more likely to be successful than with gene technology. This leaves *health* as the only legitimate goal for gene technological intervention. Without doubt, nearly all human beings regard this characteristic as highly valuable, and it also meets the criteria formulated above. It is a characteristic which definitely benefits the individual concerned, and which extends that individual's scope for acting and making decisions. The suffering which accompanies genetic diseases is so hard for those affected, and often linked with such enormous burdens for the next of kin, that it is hard to distinguish between references to a fate which should be born willingly, or the opportunity these diseases provide of practising sympathy or sufferance, and pure cynicism. Disregarding its possible abuse to date, the application of gene technology to human beings, as well as the further development of relevant procedures, are fundamentally justified when aimed at the goal of good health. This therapeutic criterion is based not merely upon the hedonistic claims of an affluent society, but also upon the legitmate claims of each human individual to self-determination and self-realisation. In the European Parliamentary recommendation quoted above, the postulated 'right to an unmanipulated genome' is relativised by specific permission for gene manipulation to be carried out for therapeutic purposes.

If the legitimacy of gene technology for therapeutic purposes is ensured, then, morally speaking, it is not very important whether somatic cell gene therapy or manipulations to the germ-line are meant. The technological procedure which is then carried out is a medical and a technological matter, and not primarily a moral one. The genome and the germ-line are parts of human nature just like the brain, the liver or the pancreas; our genetic constitution is not 'holier' than our overall biological constitution. It is immoral to intervene in the germ-line without a good reason, just as it is immoral to use technology to manipulate the brain or the liver without a good reason. But this line of argumentation can just as legitimately be reversed: if it is permissible to manipulate – with good reason – somatic parts of human nature, then it cannot be principally illegitimate to intervene in genetic parts of human nature. The decision to carry out a genetic intervention is subject to the same evaluative criteria as the decision to opt for any other form of therapy. An investigation has to determine, for example, whether the intervention is necessary in order to attain the thera-peutic goal; whether it comes up to the appropriate safety stan-dards; whether damaging side-effects outweigh the potential bene-fits of the intervention. This is my sixth conclusion: *The application of gene technology to human individuals should be deemed morally permissible, providing it is has a therapeutic objective. If this objective is taken as the decisive criterion for the moral permissibility of all such interventions, then not even germ-line manipulations may be principally rejected.*

Problems

Limiting interventions to therapeutic ones is a positive criterion for the permissibility of interventions; but this does not by any means solve all the problems involved. The therapeutic criterion is – as a result of the fluid borders of the concept of disease – not at all sharply defined. In many cases it is easy to judge the existence of a genetic disease which would justify gene therapy, for example Lesch–Nyhan syndrome, Huntington's chorea or severe mental conditions. Judgment is harder to pass in other cases of disease.

When gradual stages of handicap are at stake, for example, the question arises of how severe the handicap has to be in order to justify intervention. Is – as Fletcher has suggested (1974, pp. 12–13) – an I.Q. of less than 90 sufficient justification for technological intervention? Minor physical defects, which could possibly be treated somatically, pose another problem. We should also ask ourselves whether the therapeutic criterion would not pave the way to a general adaption to social norms: if homosexuality turned out to be genetically conditioned, could it not become a cause for therapy? Neither should we forget that in many areas there is no direct dividing line between therapy and 'improvement'. If a pre-natal intervention is capable of raising the I.Q. of a foetus from 60 to 100, why should it then be morally illegitimate to raise it another 20 or 30 points? These questions may be summarised as two objections. The first refers to the problem of drawing a line between genuine diseases and deviations from social norms; the second predicts a gradual expansion of the concept of disease to cover such deviations, so that positive eugenics are ultimately introduced in the guise of therapy. Both of these objections have to be taken seriously; they draw attention to problems regarding the therapeutic criterion, although they do not doubt its efficiency in principle.

Where to draw the line is a problem we are familiar with in various contexts: whenever we categorise and classify natural processes in the interests of intellectual order; or in the field of law and morality, when claims are distributed and rights granted. We do not hold a small child responsible for its actions, but we do an adult. In many cases it is difficult to attribute exactly the right level of responsibility to an older child or a teenager; nevertheless, we adhere to the concept of responsibility even when it is only possible to draw the line between different levels of responsibility in individual cases, and even then often with a certain vagueness and with compromises. However, it is important to make a precise distinction between the validity of moral norms or criteria and the problems surrounding their *application* in concrete cases. The above questions refer to the problems of applying the therapeutic criterion; yet these problems are of a practical and not a fundamental nature. They call for a detailed investigation of the case in question, and are often soluble only if a number of pragmatic factors are taken into consideration. This kind of question also arises in other areas of medicine where the borderline between therapy and 'improvement' is fluid. Just as bioethicists have formulated rules to deal with such problems, it is the task of GenEthicists to develop similar rules for the field of medical gene technology: to take the general therapeutic criterion and divide it up into various rules closer to the problem and to practice.

The second objection, predicting a never-ending expansion of the concept of disease, is to be treated similarly. If, for example, the World Health Organisation's famous definition of health as a state of total physical, mental and social well-being, were to be taken as a basis for gene technology, just about all deficiencies could be taken as cause to intervene. Here too, there can be no doubt that the trend could move in this direction. At the same time, it should be pointed out that this is not a problem specific to gene technology. Similar problems are raised by forms of therapy already in routine use, and they are solved – more or less successfully. Like the previous problem of where to draw the line, this is not so much a case of formulating ethical principles as of the practical difficulties involved in their application, in particular the difficulty of guaranteeing that they will be *adhered to*. Whether the feared trend towards a norming of our descendants will come about or not depends less upon the sharpness of the therapeutic criterion and more upon the 'steadfastness' of the medical profession. The same is true of the widespread fear that a steady gain in information within the field of prenatal diagnostics will lead to a further increase in intolerance towards the handicapped; each instance of genetic damage would then be regarded as an abortion or therapy which should have taken place and did not. Since not even the progress of technology can eradicate the risk of genetic damage completely, society will continue to be confronted with the fact that some of its members are born disabled. There can be no doubt regarding the moral principle that these human beings have as much right to develop their abilities as comprehensively as possible, to unfold their personalities and to be recognised by society as anybody else. Whether or not society really behaves according to this principle is, however, not only an ethical problem but also a sociological one. It depends upon the society in question, its institutions and its members, whether such principles are merely sworn to in speeches and moral treatises, or whether they are actually put into practice.

My seventh and final conclusion reads: *The therapeutic criterion does not provide a patent solution to the problems posed by gene and reproduction technology. It dismisses a number of options as immoral, but in an individual case it is only capable of providing a very general standard which has to be elaborated upon more precisely within a GenEthical framework. Its factual validity will be, however, more a matter of medical practice and social environment than a theoretical problem.*

Two limits of GenEthics

To conclude, I would like to consider the possibilities and limits of philosophy in general, and of GenEthics in particular. Maybe the result of all the deliberations within this book is disappointing. After all, neither of the main ethical positions contains the 'Archimedean point' from which a conclusive, overall evaluation of gene and reproduction technology – reaching as far as autoevolution – could be carried out. Substantialism has intricate problems with attempting to establish a fixed view of humanity, together with a system of inherently human values. Subjectivism definitely has the advantage as a basis for public GenEthics; yet the subjectivists do not have a method for constituting values which could guide an autoevolution of the future either. The first, the *theoretical limit* of GenEthics is its inability to provide a sufficiently positive orientation with regard to long-term, human genetic prospects. This conclusion is ironic in that disappointment arises in precisely a situation in which philosophy – or, more precisely, ethics – is confronted with enormous expectations regarding its orientational abilities.

> In any case, the idea of making over man is no longer fantastic, nor interdicted by an inviolable taboo. If and when *that* revolution occurs, if technological power is really going to tinker with the elemental keys on which life will have to play its melody in generations to come (perhaps the only such melody in the universe), then a reflection on what should determine the choice – a reflection, in short, on the image of

man – becomes an imperative more urgent than any ever inflicted on
the understanding of mortal man.

(Jonas 1979, p. 41)

There are many reasons to believe that these expectations will
never be realised. Firstly, it is extremely unlikely that 'metaphysical admissibility' (ibid.) will ever be able to reverse the loss of
objective teleology at the beginning of the Modern Age. Yet without a Nature which is objectively purposeful, the human being has
no way of orientating its behaviour according to a given goal
within the structure of the universe or within human nature. If the
modern human being is no longer able to fall back on an objective
'good life', instead having to set its own goals, then the notion of
an absolute system of values loses its footing. Contemplation of
the 'humanly desirable' and the 'image of man', as called for by
Jonas, would end in the dogmatisation of a particular ideal in life.
Although – as the result of individual emancipation from political
authoritarianism and heteronomous morality – it represents a
social achievement, the moral pluralism of modern societies is not
only a social fact. It also proves to be the necessary product of a
metaphysical historical process: to the same extent with which
modern metaphysics rejects the anchoring of moral values and
norms in ontology because of the deteleologicalisation of Nature, it
has to comprehend the constitution of these values and norms as
the independent and confident work of individuals, who freely
decide upon the shaping of their lives. It is then nothing but consistent for Gert to propose a precise definition of morality's
bounds of validity, declaring morality as having 'no final goal'
(1973, p. 149), but as merely desiring to ensure that each human
being has the individual scope to act and to make decisions. And if
we are unable to reach consensus about a comprehensive morality
with our contemporaries, can we really expect our descendants in
fifty, a hundred, or even thousands of years' time to agree with us
about what is 'humanly desirable'? It is far more likely that they
will design a 'view of humanity' which is just as different from
ours as ours is from that of the 18th century or the Middle Ages.

Secondly, we have to ask whether we want philosophy – metaphysics or ethics – to play this kind of rôle. The constitution of
values, the setting of goals and the establishment of what is

'humanly desirable' would form the baseline for human forms of life, just as designing 'views of humanity' would; this kind of morality would determine how human beings are to live. Yet philosophers cannot, and should not, make this kind of decision. A resuscitation of the Platonic philosopher kings who, with their supposedly privileged access to the truth, would have the power to enforce a commonly binding morality, would hardly be compatible with the principles of a democratically ordered society. Just as in a democracy the ability of political arguments and decisions to find consensus 'may not be measured exclusively, nor even primarily, according to theoretically defined truth' (Schnädelbach 1986, p. 44), the formation of a new morality should pay more attention to the public, to public discussion and consensus, than to the authority of philosophers or scientists. The GenEthics which we are in need of cannot and must not be 'invented' by experts, but must crystallise gradually from a process of public and communal debate. This is to be emphasised more than anything – more than a refutation of the claims by philosophers – as a refutation of the presumptuousness of scientists, who present their moral and political convictions as the unequivocal results of an impartial search for truth, immunising these convictions further with a reference to their specialist competence. Eugenics – whatever its special form – would also become more than just scientific methodology: namely overall social politics, which would have to be politically legitimised and answered for. Because of the authority which, despite manifold criticism, scientists have within our society, scientism – the claim that moral values may be deduced from scientific insights – should be regarded as dangerous.

All this does not mean that philosophers could not make any contribution to a public debate on the structure and content of GenEthics. Even if the approaches which have been suggested, discussed, developed and rejected over more than two thousand years of traditional ethical philosophy are not a collection of recipes for ready solutions, it would be foolish to leave unexploited the philosophical assets which have been accumulated over such a long period of time. The discipline of philosophy has at its disposal trained, analytical competence and a tried and tested apparatus of critical reflection, which could be useful in the solving of current problems. Philosophy could, for example, contribute by: (1) providing clarity regarding the goals and the 'point' of morality; (2) formulating criteria for the validity for moral arguments and then distinguishing justified claims to validity from dogmatic assertions of validity; (3) analysing the meaning of concepts and shedding light on the prerequisites of controversial moral positions, often left unspoken, in order to dispel misunderstandings, to make agreement easier, or at least to pinpoint areas of disagreement in order to open them up for discussion. The contributions to be made by philosophy are thus primarily analytical. Philosophers can formulate criteria of rationality and morality, and endeavour not to treat them as the esoterical possession of an élite, but to make them commonly accessible as goods belonging to the public. Whether, and to what extent, the public then accepts such an offer, whether, and to what extent, public debate then adheres to the criteria for rationality worked out by the philosophers, and accepts their moral standards for a GenEthics, is not a philosophical problem, but a political one. The second, *practical limit* of GenEthics is this inability to ensure that the norms and criteria developed within its framework will find social acceptance.

However, this non–identity of philosophical reflection and social practice could also mean an opportunity. It is one of the prerequisites if such reflection is not to be mere theoretical expression of current practice, but *critical*. The GenEthics of the future should take note of this chance to be critical; it must become more than just a source of legitimacy for a technological development which will continue whatever. Despite first appearances, the theoretical limitation of GenEthics is not a hinderance to its critical potency or its function. Even if we are unable to evaluate technological development in its entirety, we still have the chance to evaluate *each individual step* along the way.

Bibliography

Aristotle (1883). *Politics/ The Politics of Aristotle*, Book VII (pp. 309–37). Translated with an analysis and critical notes by J. E. C. Welldon. London: MacMillan & Co.

– (1954). *Ethica Nicomachea/ The Nicomachean Ethics of Aristotle.* Translated and introduced by Sir David Ross. London: Oxford University Press.

Augenstein, L. (1969). *Come, Let us Play God.* London: Harper & Row.

Bainbridge, I. (1982). With child in mind: the experience of a potential IVF mother. In *Test-Tube Babies. A Guide to Moral Questions, Present Techniques and Future Possibilities*, ed. William and Peter Singer, pp. 119–27. Melbourne: Oxford University Press.

Bayertz, K. (1987). Increasing responsibility as technological destiny? Human reproductive technology and the problem of meta-responsibility. In *Technology and Responsibility*, ed. P. T. Durbin, *Philosophy and Technology*, Vol. 3, p. 135–50. Dordrecht: D. Reidel.

– (1990). Biology and beauty: science and aesthetics in fin-de-siècle Germany. In *Fin-de-Siècle and its Legacy.* ed. M. Teich and R. Porter, pp. 278–95. Cambridge: Cambridge University Press.

– (1992). Techno-thanatology. Moral consequences of introducing brain criteria for death. In *Journal for Philosophy and Medicine*, Vol. 17, pp. 407–17.

– (ed.) (1994). *The Concept of Moral Consensus.* Dordrecht: Kluwer Academic Publishers.

Beauchamp, T. L. & Childress, J. F. (1989). *Principles of Biomedical Ethics.* 3rd edition. Oxford: Oxford University Press.

Benda, E. (1985). Erprobung der Menschenwürde am Beispiel der Humangenetik. In *Retortenbefruchtung und Verantwortung. Anthropologische, ethische und medizinische Aspekte neuer Fruchtbarkeitstechnologien*, ed. P. Petersen, pp. 125–59. Stuttgart: Urachhaus.

Benn, G. (1968a). Geist und Seele künftiger Geschlechter. In *Gesammelte Werke*, D. Wellershoff. Bd. 3, *Essays und Aufsätze*, pp. 794–801 Wiesbaden: Limes.

– (1968b). Züchtung II. In *Gesammelte Werke*, D. Wellershoff. Bd 3, *Essays und Aufsätze*, pp. 857–60 Wiesbaden: Limes.

Benz, E. (1961). Das Bild des Übermenschen in der europäischen Geistesgeschichte. In *Der Übermensch. Eine Diskussion*, ed. E. Benz, pp. 23–161. Zürich: Rhein.

Biggers, J. D. (1983). Generation and the human life cycle. In *Abortion and the Status of the Fetus*, ed. W. B. Bondeson, H. T. Engelhardt, S. F. Spicker and Daniel H. Winship. Philosophy and Medicine, Vol. 13, pp. 31–53. Dordrecht: D. Reidel.

Bloch, E. (1959). *Das Prinzip Hoffnung*. Frankfurt: Suhrkamp.

Bodmer W.F. & Cavalli-Sforza, L. L. (1976). *Genetics, Evolution and Man*. San Francisco: W. H. Freeman & Co.

Brumlik, M. (1986). Über die Ansprüche Ungeborener und Unmündiger. Wie advokatorisch ist die diskursive Ethik? In *Moralität und Sittlichkeit. Das Problem Hegels und die Diskursethik*, ed. W. Kuhlmann, pp. 265–99. Frankfurt: Suhrkamp.

Callahan, D. (1975). Discussion: Science and the foundation of ethics. In *The Nature of Scientific Discovery. A Symposium Commemorating the 500th Anniversary of the Birth of Nicolaus Copernicus*, ed. O. Gingerich, p. 587, passim. Washington: Smithsonian Institution Press.

Campanella, T. (1885). The City of the Sun. In *Ideal Commonwealths. Plutarch's Lycurgus, More's Utopia, Bacon's New Atlantis, Campanella's City of the Sun*. With an Introduction by Henry Morley. London: George Routledge and Sons.

Cavalli-Sforza, L. L. & Bodmer, W. F. (1971). *The Genetics of Human Populations*. San Francisco: W.H. Freeman.

Chargaff, E. (1976). On the dangers of genetic meddling. In *Science*, Vol. 192 (4 June 1976), pp. 938–40.

Comfort, A. (1967). Discussion contribution. In *Man and his Future. A Ciba Foundation Volume*, ed. G. Wolstenholme. London: Churchill.

Daele, W. van den (1985). *Mensch nach Maß? Ethische Probleme der Genmanipulation und Gentherapie*. München: Beck.

– (1986). Technische Dynamik und gesellschaftliche Moral. Zur soziologischen Bedeutung der Gentechnologie. In *Soziale Welt*, Bd. 37, Heft 2/3, pp. 149–72.

– Krohn, W. (1982). Anmerkungen zur Legitimation der Naturwissenschaften. In *Physik, Philosophie und Politik. Festschrift für Carl Friedrich von Weizsäcker zum 70. Geburtstag*, ed. K. M. Meyer-Abich, pp. 416–29. München: Hanser.

Darwin, C. (1974). *The Descent of Man and Selection in Relation to Sex.* Revised edition. Chicago: Rand, McNally & Co. Reprint of the 1874 edition. Republished by Gale Research Company, Book Tower, Detroit, 1974.

– (1988). *The Origin of Species.* London: Pickering. [Originally published 1876.]

Delgado, J. M. R. (1969). *Physical Control of the Mind: Towards a Psychocivilized Society.* New York: Harper & Row.

Descartes, R. (1953). *A Discourse on Method.* Translated by John Veitch. London: J. M. Dent & Sons.

Devereux, G. (1976). *A Study of Abortion in Primitive Societies. A Typological, Distributional and Dynamic Analysis of the Prevention of Birth in 400 Preindustrial Societies.* Revised edition. New York: International University Press.

Diderot, D. (1966). *Rameau's Nephew and d'Alembert's Dream.* Translated with introduction by L.W. Tancock. Harmondsworth, Middx: Penguin Books.

Diedrich, K. & Krebs, D. (1983). Extrakorporale Befruchtung und Embryotransfer in der gynäkologischen Praxis. In *In-vitro-Fertilisation und Embryotransfer (Retortenbaby). Grundlagen, Methoden, Probleme und Perspektiven*, ed. Ulrich Jüdes, pp. 25-43. Stuttgart: Wissenschaftliche Verlagsgesellschaft.

Dobzhansky, T. (1962). *Mankind Evolving. The Evolution of the Human Species.* New Haven, Conn: Yale University Press.

Eibach, U. (1983). *Experimentierfeld: Werdendes Leben. Eine ethische Orientierung.* Göttingen: Vandenhoeck & Ruprecht.

Eisenberg, L. (1976). The outcome as a cause: predestination and human cloning. In *The Journal of Medicine and Philosophy*, Vol. 1, no. 4, pp. 318–31.

Elias, N. (1981). *Über den Prozeß der Zivilisation. Soziogenetische und psychogenetische Untersuchungen*, Bd. 1. Frankfurt: Suhrkamp.

Engelhardt, H. T.. (1982). Bioethics in pluralist societies. In *Perspectives in Biology and Medicine*, Vol. 26, No. 1 (Autumn 1982), pp. 64–78.

– (1986). *The Foundations of Bioethics.* Oxford: Oxford University Press.

Etzioni, A. (1973). *Genetic Fix*. New York: Macmillan.

Feen, R. H. (1983). Abortion and exposure in Ancient Greece: assessing the status of the fetus and 'newborn' from Classical sources. In *Abortion and the Status of the Fetus*, ed. W. B. Bondeson, H. T. Engelhardt, S. F. Spicker and D. H. Winship. Philosophy and Medicine, Vol. 13. Dordrecht: D. Reidel.

Fletcher, J. (1972). Indicators of humanhood: a tentative profile of Man. In *The Hastings Center Report*, Vol. 2, No. 5, pp. 1–4.

– (1974). *The Ethics of Genetic Control. Ending Reproductive Roulette*. Garden City, NY: Anchor Press.

Fraling, B. (1984). Discussion contribution. In G*entechnologie, Chancen und Risiken. Ethische und rechtliche Probleme der Anwendung zellbiologischer und gentechnischer Methoden am Menschen. Dokumentation eines Fachgesprächs im Bundesministerium für Forschung und Technologie*, pp. 66–8. München: J. Schweitzer.

Frankena, W. K. (1967). The Naturalistic Fallacy. In *Theories of Ethics*, Oxford Readings in Philosophy, ed. P. Foot, pp. 50–63. Oxford, Oxford University Press.

– (1973). *Ethics*. 2nd edition. Englewood Cliffs, NJ: Prentice-Hall.

Freud, S. (1969). *Civilization and its Discontents*. Translated by Joan Riviere. Revised and edited by James Strachey. London: The Hogarth Press & Institute of Psycho-Analysis.

Gert, B. (1973). *The Moral Rules. A New Rational Foundation for Morality*. New York: Harper & Row.

Glover, J. (1984). *What Sort of People Should There Be? Genetic Engineering, Brain Control and their Impact on our Future World*. Harmondsworth, Middx: Penguin Books.

Goethe, J. W. von (1926). *Faust*. Translated into English verse in the original metres with commentary notes by W. H. van der Smissen. London: J.M. Dent & Sons.

Grobstein, C. (1981). *From Chance to Purpose. An Appraisal of External Human Fertilization*. London: Addison-Wesley Publishing Company.

Gründel, J. (1983). Theologisch–ethische Beurteilung der extrakorporalen Befruchtung und des Embryotransfers beim Menschen – Gedanken eines katholischen Theologen. In *In-vitro-Fertilisation und Embryotransfer (Retortenbaby). Grundlagen, Methoden, Probleme und Perspektiven*, ed. U. Jüdes, pp. 249–72. Stuttgart: Wissenschaftliche Verlagsgesellschaft.

Habermas, J. (1983). Diskursethik – Notizen zu einem
Begründungsprogramm. In *Moralbewußtsein und kommunikatives
Handeln*, pp. 53–125. Frankfurt: Suhrkamp.
– (1984). Über Moralität und Sittlichkeit – Was macht eine
Lebensform 'rational'? In *Rationalität. Philosophische Beiträge*, ed.
H. Schnädelbach, pp. 218–35. Frankfurt: Suhrkamp.
– (1986). Moralität und Sittlichkeit. Treffen Hegels Einwände gegen
Kant auch auf die Diskursethik zu? In *Moralität und Sittlichkeit. Das
Problem Hegels und die Diskursethik*, ed. W. Kuhlmann, pp. 16–37.
Frankfurt: Suhrkamp.
Haeckel, E. (1892). *The History of Creation. Or: The Development of the
Earth and its Inhabitants by the Action of Natural Causes. A Popular
Exposition of the Doctrine of Evolution in General, and of that of
Darwin, Goethe and Lamarck in Particular.* Translated in two volumes
by E. Ray Lankaster. Vol. I. London: Kegan, Paul, French, Trübner
& Co.
Haldane, J. B. S. (1924). *Daedalus or Science and the Future.* A paper
read to the heretics, Cambridge, on Feb. 4th 1923. London: Kegan
Paul, Trench, Trübner & Co.
– (1967). Biological possibilities for the human species in the next ten
thousand years. In *Man and his Future. A Ciba Foundation Volume*,
ed. G. Wolstenholme, pp. 337–61. London: Churchill.
Harman, G. (1977). *The Nature of Morality. An Introduction to Ethics.*
New York: Oxford University Press.
Hegel, G. W. F. *Ästhetik.* (Undated). Edited by Friedrich Bassenge.
2 Volumes. Frankfurt: Europäische Verlagsanstalt.
– (1942). *Hegel's Philosophy of Right.* Translated with notes by
T. M. Knox. Oxford: Clarendon Press.
Helmholtz, H. von (1893). The Recent Progress of the Theory of
Vision. In *Popular Lectures on Scientific Subjects.* Translated by
E. Atkinson. London: Longmans, Green & Co.
Herder, J. G. (1965). *Ideen zur Philosophie der Geschichte der Menschheit.*
Edited by Heinz Stolpe. 2 Volumes. Berlin: Aufbau.
Hertwig, O. (1921). *Zur Abwehr des ethischen, des sozialen, des politischen
Darwinismus.* 2nd edition. Jena: G. Fischer.
Himes, N. E. (1970). *Medical History of Contraception.* New York:
Schokken Books.
Hoebel, B. G. (1983). Neurogene und chemische Grundlagen des

Glücksgefühls. In *Der Beitrag der Biologie zu Fragen von Recht und Ethik*, ed. M. Gruter and M. Rehbinder, pp. 87–109. Berlin: Duncker & Humblot.

d'Holbach, P. T. (1960). *System der Natur oder Von den Gesetzen der physischen und der moralischen Welt*. Berlin: Aufbau.

Huxley, A. L. (1977). *Brave New World*. London: Triad Grafton.

Huxley, J. (1947). Eugenics and society. In *Man in the Modern World*, p. 22-54. London: Chatto & Windus.

– (1964). Eugenics in evolutionary perspective. In *Essays of a Humanist*, pp. 251–80. London: Chatto & Windus.

– (1967a). The future of Man – evolutionary aspects. In *Man and his Future. A Ciba Foundation*, Volume, ed. G. Wolstenholme, pp. 1-22. London: Churchill Ltd.

– (1967b). Discussion contribution. In *Man and his Future. A Ciba Foundation Volume*, ed. G. Wolstenholme, pp. 331–4. London: Churchill Ltd.

Instruction 1987. Instruction on Respect for Human Life in its Origin and on the Dignity of Procreation. Replies to Certain Questions of the Day. Congregation for the Doctrine of the Faith. Vatican City, 1987.

Jacob, F. (1983). *Das Spiel der Möglichkeiten. Von der offenen Geschichte des Lebens*. München: Piper.

Jaeger, W. (1973). *Paideia. Die Formung des griechischen Menschen*. Berlin: de Gruyter.

Jonas, H. (1974). Biological engineering – a preview. In *Philosophical Essays. From Ancient Creed to Technological Man*, pp. 141–67. Englewood Cliffs, NJ: Prentice-Hall.

– (1979). In *The Hastings Center Report*, Vol. 9, No. 4, pp. 34–43.

– (1984). *The Imperative of Responsibility. In Search of an Ethics for the Technological Age*. Chicago: University of Chicago Press. [Originally published in German in 1979 as *Das Prinzip Verantwortung*.]

– (1985). Mikroben, Gameten und Zygoten: Weiteres zur neuen Schöpferrolle des Menschen. In *Technik, Medizin und Ethik. Zur Praxis des Prinzips Verantwortung*, pp. 204–18. Frankfurt: Insel.

Jüdes, U. (1983). Einführung: Eingriffe in die Fortpflanzung. In *In-vitro-Fertilisation und Embryotransfer (Retortenbaby). Grundlagen, Methoden, Probleme und Perspektiven*, ed. U. Jüdes, pp. 13–23. Stuttgart: Wissenschaftliche Verlagsgesellschaft.

Kant, I. (1949). *Critique of Practical Reason and Other Writings in Moral*

Philosophy. Translated and edited by L. W. Beck. Chicago: University of Chicago Press.

– (1963a). Review of Moscati's paper on the difference in the structure of Man and animals [1771]. In *Kant*, by Gabrielle Rabel, p. 95. Oxford: Clarendon Press.

– (1963b). Ideals for a universal history of mankind with a view to world citizenship [1784]. In *Kant*, by Gabrielle Rabel, pp. 134–9. Oxford: Clarendon Press.

Kass, L. R. (1972). New beginnings in life. In *The New Genetics and Future of Man*, ed. M. P. Hamilton, pp. 14–63. Grand Rapids, Mich: William B. Eerdmans.

Kaufmann, W. (1974). *Nietzsche. Philosopher, Psychologist, Antichrist*. 4th edition. Princeton, NJ: Princeton University Press.

Kieffer, G. H. (1979). *Bioethics: A Textbook of Issues*. Reading, Mass: Addison–Wesley.

Kondylis, P. (1981). *Die Aufklärung im Rahmen des neuzeitlichen Rationalismus*. Stuttgart: Klett-Cotta.

Koyré, A. (1970). *From the Closed World to the Infinite Universe*. 2nd printing. Baltimore: The John Hopkins Press.

Kuhse, H. & Singer, P. (1985). *Should the Baby Live? The Problem of Handicapped Infants*. Oxford: Oxford University Press.

Lappé, M. (1979). *Genetic Politics. The Limits of Biological Control*. New York: Simon & Schuster.

Lederberg, J. (1966). Experimental Genetics and Human Evolution. In *Bulletin of the Atomic Scientists*, October 1966, pp. 4–11.

– (1967a). Biological future of man. In *Man and his Future. A Ciba Foundation Volume*, ed. G. Wolstenholme, pp. 263–73. London: Churchill Ltd.

– (1967b). Discussion contribution. In *Man and his Future. A Ciba Foundation Volume*, ed. G. Wolstenholme, pp. 362–83. London: Churchill Ltd.

– (1970). Orthobiosis: the perfection of Man. In *The Place of Values in a World of Facts*, ed. A. Tiselius, p. 29–58. Stockholm: Almquist and Wiksell.

Leibbrand, W. & Wettley, A. (Undated). *Der Wahnsinn. Geschichte der abendländischen Psychopathologie*. Freiburg: Alber.

Lem, S. (1976). *Summa technologiae*. Frankfurt: Insel.

– (1980). *Phantastik und Futurologie*. Teil. 2. Frankfurt: Insel.

Lenz, W. (1984). Discussion contribution. In *Gentechnologie, Chancen und Risiken. Ethische und rechtliche Probleme der Anwendung zellbiologischer und gentechnischer Methoden am Menschen*, pp. 69–70. Documentation of an experts' discussion in the German Ministry for Research and Technology. München: J. Schweitzer.

Leroi-Gourhan, A. (1980). *Hand und Wort. Die Evolution von Technik, Sprache und Kunst*. Frankfurt: Suhrkamp.

Löw, R. (1983). Gen und Ethik. Philosophische Überlegungen zum Umgang mit menschlichem Erbgut. In *Die Verführung durch das Machbare. Ethische Konflikte in der modernen Medizin und Biologie*, ed. P. Koslowski, P. Kreuzer and R. Löw, pp. 33–48. Stuttgart: Hirzel.

MacKay, D. M. (1967). Discussion contribution. In *Man and his Future. A Ciba Foundation Volume*, ed.y G. Wolstenholme, pp. 274–98. London: Churchill Ltd.

Mackie, J. L. (1977). *Ethics: Inventing Right and Wrong*. Harmondsworth, Middx: Penguin Books.

McKeown, T. (1976). *The Rôle of Medicine: Dream, Mirage or Nemesis?* London: Nuffield Provincial Hospitals Trust.

Markl, H. (1982). Untergang oder Übergang – Natur als Kulturaufgabe. In *Mannheimer Forum 82/83*, pp. 61–98.

Marx, K. & Engels, F. (1965). *The German Ideology*. London: Lawrence & Wishardt.

Mayr, E. (1982). *The Growth of Biological Thought. Diversity, Evolution and Inheritance*. Cambridge, Mass: The Belknap Press of Harvard University Press.

Medawar, P. B. (1955). The imperfections of Man. In *The Uniqueness of the Individual*, pp. 122–33. London: Methuen.

– (1961). *The Future of Man. BBC Reith Lectures 1959*. New York: Basic Books, Inc.

– (1967). Discussion contribution. In *Man and his Future. A Ciba Foundation Volume*, ed. G. Wolstenholme, pp. 274–98. London: Churchill.

Meyer-Abich, K. M. (1984). *Wege zum Frieden mit der Natur. Praktische Naturphilosophie für die Umweltpolitik*. München: Hanser.

Mill, J. S. (1969a). Utilitarianism [1861]. In *Essays on Ethics, Religion and Society. Collected Works of John Stuart Mill*, Vol. X, pp. 203–60. Toronto: University of Toronto Press.

– (1969b). Nature [1874]. In *Essays on Ethics, Religion and Society. Collected Works of John Stuart Mill*, Vol. X, pp. 373–402. Toronto: University of Toronto Press.

Monod, J. (1972). *Chance and Necessity. An Essay on the Natural Philosophy of Modern Biology.* Translated from the French by A. Wainhouse. London: Collins.

Moscovici, S. (1982). *Versuch über die menschliche Geschichte der Natur.* Frankfurt: Suhrkamp.

Muller, H. J. (1936). *Out of the Night. A Biologist's View of the Future.* London: Gollancz.

– (1967). Genetic progress by voluntarily conducted germinal choice. In *Man and his Future. A Ciba Foundation Volume*, ed. G. Wolstenholme, pp. 247–62. London: Churchill.

Musil, R. (1954). *The Man without Qualities.* Translated from the German by E. Wilkins and E. Kaiser. London: Secker & Warburg.

Nietzsche, F. (ASZ): Also sprach Zarathustra. In *Sämtliche Werke. Kritische Studienausgabe in 15 Bden*, ed. G. Colli and M. Montinari. Band 4. München: dtv and Berlin: de Gruyter, 1980.

– (*TGS*): *The Gay Science.* Translated by W. Kaufmann. New York: Vintage Books, 1974.

– (*JGB*): *Jenseits von Gut und Böse. Vorspiel einer Philosophie der Zukunft.* In *Sämtliche Werke. Kritische Studienausgabe in 15 Bden*, ed. G. Colli and M. Montinari. Band 5, pp. 9–243. München: dtv and Berlin: de Gruyter, 1980.

– (*WAG*): *Der Fall Wagner.* In *Sämtliche Werke. Kritische Studienausgabe in 15 Bden*, d. G. Colli and M. Montinari. Band 6, pp. 9–53. München: dtv and Berlin: de Gruyter, 1980.

– (1880). Nachgelassene Fragmente, Anfang 1880 bis Sommer 1882. In *Sämtliche Werke. Kritische Studienausgabe in 15 Bden*, ed. G. Colli and M. Montinari. Band 9. München: dtv and Berlin: de Gruyter, 1980.

– (1885). Nachgelassene Fragmente, Herbst 1885 bis Anfang Januar 1889. 1. Teil: Herbst 1885 bis Herbst 1887. In *Sämtliche Werke. Kritische Studienausgabe in 15 Bden*, ed. G. Colli and M. Montinari. Band 12. München: dtv and Berlin: de Gruyter, 1980.

– (1887). Nachgelassene Fragmente, Herbst 1885 bis Anfang Januar 1889. 2. Teil: November 1887 bis Anfang Januar 1889. In *Sämtliche Werke. Kritische Studienausgabe in 15 Bden*, ed. G. Colli and M. Montinari. Band 13. München: dtv and Berlin: de Gruyter, 1980.

Petersen, P. (1985). *Retortenbefruchtung und Verantwortung. Anthropologische, ethische und medizinische Aspekte neuer Fruchtbarkeitstechnologien.* Stuttgart: Urachhaus.

Plato (1956). *Protagorus*. B. Jowett's translation, extensively revised by
M. Ostwald, ed. with intro. by G. Vlastos. Indianapolis: Bobbs
Merrill Co.
– (1969). *The Republic*. Volume I, Books I–V. In *Plato in Twelve
Volumes* (Vol. Five). English translation by P. Shorey. London:
Heinemann.
Plessner, H. (1981). Die Stufen des Organischen und der Mensch.
Einleitung in die philosophische Anthropologie. In *Gesammelte
Schriften*, Vol. 4. Frankfurt: Suhrkamp.
– (1983a). Die Aufgabe der philosophischen Anthropologie. In
Gesammelte Schriften, Vol. 8, pp. 33–51. Frankfurt: Suhrkamp.
– (1983b). Die Frage nach der Conditio humana. In *Gesammelte
Schriften*, Vol. 8, pp. 136–217. Frankfurt: Suhrkamp.
– (1983c). Immer noch philosophische Anthropologie? In *Gesammelte
Schriften*, Vol. 8, pp. 235–46. Frankfurt: Suhrkamp.
Ploetz, A. (1895). *Die Tüchtigkeit unserer Rasse und der Schutz der
Schwachen*. Berlin: S. Fischer.
Rahner, K. (1967a). Experiment Mensch. In *Schriften zur Theologie*,
Vol. 8, pp. 260–285. Einsiedeln: Benzinger.
– (1967b). Zum Problem der genetischen Manipulation. In *Schriften
zur Theologie*, Vol. 8, pp. 286-321. Einsiedeln: Benzinger.
Ramsey, P. (1970). *Fabricated Man. The Ethics of Genetic Control*.
New Haven: Yale University Press.
Recommendation (1982). Translated from the German: *Recommendation
934 re. Gene Manipulation*. German Parliamentary Publication
No. 9/1373, pp. 11–13.
Remmert, H. (1980). *Ökologie. Ein Lehrbuch*. 2nd edition. Berlin:
Springer-Verlag.
Report 1985. Translated from the German: *Report by the Work-Group
In vitro Fertilisation, Genome Analysis and Gene Therapy* (Benda-
Kommission). Printed as a manuscript: Bonn.
Report 1987. Translated from the German: *Report by the Enquête-
Kommission 'Opportunities and Risks of Gene Technology'*.
Parliamentary manuscript No. 10/6775, 6 January 1987.
Rousseau, J.-J. (1984). *A Discourse on Inequality*. Translated with
introduction and notes by M. Cranston. Harmondsworth, Middx:
Penguin.
Sartre, J.-P. (1958). *Being and Nothingness. An Essay on Phenomenological
Ontology*. Translated by H. E. Barnes. London: Methuen.

– (1973). *Existentialism and Humanism.* Translated with introduction
by P. Mairet. London: Eyre Methuen.

Schäfer, L. (1986). Selbstbestimmung und Naturverhältnis des
Menschen. In *Information Philosophie* 5, pp. 4–19.

Schallmayer, W. (1903). *Vererbung und Auslese im Lebenslauf der Völker.*
Eine staatswissenschaftliche Studie auf Grund der neueren Biologie.
(*Natur und Staat, Beiträge zur naturwissenschaftlichen Gesellschaftslehre,*
Bd. 3). Jena: G. Fischer.

Schiller, F. (1967). Über die aesthetische Erziehung des Menschen in
einer Reihe von Briefen. In *Sämtliche Werke,* ed. G. Fricke and H.
G. Göpfert. 5. Band, pp. 570–669. München: Hanser.

Schmidt, O. (1873). *Descendenzlehre und Darwinismus.* Leipzig:
Brockhaus.

Schnädelbach, H. (1986). Was ist Neoaristotelismus? In *Moralität und*
Sittlichkeit. Das Problem Hegels und die Diskursethik. ed.
W. Kuhlmann, pp. 38–63. Frankfurt: Suhrkamp.

Schopenhauer, A. (1896/1977). *The World as Will and Idea.*
Volume III. Translated from the German by R. B. Haldane and
J. Kemp. 3rd edition. London: Kegan Paul, Trench, Trübner & Co.

Schweitzer, A. (Undated). *Kultur und Ethik.* In *Gesammelte Werke* in
5 Bänden. Bd. 2, pp. 95–420. München: Beck.

Shelley, M. W. (1969). *Frankenstein or the Modern Prometheus.* Edited
with an introduction by M.K. Joseph. London: Oxford.

Singer, P. (1979). *Practical Ethics.* Cambridge: Cambridge University
Press.

Snowden, R., Mitchell, G. D. & Snowden, E.M. (1983). *Artificial*
Reproduction: A Social Investigation. London: George Allan & Unwin.

Soupart, P. (1983). Present and possible future research in the use of
human embryos. In *Abortion and the Status of the Fetus,* ed.
W. B. Bondeson, H. T. Engelhardt, S. F. Spicker and
D. H. Winship, pp. 67–104. Philosophy and Medicine, Vol. 13.
Dordrecht: D. Reidel.

Spaemann, R. & Löw, R. (1981). *Die Frage Wozu? Geschichte und*
Wiederentdeckung des teleologichen Denkens. München: Piper.

The Holy Bible (1856). Containing the Old and New Testaments.
Printed at the Oxford University Press for the British and Foreign
Bible Society.

Tooley, M. (1983). *Abortion and Infanticide.* Oxford: Clarendon Press.

Trotnow, S. (1984). Diskussionsbeiträge. In *Gentechnologie, Chancen und*

Risiken. Ethische und rechtliche Probleme der Anwendung zellbiologischer und gentechnischer Methoden am Menschen. Dokumentation eines Fachgesprächs im Bundesministerium für Forschung und Technologie, pp. 51-57 and passim. München: J. Schweitzer.

Tugendhat, E. (1984a). Antike und moderne Ethik. In *Probleme der Ethik*, pp. 33–56. Stuttgart: Reclam.

– (1984b). Drei Vorlesungen über Probleme der Ethik. In *Probleme der Ethik*, pp. 57–131. Stuttgart: Reclam.

Vitzthum, W. Graf (1987). Gentechnologie und Menschenwürde-argument. In *Zeitschrift für Rechtspolitik*, 20. Jahrgang, Februar 1987, pp. 33–7.

Vogel, F. & Motulsky, A. G. (1986). *Human Genetics. Problems and Approaches.* 2nd edition. New York: Springer-Verlag.

Walters, W. A. W. (1982). Cloning, ectogenesis and hybrids: things to come? In *Test-Tube Babies. A Guide to Moral Questions, Present Techniques and Future Possibilities*, ed. W. Walters and P. Singer, pp. 110–18. Melbourne: Oxford University Press.

Warnock, G. J. (1967). *Contemporary Moral Philosophy*. London: MacMillan.

Weber, M. (1947). *Gesammelte Aufsätze zur Religionssoziologie.* Tübingen: Mohr.

Weingart, P. (1984). Eugenic Utopias: blueprints for the rationalization of human evolution. In *Nineteen Eighty-Four: Science between Utopia and Dystopia*, ed. E. Mendelsohn and H. Nowotny, pp. 173–87. Dordrecht: D. Reidel.

– Kroll, J. & Bayertz, K. (1988). *Rasse, Blut und Gene. Geschichte der Eugenik und Rassenhygiene in Deutschland.* Frankfurt: Suhrkamp.

Index of Names

General Index

germ line 311
germinal choice 53–6, 64–5
goals in reconstructing the human
species
individual 263–8, 273–4
process without 273–300
God 100, 101, 104–5
image of 100, 101, 117
playing 173–97
Greek mythology 174

handicap, severity and
intervention 315
happiness 230–3, 244, 262–3,
279–80
see also utilitarianism
harm (evil) 239–41, 251–6
definition 259
moral 255
health 234, 279, 313, 316
holiness 116–19, 129, 131–2
non-inviolability 129–32
problems with teleology 164–7
holy war against human nature
93–5
homunculi 27–9
human being (*Homo sapiens*)
alterations of human
organism 71–2
animal rationale 299
body, invasion by human
technology 71
characteristics 100
as the creator 174–5
definition 99, 101, 217
dignity 128, 146, 255, 256
equality 46–7
in God's image 100, 101, 117
human ability 148–9
insubstantiality 105–10
interests and autonomy 170–2
limitations 203–4, 205
naturalisation of 60–2
non-adaption of 60–2
outside control 201–4
qualification for 193
genetic endowment 193
positive and negative
criteria 193–4
relationship to Nature 22, 61,
103–5

spirit 100–3, 118–19
substance 128
see also human nature
human genome 59, 79, 265
human nature 16, 99–123
as an outside world 201–4
body and spirit 100–3
control over, *see* control
effect of technology 113–14
evaluation 204–9
imperfection of 206–7
inadequacies 206
incompleteness 205
insubstantiality 105–10
justification 143
as a normative category 110–14
open relationship to
Nature 103–5
(problem of) defining 103,
112–13
sexuality 45, 121–3, 132–5
subjectivity, basis for 105–10,
201–21
technology's destruction 1
see also subjectivity
humanism, utilitarian 231
Huntington's chorea 225, 314
hybrid, human–animal 86, 93, 120,
268, 310

ideals in life, *see* life
imperative of responsibility 186–7
imperfections of human
nature 206–7
improvement
of the human race 70
of individual human
characteristics 29–30
in vitro fertilisation, *see* fertilisation
inadequacies of human
nature 206–7
infanticide 34, 193
'inferior' individuals
manipulation, molecular 66
sterilisation 44
infertility, and desire for
children 91–2
inheritance of human
characteristics 29–30
germinal choice 53–6, 64–5
mutation 51–3